Metastatic Tumors of the Central Nervous System

KINTOMO TAKAKURA, M.D.
KEIJI SANO, M.D.
SHUNTARO HOJO, M.D.
ASAO HIRANO, M.D.

IGAKU-SHOIN Tokyo·New York

Authors

Kintomo Takakura, M.D.
Professor and Chairman, Department of Neurosurgery
Faculty of Medicine, University of Tokyo, Tokyo

Keiji Sano, M.D.
Emeritus Professor, Department of Neurosurgery
Faculty of Medicine, University of Tokyo, Tokyo

Professor and Chairman, Department of Neurosurgery
Faculty of Medicine, Teikyo University, Tokyo

Shuntaro Hojo, M.D.
Department of Neurosurgery
Faculty of Medicine, University of Tokyo, Tokyo

Former Fellow, Division of Neuropathology, Department of
Pathology, Montefiore Hospital and Medical Center, New York

Asao Hirano, M.D.
Head, Division of Neuropathology, Department of Pathology
Montefiore Hospital and Medical Center, New York

Professor, Department of Pathology and Neuroscience
Albert Einstein College of Medicine, New York

Published and distributed by
IGAKU-SHOIN Ltd.,
    5-24-3 Hongo, Bunkyo-ku, Tokyo
IGAKU-SHOIN Medical Publishers, Inc.,
    1140 Avenue of the Americas, New York, N.Y. 10036

Library of Congress Cataloging in Publication Data

Main entry under title:

Metastatic tumors of the central nervous system.

    Bibliography: p.
    Includes index.
    1. Central nervous system—Cancer.   2. Metastasis.
I. Takakura, Kintomo, 1932–   . [DNLM: 1. Central
nervous system diseases.   2. Nervous system neoplasms.
3. Neoplasm metastasis.   WL 358 M587]
RC280.N43M47   616.99′48   81–18635
ISBN 0–89640–067–0   AACR2

Printed and bound in Japan

In Memory of Our Patients

PREFACE

By that destiny, to perform an act
Whereof what's past is prologue, what to come . . .
William Shakespeare
(Tempest II, 1)

Metastatic tumors of the central nervous system are manifestations of advanced cancers. Once symptoms, such as headache, convulsive seizures or hemiparesis appear, patients cannot expect to return to their previous environment. Rapid progression of the disease diminishes their nervous and mental functions day by day. Patients can expect only a few months of life even if they receive full medical care. Only in exceptional cases, can the patients escape from the nails of Harpies. Recent advances in oncology, however, have made better treatment possible, allowing the life span of cancer patients to be extended. Since in many cases primary sites of cancer can now be cured, the number of patients with metastatic brain tumors requiring neurosurgical treatment has gradually been increasing in recent years. It is well known that one of the main causes of death in lung cancer patients is the metastasis of the cancer to the brain. If brain metastasis could be properly treated, the overall therapeutic results of lung cancer treatment would be improved. Many neurosurgeons have neglected the treatment of metastatic brain tumors simply for the reason that it is not rewarding. While there are many who are not enthusiastic about treatment, there are other neurosurgeons who devote themselves to tiresome works of therapy. Although very rare, there have been cases in which the patient miraculously recovered and returned to an active social life.

The recent advance in computed tomography has completely changed the diagnostic process of metastatic brain tumors. It has now become possible to easily and accurately clarify the real features and characteristics of tumors. Every primary cancer has its own characteristic biological behavior. Sensitivity to radiation and chemotherapeutic agents also differs. Not only the patient's subjectability to surgery but to other modes of treatment, radiation, chemotherapy or immunotherapy should also be established on the basis of the biological properties of the tumor. Furthermore, it is essential that physicians take into consideration the social background and problems of the patients and their families. What can we physicians do for them? Sometimes we are too ambitious to treat them, and sometimes we are too pessimistic to do anything. In almost every case, our attempt ends in failure. We have been successful only in exceptional cases. Nevertheless, we feel it our duty at least to relieve the patients of their agony.

What physicians should do for patients is one of the objectives of the current study, which is being undertaken jointly by researchers in Japan and the United States. All phases of work involving neuropathological studies of metastatic brain tumors described in Chapter II were undertaken at Montefiore Hospital in New

York, while all other clinical studies of diagnosis and treatment were made at the University of Tokyo and the National Cancer Center in Tokyo. The pathological data presented here is based upon more than 8,000 autopsies of cancer patients in hospitals in New York and Tokyo. The clinical data is a summary of 616 cases treated during the past 20 years in Tokyo.

It is our earnest hope that the results of our studies will contribute to the advancement of the treatment of metastatic tumors of the central nervous system in the future.

The authors are grateful to Dr. Leopold G. Koss, Chairman, Department of Pathology, Montefiore Hospital and Medical Center, for his support given us in this undertaking. We must also acknowledge our debt to Dr. Harry M. Zimmerman and the staff of the Department of Pathology of Montefiore Hospital and Medical Center who over the past 25 years have provided data and material on which this study was based.

Our work was accomplished with the cooperation of many doctors, colleagues and collaborators. We also acknowledge the kind cooperation of Drs. Masao Matsutani, Isao Terao, Takeshi Kohno, Nobuyuki Shitara, Masayoshi Miki, Kazuhiro Nomura, Hiroshi Yamamoto, Tatsuya Kondoh, Akira Teraoka, Yuichi Ueda, Hiroshi Segawa, Masakatsu Nagai, Yoshiaki Mayanagi, Isamu Saito, Masumi Yoshioka, Tadayuki Maehara, Atsuo Akanuma, Takeshi Yoneyama, Toshiro Ogata, Keiichi Suemasu, Akio Naruke, Yasuo Koyama, Toshio Kitagawa, Kiichi Seto, Yukio Shimosato, Yukitaka Ushio, Susumu Wakai, Toshio Kumanishi, Masamichi Hara, Makoto Iwata, Kiyoharu Inoue, Shigetoshi Kuroda and Motoharu Sugiyama. We are very grateful to Dr. Shichiro Ishikawa, Director of the National Cancer Center, for his continuous aid for this work. We thank Drs. Josefina Llena and Herbert Dembitzer for their help in the preparation of the manuscript for Chapter II. The assistance of Miss Mitsuko Yamazaki, Mrs. Motoko Nagashima and Mrs. Eiko Kakinuma is also greatly appreciated. We acknowledge Dr. Takayoshi Matsui's suggestion that this study be jointly undertaken between the Division of Neuropathology at Montefiore Hospital and the Department of Neurosurgery of the University of Tokyo. Finally, we also wish to express our appreciation to Messrs. Minoru Sakamoto, Shigekazu Suginoo, Takayoshi Ishihara and Hideo Okada of Igaku-Shoin for their assistance in the editing and technical preparation of this book.

September 1981

The Authors

CONTENTS

I. INTRODUCTION

Metastasis is a vicious characteristic of malignant neoplasms. It is said that cancers are curable if metastasis can be prevented and controlled. The brain, which physically and mentally controls all human behaviors and functions, is unfortunately one of the predominant target organs for the metastasis of tumor cells. When the central nervous system is affected by a neoplasm, the patient suffers grievous agonies such as severe headaches, nausea, convulsive seizures or gradually developing weakness of nervous functions. It is miserable not only for the patients themselves, but also for their families. The number of metastatic brain tumor patients in neurosurgical clinics has, however, been increasing the past ten years concurrent with the advances in the treatment of cancer in primary sites.

It is extremely difficult to find initial reports of metastatic brain tumors in medical literature. It is believed that the first case was reported by Schraut in 1853 (cited by Simionescu, 1960). During the 19th century, the metastatic brain tumor was a subject of study for neurologists and pathologists. A few cases of primary carcinoma of the brain were reported (Gedge-Latham, 1869; Rustizky, 1874; Russel, 1876; Coats, 1888). These cases, however, might have been varieties of tumors such as gliomas or sarcomas (Hassin, 1919). Precise descriptions of symptoms and the histopathology of metastatic brain tumors appeared in several kinds of literature at the beginning of this century. Siefert (1903) reported four cases, and Gutmann (1904) reported two cases of metastatic brain tumors. During the same period, statistic analyses of intracranial metastases of tumors were reported by Bucholz (1898), Gallavardin and Varay (1903), Fischer-Defoy (1905), Kaufman (1906) and Krasting (1906). Statistics in the early days, however, were not fully reliable since there were no definite differential criteria defining glioblastoma, sarcomas and small cell carcinoma of the lung. Not suspecting the presence of intracranial lesions in a number of cases, pathologists in those days failed to fully examine the central nervous system. Gallavardin and Varay (1903) reported that the incidence of metastatic brain tumors was very rare, being only 0.1 per cent of all cases autopsied.

The most reliable statistics in that period were those reported by Krasting (1906). He found 53 cases (5.6%) of metastatic brain tumors in his series of 935 verified cases of cancer out of a total of 12,730 autopsies. His findings drew attention to the fact that the brain is one of the predominant target organs for cancer metastasis. He concluded that sarcoma metastasized three times more than carcinoma, but the sarcoma based on his criteria probably included many cases of glioblastoma. Since then histopathological studies of metastatic brain tumors have become increasingly precise and accurate. Besides solid-type parenchymal metastasis, meningeal infiltration of cancer cells has also been attracting attention. In the past, these cases were thought to be a toxemic pathophysiological states of cancer caused by so-called "cancer toxins" (Oppenheim, 1888). Nonne (1900) and Siefert (1903) shared this view. It was later found, however, that the dura or pia-arachnoid is so infiltrated as to cause various nervous symptoms. Two types of infiltration were described. Westenhöffer (1903), Dahmen (1905), and Lissauer (1911) reported cases of pachymeningitis carcinomatosa in which only the dura mater affected resembled so-called hemorrhagic internal pachymeningitis. The other form, which did not involve the dura but involved the arachnoid was reported by Nonne (1902), Siefert (1902), Krause (1903, 1908), Saxer (1903), Scholz (1905), Stadelman (1908), and Schwarz and Bertels (1911) as meningitis carcinomatosa. Hassin (1919), and Hassin and Singer (1922) described the histopathology of these two forms of intracranial metastasis of cancer.

Since the beginning of this century, numerous papers have been written concerning the pathology, symptomatology and statistic analysis of metastatic tumors of the central nervous system. A historical review will be outlined in each section of this monograph.

From a clinical point of view, Globus and Selinsky (1927) reported 12 cases of metastatic brain tumors. They analyzed their cases precisely and described clinical features with a necropsy record. Meagher and Eisenhardt (1931) accumulated clinical cases at the surgical clinic of Harvey Cushing at the Peter Bent Brigham Hospital. Of 1,850 verified intracranial tumors, 57 (3.0%) were metastatic tumors. Of these, 44 (2.3%) were carcinomas and one fourth of them were breast cancers. They reported that the course from the initial appearance of intracranial symptoms was rapid, and that the average survival time was six months. The average postoperative survival time was six weeks, the longest period being five months. The incidence of metastatic brain tumors at the neurosurgical clinic was relatively low. In Cushing's series, the rate was 4.2 per cent (Cushing, 1932). Only selected cases of intracranial metastasis were sent to neurosurgical clinics, and many cases were never presented for surgical consideration. In autopsied cases, the incidence of intracranial metastasis was naturally higher (13.5%, Globus and Meltzer, 1942; 17%, Courville, 1945; 18%, Baker, 1942; 22%, Petit-Dutaillis et al., 1956).

The most common primary site of intracranial metastasis is the lung. This observation has been reported elsewhere since the beginning of this century.* In an earlier report by Globus (1944), 55 per cent of all intracranial metastases were secondary to lung cancer. In some clinics, breast cancer was much more predominant (Lesse and Netsky, 1954; Chu and Hilaris, 1961; Constans et al., 1973b). In Montefiore Hospital in New York and in our clinic in Tokyo, lung cancer is the predominant primary malignant tumor for intracranial metastasis. A further review of incidence will be made in the following chapters.

The period of pathological consideration of intracranial metastasis was determined by the age of studies on methods of clinical examination. Angiography and RI scintigram were for a long time the most important examinations. Electroencepha-

---

* Holzer, 1925; Shelden, 1926; Fried, 1927; Parker, 1927; Davison and Horwitz, 1930; Fried, 1930; Fried and Buckley, 1930; Putschar, 1930; Paillas, 1933; Elkington, 1935; Olson, 1935; Ochsner and DeBakey, 1941; King and Ford, 1942; Tinney and Moersch, 1944; Kiefer, 1947; Puech et al., 1947; Livingston et al., 1948; Elsaesser, 1949; Mason, 1949; Graham, 1950a, 1950b; Reingold et al., 1950; Steiner et al., 1950; Grant and Sayers, 1951; Engelman and McNamara, 1954; Halpert et al., 1954; Galluzzi and Payne, 1955; Perese, 1956; Leitholf and Kuhlendahl, 1957; Papo and Tritapepe, 1957; Pool et al., 1957; Roger and Heard, 1958; Onuigbo, 1962; Hyde et al., 1965; Hunter and Rewcastle, 1968; Roswit et al., 1968; Spiers, 1969; Line and Deely, 1971; Palma, 1972; Paillas et al., 1974b; Hojo et al., 1978. (Other reports are cited throughout this monograph).

lography often gave abnormal findings, which were not specific to any intracranial metastasis. Computed tomography (CT), however, has completely changed the method of examination.

It was almost impossible to detect, by either angiography or RI scintigram, tumors of multiple metastases and tumor nodules less than one centimeter in diameter. Computed tomography, on the other hand, can demonstrate not only the real shapes and characteristics of all multiple metastatic nodules, but also the features of brain edema caused by tumors. Surgical indications for intracranial metastasis can, therefore, be established in a rational way. The regression of the tumor size can be ascertained after various forms of treatment, such as radiotherapy and chemotherapy. Since the sensitivity of the tumor to radiation or chemotherapeutic agents can be checked, it is possible to design the most suitable therapeutic regimen for each case. In the chapter on clinical examinations in this monograph, emphasis is placed on CT findings of intracranial metastasis.

Treatment for intracranial metastatic tumors started at the beginning of this century (Cushing, 1937). Cushing observed some favorable cases after craniotomy, especially in patients with hypernephroma. Nevertheless, most other neurosurgeons, such as Grant (1926) and Dandy (1932), were opposed to surgical management because of its short life expectancy. There have always been both optimistic and pessimistic views regarding the surgical treatment of intracranial metastasis of malignant tumors. Despite the dominating pessimistic views, many successful cases of surgical management have evidently been reported. Radiotherapy was also introduced for the treatment of intracranial metastasis. Lenz and Freid (1931) reported the results of radiotherapy on five patients suffering from intracranial metastasis from breast cancer. Four out of the five patients demonstrated encouraging effects. A large series of radiotherapy for intracranial metastases was reported by Memorial Hospital in New York (Chao et al., 1954; Chu and Hilaris, 1961; Nisce et al., 1971). Nisce and others summarized the results of a total of 816 cases treated by conventional radiotherapy. In 80 per cent of the cases, improved symptoms were noted, but the mean duration of remission was only five months. A large number of papers describing the results of surgery and radiotherapy have been published. The recent trend in radiotherapy is short-term, high-dose treatment. This concept has been adopted for quick palliation of metastatic tumors since it shortens the period of hospitalization for patients with limited life expectancies. Potentiation of radiotherapy by several radio-sensitizers or by synchronization of the tumor cell cycle has recently been introduced, showing better suppressive effects on metastatic tumors. Quite recently chemotherapy has been utilized for treatment. Many chemotherapeutic agents were clinically studied in the Phase II studies, but only a few have shown definite effectiveness. Among them, nitrosourea compounds and tegafur have proved effective for intracranial metastasis of cancer and prolonged the survival time of the patients. Glucocorticoid administration for intracranial metastatic tumors has also brought an enormous benefit to the patients. Glucocorticoids can subside clinical symptoms due to brain edema and relieve the patients of their suffering, even though its effects may last only for a short period. Concomitant use of glucocorticoids with some chemotherapeutic agents has extended the survival time of patients much longer than expected. Since the immunocompetence of cancer patients deteriorates, the potentiation of immunological functions has recently been introduced for treatment.

Metastatic tumors of the central nervous system are pathophysiological manifestations of advanced and disseminated malignant tumors. Difficulties involved in the treatment for metastatic tumors of the central nervous system are dependent on complicated pathophysiological features as follows:

1. The majority of patients with metastatic tumors in the central nervous system also have other disseminated tumors (primary or metastatic) in various organs. The presence of tumors in the lung or the liver is especially a limiting factor in treatment. It should, however, be noted that great advances have been made in the treatment of metastatic lung and liver cancer in recent years. Cases of long-term survivors after surgery for such metastatic tumors have been reported. In the coming years, the mean survival time of these patients is expected to dramatically increase over the present mean survival time.

2. The incidence of multiple metastases, diffuse or disseminated infiltration to the meninges or arachnoid, is higher than that of single and solitary types of metastases. The latter can be removed by surgery. In the former types, surgical management is, however, generally not indicated.

3. Severe brain edema usually develops in tissue adjacent to metastatic tumors. It causes a rapid increase in intracranial pressure and damages the brain or the spinal cord. Pulmonary dysfunction due to tumors causes hypoxia and accelerates the expansion of brain edema.

4. Each primary tumor has its own biological characteristics. Sensitivity to radiation or chemotherapeutic agents differs for each type of tumor. For instance, choriocarcinoma is quite sensitive to Actinomycin D and methotrexate. Lung adenocarcinoma, however, is sensitive to neither.

5. The vertebral column is a predominant site for bone metastasis of cancer. The spinal cord is easily compressed, and irreversible spinal cord destruction occurs rapidly in a few days or weeks.

6. The immunocompetence of patients with metastatic tumors of the central nervous system notably deteriorates compared with that of primary brain tumor patients.

II. PATHOLOGY OF METASTASES AFFECTING THE CENTRAL NERVOUS SYSTEM

GENERAL ASPECTS

The results of the survey to be reported here were drawn exclusively from autopsies performed at Montefiore Hospital from 1950 through 1974; a period of 25 years. During this time 3,849 autopsies were performed in which primary malignant tumors were discovered outside the central nervous system. Among them, there were some in which two, three, or even more primary malignant lesions were present, so that the total number of primary malignant tumors recorded was 3,958. Primary lymphoma and sarcoma of the central nervous system were excluded from this study. The brain was examined in 3,824 cases (99.4%) and the spinal cord in 485 cases (12.6%). The racial composition of these cases included 90.3 per cent Caucasian, 7.7 per cent black, 1.9 per cent Latin-American, 0.2 per cent Oriental, and a few of indeterminate racial backgrounds.

The frequency of metastases to the central nervous system and the site of predilection for each type of primary tumor are best presented in tabular form. Tables II-1 and 2 and Figure II-1 show the frequency of metastases and the site of predilection for various kinds of carcinomas and sarcomas (3,359 cases). Table II-3 and Figure II-2 present the same information for lymphomas, leukemias and multiple myeloma (599 cases). In our material, the frequency of CNS involvement (including the dura mater and the pituitary gland) by tumors, carcinoma or sarcoma, was 29 per cent. The frequency of CNS involvement for patients with lymphoma, leukemia and multiple myeloma was 34 per cent. These figures are relatively high compared with several other reports (Table II-4).

The data presented here is in substantial agreement with that reported by the American Cancer Society in 1978. Comparison of our observations with those reported by others is limited by several factors. Data derived from neurosurgical clinics are based, for the most part, on evidence derived from surviving patients, and therefore show a much lower rate of metastases to the central nervous system. The differences between our data and those reported from other autopsy series (Table II-5) may be explained on various grounds. Racial and environmental differences among the patient population may account for some of these differences. The skill and thoroughness of the autopsy examination may also have an important impact on the findings. Finally, a marked increase in the rate of metastases may have occurred since the middle part of the century. This is suggested by a comparison of early studies listed in Table II-4 (including Rau, 1921 and Baker, 1942) with more recent studies. The increase may be related to the longer survival time of cancer

Table II-1 Primary site and location of metastases (Number of cases).

Location of metastasis	Primary site												
	Lung	Breast	G.I. tract	Urinary tract	Mela-noma	Pros-tate	Head & neck	Female repro-ductive system	Sar-comas	Liver, Biliary tract & Pancreas	Thyroid	Others	Total
Brain parenchyma	266	111	43	34	34	10	10	5	10	14	9	9	555
Leptomeninges	25	30	4	1	15	3	3	3	2	1	0	3	90
Cranial nerves	4	10	0	1	0	0	8	0	0	0	0	0	23
Dura mater	54	164	21	9	22	15	12	8	6	3	4	5	323
Pituitary gland	46	103	12	5	7	7	11	5	3	3	1	2	205
Intracranial	**316**	**267**	**64**	**42**	**45**	**24**	**28**	**16**	**15**	**17**	**13**	**13**	**860**
Spinal cord	6	2	0	0	1	0	0	0	0	0	0	0	9
Spinal nerves	10	4	4	3	2	1	1	1	1	0	1	0	28
Spinal epidural tissue	41	26	16	12	2	14	1	4	11	5	3	5	140
In the vertebral canal	**51**	**35**	**17**	**12**	**12**	**14**	**2**	**6**	**12**	**5**	**3**	**6**	**175**
Total CNS & its coverings	**349**	**278**	**76**	**52**	**47**	**37**	**29**	**21**	**20**	**22**	**15**	**17**	**963**
Total number of Patients	774	526	773	199	69	140	155	236	68	293	54	72	3,359

The sum of the intracranial and intra-vertebral canal metastases is higher than the number of total intracranial metastasis. This is due to the fact that a single primary tumor may metastasize to more than one location within the central nervous system. For example, a primary in the lung may metastasize to both the parenchyma and to the dura mater in the same patient. This case would then be included in both categories but only once under "Total intracranial." Metastases include both distant spread and direct invasion.

Table II-2 Primary site and location of metastases (Frequency in percentage).

Location of metastasis	Primary site												
	Lung	Breast	G.I. Tract	Urinary tract	Mela-noma	Pros-tate	Head & neck	Female repro-ductive system	Sar-coma	Liver, Biliary tract & Pancreas	Thyroid	Others	Total
	N=774	N=526	N=750	N=199	N=69	N=140	N=155	N=236	N=68	N=293	N=54	N=72	N=3,359
Brain parenchyma	*34.4	21.1	5.5	17.1	49.2	7.1	6.5	2.1	14.7	4.8	16.7	12.5	16.5
Leptomeninges	3.2	5.7	0.5	0.5	21.7	2.1	1.9	1.3	2.9	0.3	0.0	4.2	2.7
Cranial nerves	0.5	1.9	0.0	0.5	0.0	0.0	5.2	0.0	0.0	0.0	0.0	0.0	0.7
Dura mater	7.0	31.2	2.7	4.5	31.9	10.7	7.7	3.4	8.8	1.0	7.4	6.9	9.6
Pituitary gland	5.9	20.0	1.6	2.5	10.1	5.0	7.1	2.1	4.4	1.0	1.9	2.8	6.1
Intracranial	**40.8**	**50.8**	**8.3**	**21.1**	**65.2**	**17.1**	**18.1**	**6.8**	**22.1**	**5.8**	**24.1**	**18.1**	**25.6**
Spinal cord	0.8	0.4	0.0	0.0	1.4	0.0	0.0	0.0	0.0	0.0	0.0	0.0	0.3
Spinal nerves	1.3	0.8	0.5	1.5	2.9	0.7	0.6	0.4	1.5	0.0	1.9	0.0	0.8
Spinal epidural tissue	5.3	4.9	2.1	6.0	2.9	10.0	0.6	1.7	16.2	1.7	5.6	6.9	4.2
In the vertebral canal	**6.6**	**6.7**	**2.2**	**6.0**	**17.4**	**10.0**	**1.3**	**2.5**	**17.6**	**1.7**	**5.6**	**8.3**	**5.2**
Total CNS & its coverings	**45.1**	**52.9**	**9.8**	**26.1**	**68.1**	**26.4**	**18.7**	**8.9**	**29.4**	**7.5**	**27.8**	**23.6**	**28.7**

N: Number of cases = 100% (See Table II-1)
   For each primary site, the frequency of metastases was expressed as a percentage value.
* Example: At autopsy, 34.4% of patients who died of lung cancer had metastases in the parenchyma of the brain.

$$\frac{266 \text{ (Number of patients with parenchymal metastases from lung cancer)}}{774 \text{ (Number of cases with lung cancer)}} \times 100 = 34.4\% \text{ (See Table II-1)}$$

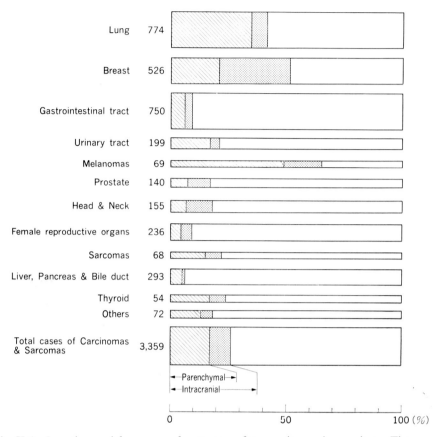

Fig. II-1 Location and frequency of metastases from various primary sites. The number of cases of each primary origin is shown in the vertical column, while the frequencies of intraparenchymal and intracranial involvement are shown on the horizontal axis.

Table II-3 Location of metastases of malignant lymphoma, leukemia and multiple myeloma. Number of cases and frequency (%).

Location of involvement	Lymphoma		Leukemia		Multiple myeloma		Total	
Brain parenchyma	18	(5)*	15	(8)	1	(1)	34	(5.7)
Leptomeninges	38	(11)	40	(22)	0		80	(13.4)
Dura mater	27	(8)	33	(18)	15	(19)	75	(12.5)
Pituitary gland	40	(12)	51	(28)	5	(6)	96	(16.0)
Intracranial	**74**	**(22)**	**89**	**(48)**	**18**	**(23)**	**181**	**(30.2)**
Spinal epidural	22	(7)	5	(3)	5	(6)	32	(5.3)
In the vertebral canal**	**31**	**(9)**	**8**	**(4)**	**5**	**(6)**	**44**	**(7.3)**
Total CNS and its coverings	**90**	**(27)**	**92**	**(50)**	**22**	**(28)**	**204**	**(34.1)**
Total number of patients	335	(100%)	184	(100%)	80	(100%)	599	(100%)

* Example:

$$\frac{18 \text{ (Number of cases with parenchymal involvement by lymphoma)}}{335 \text{ (Number of cases with lymphoma)}} \times 100 = 5\%$$

** This includes involvement of spinal epidural, spinal roots and spinal cord itself.

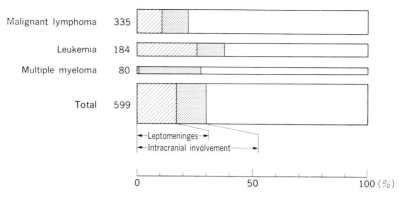

Fig. II-2 Frequency of intracranial and leptomeningeal involvement in lymphoma, leukemia and multiple myeloma. A graphic presentation of Table II-3. The column for leptomeningeal involvement includes some cases of parenchymal involvement.

Table II-4 Reports of frequency of CNS metastases at autopsy.

Authors	Frequency %	Cases with CNS lesions / Number of Patients	Sites analyzed**	Inclusion of direct invasion	Inclusion of lymphoma or leukemia
Krastings (1906)	5.7	53/935	C, V	Yes	Yes
Neustaedter (1944)	2.3	153/6761	C, V	No	No
Abrams et al. (1950)	17.6	43/244	B	No	No
Lesse & Netsky (1954)	34.7	207/595	C, V	Yes	Yes
Earle (1954)	11.1	167/1498*	C	Yes	Yes
Toyokura et al. (1957)	5.8	49/839	C	No	No
Chason et al. (1963)	18.2	200/1096	C, V	No	No
Aronson et al. (1964)	16.5	397/2406	C, V	No	Yes
Koyama & Takakura (1969)	12.0	127/1060	C	Yes	No
Present series (1978)	28.6	963/3359	C, V	Yes	No

*   Adult men only.
** B: brain, C: intracranial, V: vertebral canal.

patients, and to treatment, such as radiotherapy or chemotherapy. The relationship between the rate of metastases and chemotherapy will be discussed later.

Overall, the most common sites of primary tumors which produced secondary tumors in the CNS and its coverings were the lung and breast, followed by the gastrointestinal tract, urinary tract and melanomas. These five primaries accounted for 85 per cent of all metastatic tumors of the CNS (Table II-6, Fig. II-3).

Our results are generally in keeping with those reported by others, although some differences may be seen, as shown in Table II-7.

Table II-5 Reports of frequency of CNS metastases arranged according to the various primary sites.

	Krasting 1906	Baker 1942	Abrams et al. 1950**	Lesse and Netsky 1954	Earle 1954***	Toyokura et al. 1957	Chason et al. 1963	Aronson et al. 1964	Koyama and Takakura 1969	Present series 1978
	0%									
Lung	0	13	43	50	29	28	37	42	27	45
Breast	19	16	29	57		12	37	25	24	53
G.I. tract	1.3	3.3*	8.3*	9.7	2.8	2.9*	5.5	6.0	2.9	10
Urinary tract	9			27	13		16	8.3		26
Melanoma				53	92		91	57	30	68
Prostate	22	4.3		31	1.2		9.5	5.8		26
Head & neck	25			50	23		14	14	21	19
Female reproduct. syst.	6			7			6.4	5.2	1.7	8.8
Sarcoma	13			20	15	5		24	9.4	29
Liver, biliary duct, Pancreas	1.6			11	4.7	1.6	8	6.0	0	7.5
Thyroid	9			60	14		14			28
Others										8.3
Total of carcinomas & Sarcomas	4.8		18	33	11	5.8	18	16	12	29
Lymphoma	13			38				0	9.0	27
Leukemia				44				18	22	50
Multiple myeloma				45						28

* Gastric carcinoma.   ** Brain metastasis.   *** Adult men only.

Table II-6 Primary sites and location of metastases (Percentage of total number of metastases in each intracranial tissue).

Location of metastasis	Primary site											
	Lung	Breast	G.I. tract	Urinary tract	Mela-noma	Prostate	Head & neck	Female repro-ductive system	Sarcoma	Liver, biliary tract & pancreas	Thyroid	Others
Brain parenchyma N = 555	*47.9	20.0	7.7	6.1	6.1	1.8	1.8	0.9	1.8	2.5	1.6	1.6
Leptomeninges N = 85	27.8	33.4	4.5	1.1	16.7	3.3	3.3	3.3	2.2	1.1	0.0	3.3
Dura mater N = 323	16.7	50.8	6.5	2.8	6.8	4.6	3.7	2.5	1.9	0.9	1.2	1.5
Pituitary gland N = 205	22.4	50.2	5.9	2.4	3.4	3.4	5.4	2.4	1.5	1.5	0.5	1.0
Intracranial N = 860	**36.7**	**31.0**	**7.4**	**4.9**	**5.2**	**2.8**	**3.3**	**1.9**	**1.7**	**2.0**	**1.5**	**1.5**
Spinal epidural tissue N = 140	29.3	18.6	11.4	8.6	1.4	10.0	0.7	2.9	7.9	3.6	2.1	3.6
In the vertebral canal N = 180	**29.1**	**20.0**	**9.7**	**6.9**	**6.9**	**8.0**	**1.1**	**3.4**	**6.9**	**2.9**	**1.7**	**3.4**
Total CNS & its coverings N = 963	**36.2**	**28.9**	**7.9**	**5.4**	**4.9**	**3.8**	**3.0**	**2.2**	**2.1**	**2.3**	**1.5**	**1.8**

N: Number of cases with metastasis = 100%

* Example:

$$\frac{266 \text{ (Number of cases with parenchymal metastases from lung cancer)}}{555 \text{ (Total number of cases with parenchymal metastases)}} \times 100 = 47.9\%$$

(See Table II-1)

Table II-7 Reports of primary sites* of metastases in the CNS. Percentage of total cases of CNS metastases.

Primary sites	Baker 1942 N = 114	Meyer & Reah 1953 N = 216	Lesse & Netsky 1954 N = 192	Toyokura et al. 1957 N = 49	Simionescu 1960** N = 195	Chason et al. 1963 N = 200	Vieth & Odom 1965a** N = 313	Koyama & Takakura 1969 N = 112	Present series 1978 N = 963
Lung	21.0	54.1	27.4	36.7	38.1	61.0	27.5	37.5	36.2
Breast	21.0	9.3	39.0	6.1	22.6	5.0	16.3	16.1	28.9
G.I. tract	11.4	9.3	6.0	14.3	3.6	7.5	5.1	8.9	7.9
Urinary tract	10.5	0.9	5.4	4.1	8.2	5.0	7.0	0.0	5.4
Melanoma	***7.8	1.4	1.6	0.0	***6.2	5.0	15.7	2.7	4.9
Prostate	0.9	2.3	2.7	0.0	0.6	4.5	0.0	0.0	3.8
Head & neck	2.6	7.4	2.2	4.1	0.0	4.0	4.5	24.1	3.0
Female reproduct. syst.	5.3	5.1	1.6	10.2	3.7	1.5	0.0	0.9	2.2
Sarcoma	0.0	2.3	1.6	10.2	1.6	0.0	2.6	2.7	2.1
Liver, biliary tract & pancreas	13.2	0.5	1.1	4.1	0.0	4.0	0.0	0.0	2.3
Thyroid	0.9	0.5	3.3	4.1	2.1	0.5	0.0	0.0	1.5
Others	14.0	3.8	0.0	6.1	12.9	2.0	21.3	6.3	1.8

N: Total number of cases with CNS metastases = 100 %
*   Excluding lymphoma, leukemia and multiple myeloma.
**   Surgical series.
*** Skin carcinoma.

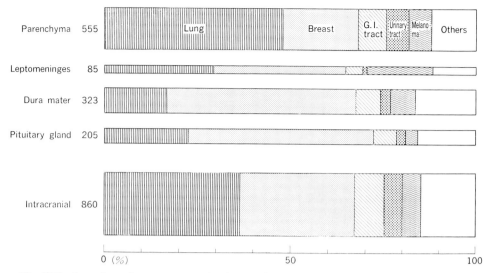

Fig. II-3   Location of metastases and primary sites.   A graphic presentation of Table II-6.

Sex

The rate of primary neoplasms in this series was approximately the same for both men and women, as was the rate of metastases to the central nervous system. As may be seen in Table II-8 and 9, lung cancer was the most common source of CNS metastases in men (56%), followed by the gastrointestinal tract and the urinary tract.   These three primary sites account for approximately 80 per cent of all metastatic lesions.   In women the breast is the most common source of metastatic lesions, accounting for 53 per cent of the total.   The lung (19%), the gastrointestinal tract (6%) and melanoma (5%) are the next most common and, together with the breast, account for over 80 per cent of the sources of metastatic lesions in women.   The rate of metastases according to the primary sites and to sex is roughly similar to those reported by others, although a few authors describe a somewhat higher percentage

Table II-8   Number of cases and percentage of total number of CNS metastases in men and women, arranged according to the primary sites.

Primary sites	Men		Women	
Lung	251	(55.5)	98	(19.2)
Breast	6	(1.3)	272	(53.2)
GI tract	46	(10.2)	30	(5.9)
Urinary tract	33	(7.3)	19	(3.8)
Melanoma	24	(5.3)	23	(4.5)
Prostate	37	(8.2)	—	(—)
Head & neck	17	(3.8)	12	(2.3)
Female reproductive organ	—	(—)	21	(4.1)
Sarcomas	6	(1.3)	14	(2.7)
Liver, biliary tract & pancreas	14	(3.1)	8	(1.6)
Thyroid	7	(1.5)	8	(1.6)
Others	11	(2.4)	6	(1.2)
Total	**452**	**(100%)**	**511**	**(100%)**

Table II-9   Number of cases with involvement
by lymphoma, leukemia and multiple myeloma
in men and women.

Primary tumors	Men	Women
Lymphoma*	51	49
Leukemia*	52	40
Multiple myeloma	10	12
Total	**113**	**101**

* See Tables II-18 and 19 for further classification of
lymphoma or leukemia.

of metastases derived from tumors of the female reproductive organs (Earle, 1954; Lesse and Netsky, 1954; Aronson et al., 1964; Paillas and Pellet 1975). This is explained by the low rate of gynecological activity at Monetefiore Hospital during the reporting period.

Age

The average age of the autopsied patients who died of malignant lesions without evidence of CNS metastases was 64. Those who had CNS involvement were substantially younger, with a mean age of 58. The average age for men with CNS metastases was about 60 years while that of women was only 56. These findings are substantially similar to other reports. The age difference between both sexes is presumably influenced by the fact that the average age at the time of death from carcinoma of the lung, the predominant source of metastases to the brain in men, is higher than that of women with breast carcinoma, the most common primary cancer in women with CNS involvement (Simionescu, 1960; Aronson et al., 1964; Vieth and Odom, 1965a; Koyama and Takakura, 1969).

Also as reported by others, over 60 per cent of the patients with CNS metastases are between 50 and 70 years of age at the time of death. Patients with sarcoma and melanoma die at substantially younger ages. The age at death of patients with lymphoma and leukemia show two peaks; one during childhood and the other in late adulthood. This is in keeping with the age distribution of these diseases.

Our findings with regard to the metastatic rate and its relationship to age are also similar to those reported by others (Fig. II-4). In general, regardless of the primary, there is a tendency towards a lower metastatic rate with advancing age (Galluzzi and Payne, 1956; Aronson et al., 1964; Koyama and Takakura, 1969). In our series, we discovered only nine patients between the ages of 86 and 90 who had CNS involvement. Their primaries were lung, kidney, prostate, leukemia and lymphoma.

Among 48 cases of malignant neoplasms in patients under 15 years of age, 27 (approximately 56%) had metastases to the CNS (Table II-10). Koyama and Takakura (1969) reported that 43 per cent of the malignant neoplasms in patients under the age of 10 metastasized to the brain. French (1948) and Vannuci and Baten (1974) reported a frequency of seven per cent and six per cent respectively of metastases in young children with cancer exclusive of leukemias. Leukemias are the major source of metastatic lesions in the CNS of young patients. Lymphomas,

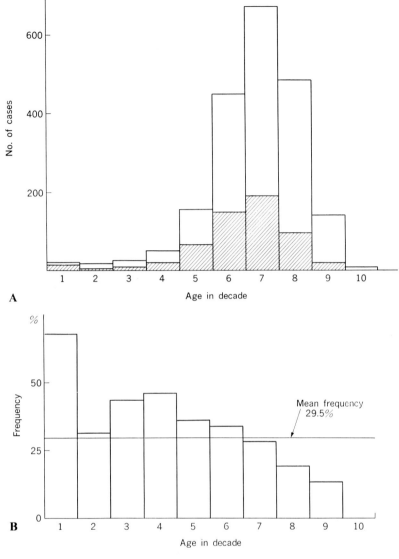

Fig. II-4 A. Age distribution of the patients with malignant neoplasms and CNS meta-stases. Total number of malignant neoplasms: total length of bars. Number of cases with CNS metastases: length of striped bars.
B. Frequency of CNS metastases and age.

Table II-10 Number of cases with metastases in the CNS in patients under 15 years old.

Primary tumors	Total number of cases	Cases with CNS metastases
Leukemia	27	17
Lymphoma	11	5
Sarcoma	5	3
Melanoma	1	1
Retinoblastoma	1	1
Others	3	0
Total	**48**	**27**

sarcomas, neuroblastomas, retinoblastomas, Wilms' tumors, melanomas and embryonal carcinomas have been reported as sources of CNS metastases in childhood (Baily et al., 1939; Cuneo and Rand, 1952; Vannucci and Baten, 1974; Matsutani et al., 1976).

DISTRIBUTION OF METASTASES ACCORDING TO THE PRIMARY SOURCE

As may be seen in Table II-2, each primary tumor shows distinct characteristics with regard to the distribution of metastases to the CNS. In the following sections we shall describe the principal features of metastases from various primary sources.

Lung

Lung cancer, which has a high frequency of CNS metastases, was observed in 45 per cent of the patients with this disease in the autopsy series, and up to 50 per cent in the reports listed in Table II-5. Other reports described the rate of metastases between 22 and 38 per cent (Meyer and Reah, 1953; Galluzzi and Payne, 1956; Halpert et al., 1960; Newman and Hansen, 1974).

Among the various intracranial tissues the brain parenchyma was involved in 34 per cent of the patients with carcinoma of the lung (Table II-2). Metastases to the leptomeninges, the dura and the pituitary gland were less frequent. Lung cancer was also one of the most frequent sources of intramedullary spinal cord metastasis but much more frequently diagnosed as spinal epidural metastasis.

The distribution of various histological types of lung cancer in each sex is shown in Table II-11. Squamous cell carcinoma and anaplastic carcinoma were more frequent in men (M: F = 7: 1 and M: F = 4.3: 1 respectively), but adenocarcinoma did not show such a distinct sex preference (M: F = 1.5 :1). The frequency of CNS metastases according to various types of lung cancer is shown in Table II-12. The rate of metastases from oat cell carcinoma was very high (70%), while squamous cell carcinoma metastasized less frequently (32%). Adenocarcinomas and anaplastic carcinomas, other than oat cell carcinoma, produce CNS metastases in 51 and 52 per cent of the cases respectively. Allowing for small differences in figures and classification, our observations are similar to those reported by others (Meyer and Reah,

Table II-11   Prevalence of lung cancer of various histological types, in men and women.

	Histological classification				
	Adeno-carcinoma	Squamous cell carcinoma	Anaplastic carcinoma*	Others**	Total
Men	123	189	186	100	598
Women	83	27	43	23	176
Total	**206**	**216**	**229**	**123**	**774**

*   Including small cell carcinoma.
**   Mixed type and unclassified carcinomas.

Table II-12 Frequency of CNS metastases from lung cancer of various histological types.

	Histological classification					
	Adeno-carcinoma	Squamous cell carcinoma	Small cell carcinoma	Anaplastic carcinoma	Others	Total
Cases with CNS metastases: A	107	70	30	97	45	349
Total number of cases: B	209	216	43	186	120	747
Frequency of metastases: A/B × 100	50.7%	32.4%	69.8%	52.2%	37.5%	45.1%

1953; Galluzzi and Payne, 1956; Strauss and Weller, 1957; Deeley and Rice Edwards, 1968; Newman and Hansen, 1974).

Lung cancer often produces neurological symptoms as its initial manifestation. In such circumstances, differentiation from primary brain tumors is important (Craig et al., 1939; Rupp, 1948; Russell and Rubinstein, 1971; Berardi, 1973). CNS metastases are sometimes considered the only evidence of metastatic spread, and therefore, become the target of surgical intervention (Flavell, 1949).

Breast

Intracranial metastases from mammary carcinoma were observed in 51 per cent of the breast cancer cases in our autopsy series. Other reports indicated a range from 12 to 57 per cent, as shown in Table II-5. A 25 per cent frequency rate was reported by Viadana et al. (1973).

The frequency of metastases from breast cancer to the dura, pituitary and leptomeninges was very high (see also p. 75, 89 and 101). The brain parenchyma had a moderate frequency of metastases, which were often the result of an extension of metastatic focus in the dura and the skull. Mammary carcinoma was also a frequent source of secondary growth in the vertebral canal, mainly in the spinal epidural tissue. Vertebral metastases were also frequent, 32 per cent in our series and 65 per cent in another series (Viadana et al., 1973). In some cases of breast cancer, CNS metastasis may appear after a long period of clinical latency (Ederer et al., 1963; Berg and Robbins, 1966). One such example is illustrated in Fig. II-65B (see p. 86).

Gastrointestinal Tract

The frequency of CNS metastases in patients with carcinomas of the gastrointestinal tract was low, namely 9.8 per cent in the present study and from 1.3 to 9.7 per cent in other reports (Tables II-5 and 13). Metastases from carcinomas of the liver, pancreas and biliary tract occured in 7.5 per cent of the patients in our series and in 1.6 to 11 per cent in other reports (Tables II-5 and 14). Metastases occurred in 12 per cent of the patients with carcinomas of the colon and rectum (Table II-13), and

Table II-13   Frequency of CNS metastases from carcinomas of gastrointestinal tract-1.

	Esophagus	Stomach	Small intestine	Colon	Rectum	Total
Cases with CNS metastases: A	7	11	0	44	14	76
Total number of cases: B	89	170	5	371	138	773
Frequency of metastases: A/B × 100	7.9%	6.5%	0%	12.0%	10.1%	7.8%

Table II-14   Frequency of CNS metastases from carcinomas of gastrointestinal tract-2.

	Pancreas	Biliary tract	Liver	Total
Cases with CNS metastases: A	17	3	2	22
Total number of cases: B	185	66	42*	293
Frequency of metastases: A/B × 100	9.2%	4.5%	5.0%	7.5%

*   Including 28 cases of hepatoma and 14 cases of adenocarcinoma.

4.8 per cent in a report by Dionne (1965).   In Japan, the incidence of gastric carcinoma is high, and consequently, the rate of brain metastases of this origin is higher than that observed in patients with colorectal carcinoma (Koyama and Takakura, 1969).   Although a high frequency of diffuse leptomeningeal carcinomatosis in stomach cancer was reported, we did not observe this event in the United States (see p. 75).   Brain metastases from tumors of the gastrointestinal tract tend to produce single nodules (Vieth and Odom, 1965a) which favor the subtentorial region (see p. 29).

Urinary Tract

Metastases to the CNS in patients with carcinomas of the urinary tract were observed in 21 per cent of our series and from 8.3 to 53 per cent in other reports (Tables II-2 and 5).   Thirty-five per cent of the patients with renal carcinoma had CNS metastases.   Sixteen per cent of patients with tumors of the lower urinary tract had CNS metastases (Table II-15).   Some cases of renal adenocarcinoma showed long survival after surgery for brain metastases (Holland, 1973; Dayes et al., 1977).   Wilms' tumors have been reported to produce brain metastases in 4 to 13 per cent of the patients (Bannayan et al., 1971; Vannuchi and Baten, 1974).   No metastases were seen in our single case of this disease.

Table II-15 Frequency of CNS metastases from carcinomas of the urinary tract.

	Kidney*	Bladder & ureter	Total
Cases with CNS metastases: A	38	14	52
Total number of cases: B	110	89	199
Frequency of metastases: A/B × 100	35%	16%	26%

* Including one case of Wilms' tumor, which was without metastasis in the CNS.

Prostate

Intracranial metastases were observed in 17 per cent of the patients with prostatic carcinoma in our series and from 1.2 to 31 per cent in other series (Tables II-2 and 5). This tumor shows a predilection for the dura (11% of the cases) and the skull. Metastasis to the brain parenchyma was observed in seven per cent of our patients, 2.4 per cent and 4.4 per cent in other series (Catane et al., 1976; Parker et al., 1978). This tumor is known to produce metastases to the vertebrae and spinal epidural tissue (Vieth and Odom, 1965a; Viadana et al., 1976). The rate of metastases in spinal epidural tissue was 10 per cent in our series.

Female Reproductive Organs

CNS metastases from carcinoma of the female reproductive organs were relatively uncommon, nine per cent in our series and from 1.7 to 6.4 per cent in other reports (Table II-5). Metastases occurred in 18 per cent of the patients with cervical cancer distributed mainly in the spinal epidural tissue or the cranial dura. The rates of CNS metastases in patients with carcinoma of the corpus of the uterus and the ovary were seven per cent and six per cent respectively (Table II-16). These tumors also

Table II-16 Frequency of CNS metastases from carcinomas of female reproductive organs.

	Cervix of uterus	Corpus of uterus*	Ovary	Total
Cases with CNS metastases: A	9	4	8	21
Total number of cases: B	51	60	125	236
Frequency of metastases: A/B × 100	18%	7%	6%	9%

* Including the fallopian tubes.

involved the lower vertebrae (Blythe et al., 1975). The rates of CNS metastases from cancer of the uterus in other reports were 0.1 and 3.4 per cent (Lipin and Davison, 1947; Takakura, 1976), while that of ovarian carcinoma was reported by Mayer et al. (1978) as 0.9 per cent.

Our autopsy series do not include any cases of choriocarcinoma. This tumor is common in Asia (Hou and Pang, 1956). Metastatic choriocarcinoma to the CNS is frequently associated with fatal intracranial hemorrhage (Vaughan, Jr. and Howard, 1962; Aguilar and Rabinovitch, 1964; Adeloye et al., 1972; Bucy and Stilp, 1972; Shuangshoti et al., 1974; Gurwitt et al., 1975; Nakahara et al., 1975).

Melanoma

There were 69 cases of malignant melanoma in this series, which was two per cent of the malignant tumors exclusive of leukemias and lymphomas. However, the frequency of metastases to the central nervous system was extremely high—65 per cent in our series and from 30 to 92 per cent in other series (Table II-5). Das Gupta and Brasfield (1964) and Beresford (1969) reported CNS metastases in 39 and 44 per cent respectively.

Melanoma shows the highest incidence of intracranial metastases among the following primary lesions; 49 per cent for parenchymal, 22 per cent for leptomeningeal and 32 per cent for dural metastasis. Beresford (1969) reported frequent (45%) involvement of the leptomeninges.

Metastases of melanoma to the brain parenchyma are characterized by multiple foci and frequent hemorrhage. Multiple foci occurred frequently in brain metastases of melanoma in our series (see p. 28), as has been reported by others (Moersch et al., 1940; Das Gupta and Brasfield, 1964; Beresford, 1969). Hemorrhage is sometimes the initial symptom of CNS metastases (Lockesley et al., 1966). Blood-stained CSF was frequently found during the clinical course in 36 per cent and 45 per cent of the patients whose CSF were examined (Madonick and Savitsky, 1951; Clifford et al., 1975).

The average age of patients with CNS metastases of melanoma was 51, lower than the mean age of patients with metastases from other primary tumors. The prognosis of patients with CNS metastasis of melanoma is nearly hopeless (Gottlieb et al., 1972; Pennington and Milton, 1975; Hayward, 1976). However, occasional cases with a long survival time have been reported (Reyes and Horrax, 1950; McCann et al., 1968; McNeel and Leavens, 1968).

Head and Neck

This group of carcinomas consists of several subgroups as shown in Table II-17. The tumors of the head and neck region sometimes invade the base of the skull and directly adjacent tissues such as the dura, the cranial nerves, the pituitary gland and the brain (Digby et al., 1941; Geist and Portmann, 1952; Hare and Crew, Jr., 1963). There were also a few cases of blood-borne metastases. The rates of dural and

Table II-17 Frequency of CNS metastases from carcinomas of the head and neck region.

	Mouth*	Nose & pharynx	Larynx	Others	Total
Cases with CNS metastases: A	9	15	4	1	29
Total number of cases: B	72	39	42	2	155
Frequency of metastases: A/B × 100	13%	39%	10%		18.7%

* Including the salivary glands.

pituitary gland involvement were eight and seven per cent respectively. Brain involvement was less frequent at seven per cent. One other report had similar findings (Meyer and Reah, 1953). Koyama and Takakura (1969) reported two cases of blood-borne metastasis and 25 cases of contiguous invasion in 103 cases of carcinomas of the head and neck region. Other authors also reported the rare occurrence of blood-borne metastases (O'Brien et al., 1971; Probert et al., 1974).

Of this group, the primary carcinomas are divided into subgroups. Nasal and pharyngeal carcinomas involved the CNS and its coverings more frequently than those that arose in the oral cavity and larynx (Table II-17). A similar result was found in other reports (Teoh, 1957; Koyama and Takakura, 1969).

Thyroid

CNS metastases from thyroid cancer occurred in 28 per cent of the patients in our autopsy series and from 9 to 60 per cent in other series (Table II-5). Thyroid cancer frequently affects bones, including the skull and the vertebrae (Turner and German, 1941; Friedman, 1943).

Sarcomas

CNS metastases of sarcoma occurred in 22 per cent of the patients in our series and from 4 to 25 per cent in other series (Table II-5). Some authors suggested that an increased rate of CNS involvement may be due to the application of chemotherapy and the accompanying extension of the life span (Marsa and Johnson, 1971; Mehta and Hendrickson, 1974; Gercovich et al., 1975).

Our cases included a variety of soft part sarcomas, such as fibrosarcoma, chondrosarcoma, rhabdomyosarcoma, liposarcoma, osteosarcoma, angiosarcoma and undifferentiated sarcoma. Zucker et al. (1978) have recently published a review on sarcoma metastasis to the CNS.

Other Tumors

Primary tumors included in this group were malignant teratoma, seminoma, thymoma, neuroblastoma, retinoblastoma and five tumors of unknown origin. These tumors are too few to establish a pattern for CNS metastasis.

Retinoblastoma invades the optic nerve and leptomeninges directly. A high incidence (75%) of intracranial involvement has been reported (Carbajal, 1959).

Neuroblastoma affects bones frequently, but metastases to the brain parenchyma are rare (Willis, 1948). The dura mater or spinal epidural tissue, on the other hand, are frequently invaded by extension of bony metastases (Kincaid et al., 1957; Carter et al., 1968).

Malignant teratomas usually arise in the testes, ovaries, retroperitoneum or the mediastinum. Two cases of this kind of tumor metastasizing to the CNS have been reported (Störtebecker, 1954; Moore et al., 1956).

Lymphomas

Lymphomas affected the CNS in 27 per cent of the patients with this group of diseases in our series and up to 38 per cent in other series (Table II-5). An apparent increase of CNS involvement accompanied by longer survival periods of the patients was reported by some authors following the application of chemotherapy (Janota, 1966; Griffin et al., 1971).

Lymphomas often involve the leptomeninges. The dura mater, spinal epidural tissue and capsule of the pituitary gland are also sites of predilection in lymphoma. In some cases, demarcated metastatic foci in the brain are associated with focal or diffuse leptomeningeal involvement.

The frequency of CNS involvement in lymphomas in this study is shown in Table II-18. The distribution of various types of lymphomas may vary according to the geographical area (Correa and O'Connor, 1973; Kumanishi et al., 1975).

Although a variety of tissues may be involved in any type of lymphoma, there are some differences in the pattern of CNS involvement based on the different types of lymphomas. Non-Hodgkin's lymphomas may infiltrate the dura and the leptomeninges and often produce a relatively circumscribed mass in the brain, with a preference for midline structures (see Fig. II-7B, p. 28). The frequency of intracranial

Table II-18 Frequency of CNS involvement in malignant lymphoma.

	Non-Hodgkin's lymphoma	Hodgkin's disease	Total
Cases with CNS involvement: A	71	19	90
Total number of cases: B	212	123	335
Frequency of involvement: A/B × 100	33%	15%	27%

involvement in patients with non-Hodgkin's lymphoma cases was reported by several authors to be from 11 to 33 per cent (Sparling et al., 1947; Whinsnault et al., 1956; Law et al., 1975; Jellinger and Radaszkiewicz, 1976). Lymphomas complicated by leukemic conversion have a higher frequency of intracranial involvement than in the absence of leukemia (Gendelman et al., 1969).

Hodgkin's disease tends to affect the dura and the spinal epidural tissue. Occasionally, it also involves the brain parenchyma and leptomeninges (Bhagwati and McKissock, 1961; Marshall et al., 1968; Mullins et al., 1971; Biran and Herishianu, 1972; Brazinsky, 1973).

Leukemias

Leukemias affect the CNS more frequently than lymphomas. The frequency in our patients was 50 per cent and was reported as 18 to 44 per cent in other series (Tables II-3 and 5). The increased rate of CNS involvement was reported with the application of chemotherapy (Evans et al., 1970), an observation that has also been demonstrated by experimental studies (Thomas et al., 1962; Perk et al., 1974; Lynch et al., 1975).

Table II-19   Frequency of CNS involvement in leukemia.

	Lymphocytic leukemia	Myelocytic leukemia	Others*	Total
Cases with CNS involvement: A	34	52	6	92
Total number of cases: B	58	109	17	184
Frequency of involvement: A/B × 100	59%	48%	35%	50%

* Polycythemia vera and unclassified leukemias.

The frequency of CNS involvement according to the type of leukemia is shown in Table II-19. Lymphocytic leukemia has a higher frequency of CNS involvement (59%) in our series than myelocytic leukemia (48%). In each group of leukemia, acute leukemia has a higher rate of CNS involvement than chronic leukemia. Similar findings have been reported by many authors; from 25 to 56 per cent frequency in lymphocytic leukemia and from 4 to 25 per cent in myelocytic leukemia (Moore et al., 1960; Shaw et al., 1960; Evans et al., 1970; Pole, 1973). Recent reports indicate a high rate of CNS involvement, approximately 50 per cent in myelocytic leukemia (Walters et al., 1972; Armentrout and Ulrich, 1974; Fleming et al., 1974).

Leptomeningeal infiltration is one of the significant features of leukemia. Proliferating tumor cells in the subarachnoid space invade the nerve roots of both cranial and spinal nerves. Tumor cells also invade the brain parenchyma by penetrating the pia mater. Tumor infiltration in the hypothalamo-hypophyseal region may cause obesity or other hormonal disturbances (Joseph and Levin, 1956; Kovacs, 1973; Pochedly, 1977a).

Dural infiltrations are very frequently observed. Most of these, however, are asymptomatic (see also p. 93). Some authors have reported cases of chloroma involving the dura, usually proceeding from acute myelocytic leukemia (Wilhyde et al., 1963; Mason et al., 1973; Stefansson and Rask, 1973; Walters, 1977; Llena et al., 1978). The capsule of the pituitary gland is another tissue frequently involved with leukemia, with a rate of 28 per cent in our series (Table II-3 and 23, p. 102) and 46 per cent in another report (Masse et al., 1973).

Besides infiltration by tumor cells, vascular lesions and secondary infections are also important. Intracerebral hemorrhage, usually due to thrombocytopenia and adverse effects of chemotherapy, may accompany tumor infiltration. This occurred in 32 per cent of the leukemic patients (Schwab and Weiss, 1935), and is a frequent cause of death (Moore et al., 1960). Infection is caused by various kinds of organisms including viruses, bacteria and fungus (Williams et al., 1959). Similar processes occur in lymphomas (Ghatak, 1975; Hirano, 1976b).

Multiple Myeloma

Multiple myelomas affecting the skull and the vertebrae may invade the dura and the spinal epidural tissues. In the present series, 28 per cent of 80 patients with multiple myeloma were observed to have CNS involvement. Most of them were affected in the dura mater (Table II-3). The dural involvement is usually limited to its outer layer, but it may extend into the subdural spaces and invade the brain parenchyma (Courville, 1948; Clarke, 1954, 1956; Silverstein and Doniger, 1963; Zimmerman, 1974; Holness and Sangalang, 1976). Cranial or spinal nerves may be compressed in their courses through the bony canals when the tumors affect the skull base or the vertebrae.

SITES OF METASTATIC INVOLVEMENT

In the following section, we describe the pathologic features of metastatic tumors in each of the intracranial tissues.

Brain Parenchyma

Metastases to the parenchyma of the brain occurred in 16.5 per cent of all the carcinomas and sarcomas found at autopsy (Table II-2). Approximately half (48%) of these metastatic lesions were derived from lung cancer (Table II-6 and Fig. II-3). The breast was the source of 20 per cent of the lesions, the gastrointestinal tract 8 per cent, the urinary tract 6 per cent, and melanoma 6 per cent. Metastases to the brain parenchyma were observed in approximately six per cent of all lymphomas and leukemias (Table II-3).

Macroscopic Findings

Metastatic deposits of carcinomas and sarcomas, regardless of primary origin, were usually spheroid in shape and formed well-demarcated discrete nodules. When the white matter was involved, however, the metastases sometimes spread in an irregular fashion.

It has been suggested (Rich, 1930; Lesse and Netsky, 1954) that because of the vascular architecture, most metastatic lesions in the brain are located at the border between the white and gray matter (Fig. II-5A). There are, however, many exceptions to this rule. For example, some areas within the gray matter, such as the basal ganglia, thalamus and hypothalamus (Figs. II-5B and 6A, B), as well as some in the white matter such as the centrum semiovale (Fig. II-6C) and the corpus callosum, are all known as sites of metastatic tumors. Some deeply seated tumors in the cerebral hemisphere can even protrude into the ventricle. In the cerebellum, tumors tended to be located in the Purkinje cell layer and superficial portions of the granule cell layer. Tumors were found in both the tegumentum and the base of the pons with approximately equal frequency.

Metastatic tumors, generally speaking, are easily recognized on gross examination. Their maximal diameters range from microscopic size to 10 cm. They often have a color and texture different from the surrounding tissue. When they are very small, they are usually somewhat more granular on the cut surface than normal parenchyma. The use of methylene blue (Hara et al., 1979) has been shown to be helpful in detecting minute tumors and ill-circumscribed lesions (Fig. II-7, Plate II-1B).

The color of the metastatic tumor nodules depends on the amount of fibrous stroma, the degree of vascular proliferation, hemorrhage, necrosis and the presence of pigments such as melanin. When the patient is jaundiced, the tumor may appear yellowish-green due to the accumulation of bilirubin. The consistency of the metastatic tumor varies, but in general, it is firmer than the soft surrounding edematous brain tissue. In the presence of a pronounced fibrous stromal reaction, the tumors appear to be white and firm.

Metastatic tumors in the brain parenchyma often form cyst-like structures. These may be a result of secretory activities (e.g. mucin) leading to the accumulation of clear or turbid fluid within the cyst. More often, the cysts are the result of central necrosis of the tumor nodule (Figs. II-8 and 9A).

Hemorrhage is a common finding associated with metastatic tumors (Figs. II-9B and 10). Small hemorrhagic foci are often found within the tumor nodule. When the hemorrhage is extensive, a hematoma may form surrounding the tumor nodule (Fig. II-9C). Massive hemorrhages are very often associated with melanoma, choriocarcinoma and carcinoma of the lung and kidney. They may occur with other tumors as well (Scott, 1975; Mandybur, 1977). Even in the absence of hemorrhage, the tumor may appear reddish-brown in color due to congested and proliferated blood vessels.

Extensive edema of surrounding tissue is usually associated with metastatic tumors. The edema may extend a considerable distance from the nodule and may result in swelling of the brain and cerebral herniation (see Plate II-1A, p. 32 and Fig. II-47A).

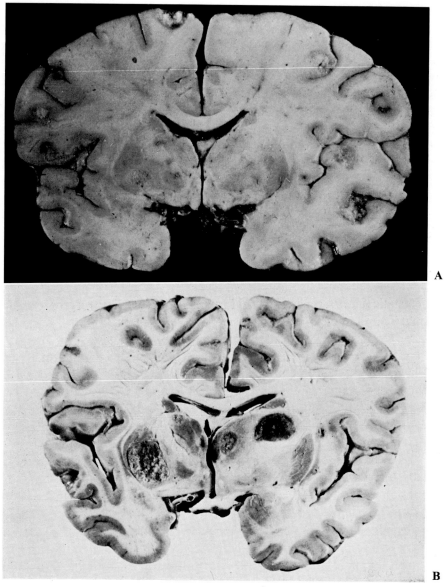

Fig. II-5 Multiple intracerebral metastases.
A. Multiple nodules located in the cortical and subcortical areas. (A 68-year-old woman, who had general weakness eight months before admission, developed headache, right homonymous hemianopsia, right hemiparesis and obtunded consciousness. Autopsy revealed a carcinoma of the adrenal gland that metastasized to the mesentery, cerebrum, cerebellum, spinal cord and dura mater. MH 18004.)
B. Multiple nodules located in the thalami and basal ganglia. (A 53-year-old woman, who had backache 15 months before admission, developed hypesthesia of all four extremities. Autopsy revealed anaplastic adenocarcinoma of the lung with metastases in various organs including the cerebrum and pituitary gland.   MH 12151.)

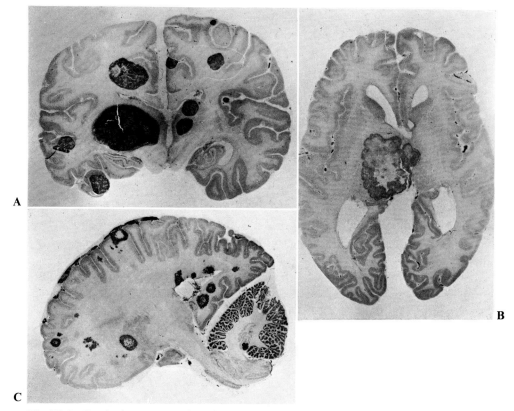

Fig. II-6 Cerebral metastases in Nissl preparations. Metastatic lesions are clearly seen. The margin of the tumor is well demarcated and the necrotic center is evident due to the pale stain.

A. (A 40-year-old man, who had dyspnea for one and a half years before admission, developed hallucinations. Autopsy, performed three months later, revealed adenocarcinoma of the lung with multiple metastases in the cerebrum and cerebellum. MH 6967.)

B. (A 63-year-old man developed right hemiparesis. Autopsy, performed six months later, revealed carcinoma of the adrenal gland with a metastasis in the left thalamus, which extended to the thalamus of the opposite side. MH 8311.)

C. (A 54-year-old woman, who was operated on for breast carcinoma two years before her last admission, developed left hemiparesis. Autopsy revealed metastases in the dura mater, leptomeninges, cerebrum and cerebellum. MH 9851.)

The macroscopic appearances of metastatic lymphoma and leukemia are quite different from those of carcinoma and sarcoma. Lymphoma may form tumors in the brain parenchyma similar to carcinoma but, in contrast, their borders are generally poorly defined and irregular. Furthermore, they tend to occur in midline structures such as the corpus callosum, septum pellucidum, fornix, basal ganglia, thalamus and centrum semiovale (Fig. II-7B and Plate II-1B, p. 32; Zimmerman, 1971, 1974, 1975). Due to the poorly defined boundaries, the demarcation of the tumors may be difficult to determine in gross examination. The tumors tend to have a tan color and their cut surface is soft and granular.

Leukemia often produces multiple hemorrhagic nodules (Fig. II-11), besides the usual form of infiltration of the leptomeninges. Even in the absence of metastases to the brain, lymphomas and leukemias are often associated with hemorrhage and infection.

The number of metastatic nodules varies depending on the thoroughness of the examination. Sometimes 50 or more independent nodules can be observed scattered throughout the brain (Plate II-2A p. 32 and Figs. II-5 and 6). In general, for carcinomas and sarcomas, approximately one third of the cases showed only a single nodule, one third showed between two and five, and the remaining one third showed six or more (Table II-20). In other reports, single metastasis is found in 23 to 35 per cent of the cases (Earle, 1954; Lesse and Netsky, 1954; Störtelbecker, 1954; France, 1975). On the other hand, there seems to be substantial differences in the number of metastases that may be expected from different primaries. More than half of the metastatic melanomas had six or more nodules (Fig. II-10). Carcinomas of the gastrointestinal tract and urinary tract, on the other hand, tend to produce a single metastasis (Table II-20 and France, 1975; Paillas and Pellet, 1975).

The distribution of nodules within the brain parenchyma was studied by examining the location of 743 easily recognizable nodules in brains containing one to five nodules. Seventy-seven per cent of the studied nodules were found in the supratentorial region, and in 23 per cent the infratentorium was involved (Table II-21). When the weight distribution of these two regions is considered [88% supratentorial and 12% subtentorial, (Blinkof and Glezer, 1968)], it is apparent that there are actually more metastatic nodules per gram of brain tissue found in the subtentorial region.

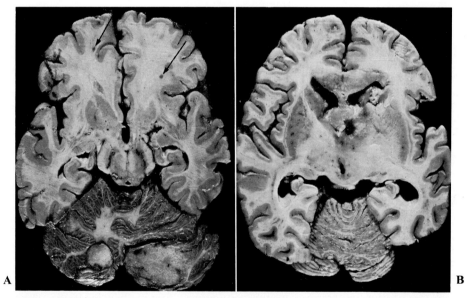

A   **B**

Fig. II-7   Horizontal section corresponding to CT scan. (15° from the canthomeatal line.)
A.   Two large metastatic foci are seen in the cerebellar hemispheres. Small multiple tumor nodules are seen in the frontal lobes (arrows). (A 60-year-old woman developed walking difficulty. Autopsy revealed squamous cell carcinoma of the lung that metastasized to the liver, lymph nodes and brain parenchyma. OS 1804.)
B.   Malignant lymphoma involving midline structures especially around the third ventricle and anterior horn. (A 61-year-old man, who had lymphoma of the nasopharynx and was treated with surgery and radiation therapy three years previously, developed paralysis of the third through twelfth cranial nerves and died six months later. Autopsy revealed reticulum cell sarcoma involving the leptomeninges and brain parenchyma. Small lesions were also found in the submucosa of the colon. MH 78191.) (From Hara et al., 1979.)

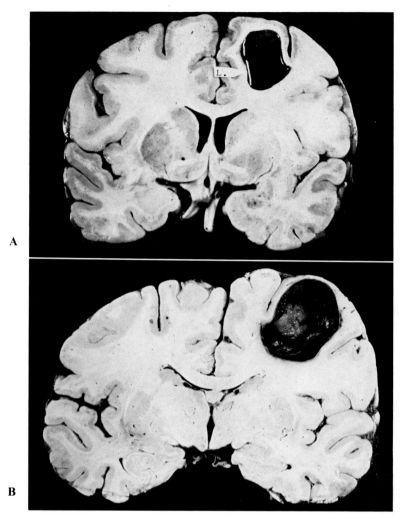

Fig. II-8   Necrotic metastatic lesions.
A.   (A 38-year-old woman was operated on for lung carcioma one year before admission.
No neurological deficits were noted.   Autopsy revealed oat cell carcinoma of the lung which
metastasized to the liver, pancreas, cerebrum, (single cystic lesion) and the dura mater.   MH
22242.) (From Hirano et al., 1980.)
B.   (A 64-year-old woman, who was operated on for carcinoma of the maxillary sinus three
years before her last admission, developed generalized seizures, then right hemiparesis and
speech difficulties.   Autopsy, performed one and a half months later, revealed squamous cell
carcinoma metastasized to the lymph nodes and adrenal gland.   The cerebrum contained
several metastatic nodules including one large mass.   MH 21396.)

Other authors reported similar results (Meyer and Reah, 1953; Ask-Upmark, 1956;
Chason et al., 1963; France, 1975).   Our recent clinical data on this subject are shown
in p. 119 in next chapter.

   Actually, the distribution of metastatic nodules is sometimes even more skewed
in favor of the infratentorial region depending on the tumor types.   Metastases of
melanomas and carcinomas of the urinary tract were distributed roughly in proportion to the relative weight of the two areas.   On the other hand, approximately
40 per cent of the nodules derived from tumors of the gastrointestinal tract were

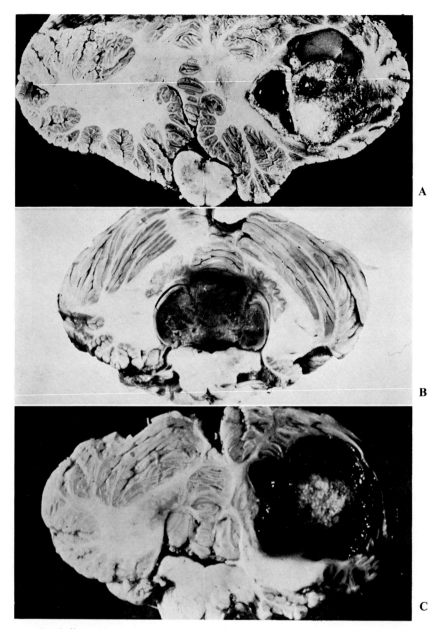

Fig. II-9 Cerebellar metastases.
A. (A 71-year-old woman, who was operated on for breast carcinoma two years before admission, developed right hemiparesis and disturbance of consciousness in the course of hospitalization. Autopsy revealed metastases in the lungs, lymph nodes, cerebrum, cerebellum and other organs. MH 13231.)
B. (A 57-year-old man who complained of generalized weakness and dyspnea. Autopsy revealed anaplastic carcinoma of the lung that metastasized to the liver, kidney, cerebrum, cerebellum and other organs. MH 11893.)
C. (A 68-year-old man, diagnosed as having a lung tumor two years before admission, suddenly became unconscious. Bloody cerebrospinal fluid was observed. Autopsy revealed adenocarcinoma of the prostate with metastases to the lungs, liver, cerebrum, cerebellum, posterior lobe of the pituitary gland, and other organs. MH 18115.) (From Hirano et al., 1980.)

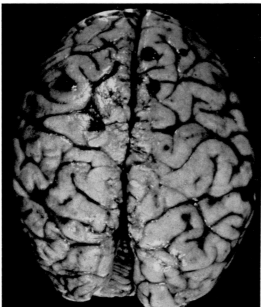

Fig. II-10 Hemorrhagic metastatic tumors.

A and **B** (A 44-year-old man, who was operated on for melanoma of the skin of his back half a year prior to admission, developed generalized seizures and mental changes. Autopsy, which was performed one year later, revealed metastases in many organs. The brain parenchyma, pituitary gland and dura mater contained multiple tumor nodules. MH 19968.) (A: From Hirano et al., 1980)

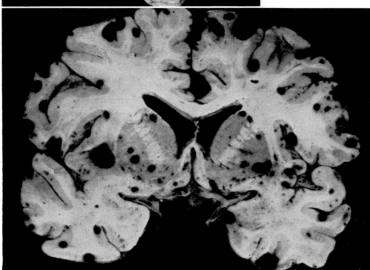

found in the infratentorial region.   Metastasis per unit volume of the brain from carcinomas of the lung and breast were also somewhat more common in this region.

The brain stem seems to be the preferred site of metastases in relation to its weight, when compared with the cerebrum or cerebellum.   In our series, 4.4 per cent of the studied nodules were found in the brain sten (Table II-22).   Hunter and Rewcastle (1968) reported an incidence of 11.7 per cent of metastases to the brain stem.   This subject has been studied by a number of other researchers (Davison and Spiegel, 1945; Netsky and Strobos, 1952; McFarland and Truscott, 1961; Derby and Guiang, 1975; Ogawa et al., 1977).

There seems to be no difference between the left and right cerebral hemispheres in the distribution of metastatic nodules from carcinomas and sarcomas.   The distribution of nodules among the various cerebral lobes showed no special area of

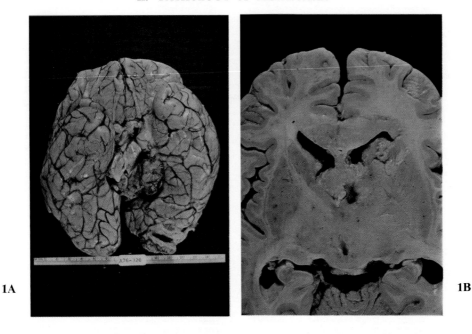

1A   1B

Plate II-1A   An adenocarcinoma of the rectum which spread to the left occipital lobe.   The inferior surface of the left occipital lobe and the temporal lobe show marked edema.   The herniated left parahippocampal gyrus and the uncus are necrotic.   The midbrain is compressed and deformed.   (MH 76326.)

Plate II-1B   Malignant lymphoma (reticulum cell sarcoma) involving the midline structure of the brain.   Note the enlarged septum pellucidum and the fornix.   (Methylene blue stain, MH 78191.) (From Hara et al., 1979.)

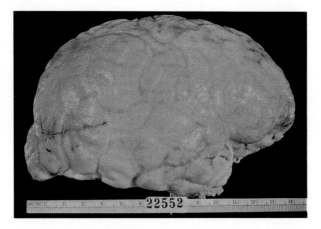

Plate II-1C   Lymphocytic leukemia cells infiltrating the leptomeninges, which has become white and opaque.   (MH 22552.)

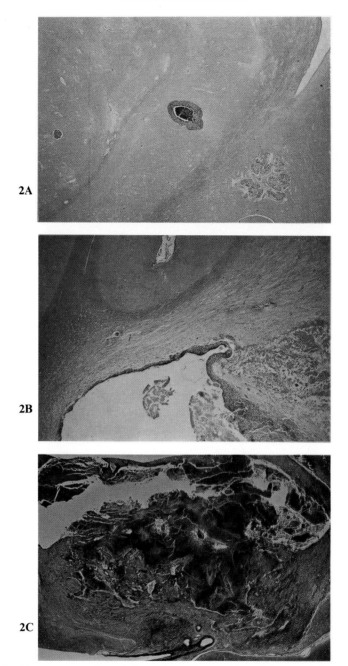

2A

2B

2C

Plate II-2A   Three metastatic nodules are seen in a section of Ammon's horn.   Small metastatic nodules were disseminated throughout the entire brain.   Metastatic breast carcinoma in the cerebrum.   (H & E × 4.29, MH 21041.)

Plate II-2B   A metastatic lung carcinoma in the cerebrum replaced by connective tissue after radiation therapy.   The fibrous tissue (green) surrounds the necrotic area.   (Masson trichrome × 3.25, MH 21117.)

Plate II-2C   The center of the metastatic tumor is necrotic.   Only a thin layer of neoplasm is visible at the periphery.   The surrounding white matter shows marked edema and desstruction of myelin.   Anaplastic carcinoma of the lung.   (Luxol fast blue — periodic acid Schiff × 3.25, MH 20256.)

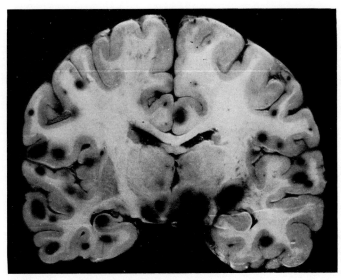

Fig. II-11   Intracerebral hemorrhage.
These multiple hemorrhagic lesions were associated with acute lymphocytic leukemia. (A 17-year-old boy, who received radiotherapy and
chemotherapy for leukemia for one year, developed meningeal irritation.
The autopsy, four months later, revealed tumor involvement of the leptomeninges and brain parenchyma, in addition to intracerebral hemorrhage.
MH 18260.)

Table II-20   Number of metastatic nodules in the brain parenchyma,
arranged according to the primary sites.

	Number of Nodules						Percentage of cases with single nodule A/N × 100 (%)	Percentage of cases with multiple nodules over 5. B/N × 100 (%)
	1 (A)	2	3	4	5	over 5 (B)		
Lung (N = 266)	74	50	32	17	7	74	28	28
Breast (N = 111)	34	16	10	4	3	43	31	39
G.I. tract (N = 43)	20	10	4	1	3	5	47	12
Melanoma (N = 34)	8	2	1	4	1	18	24	53
Urinary tract (N = 67)	15	5	3	2	3	6	44	18
Others (N = 67)	28	9	10	3	2	15	42	22
Total number of cases (N = 555)	179	92	60	45	19	163	32	29

N: Number of cases with metastases in the brain parenchyma.

definite predilection in our study, although there was a slightly lower frequency of
metastases in the temporal lobe when compared to the parietal and occipital lobes
(Table II-22 and Fig. II-12).   Some researchers have concluded that there is no pre-
ferential site within the cerebrum (Simionescu, 1960; Rhoton, Jr., et al., 1966; Willis,
1973; Arseni and Constantinescu, 1975; France, 1975) while others indicated that
the parietal lobe, the location irrigated by terminal branches of the middle cerebral
artery, was more often involved (Kindt, 1964; Vieth and Odom, 1965a; Paillas and
Pellet, 1975).

Table II-21 Distribution of metastatic nodules in the brain parenchyma, arranged according to the primary sites (1).

Primary sites and total number of nodules examined	Number and rate of supratentorial nodules	Number and rate of infratentorial nodules
Lung (N = 373)	291 (78%)	82 (22%)
Breast (N = 117)	83 (71%)	34 (29%)
G.I. tract (N = 71)	42 (59%)	29 (41%)
Melanoma (N = 36)	31 (86%)	5 (14%)
Urinary tract (N = 57)	53 (93%)	4 (7%)
Others (N = 89)	75 (84%)	14 (16%)
Total (N = 743)	**575 (77%)**	**168 (23%)**

N: Number of nodules examined = 100%
Location of metastatic nodules were examined in 743 nodules. The precise location is shown in Table II-22.

Table II-22 Distribution of metastatic nodules in the brain parenchyma (2).

Location of nodules	Number of nodules	Ratio to total supratentorial nodules (624) = 100%
Frontal lobe	205	33%
Temporal lobe	77	12
Parietal lobe	123	20
Occipital lobe	123	20
Basal ganglia	34	5
Thalamus & hypothalamus	23	4
(In the cerebrum)*	39	6
Midbrain	6	
Pons	25	
Medulla oblongata	1	
Cerebellum	142	

*   Details of location of the nodules are not available.

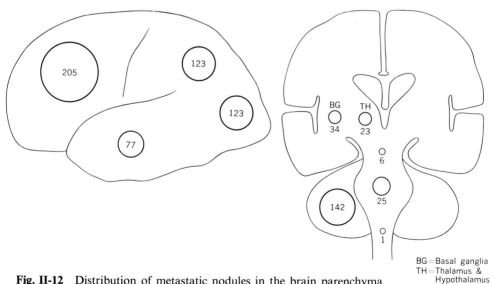

BG = Basal ganglia
TH = Thalamus & Hypothalamus

Fig. II-12 Distribution of metastatic nodules in the brain parenchyma. A diagramatic presentation of Table II-22.   Number indicates the number of metastatic nodules.

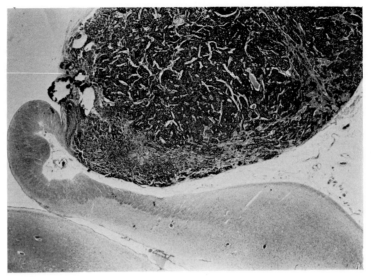

Fig. II-13 Metastasis in the pineal body from a carcinoma of the lung.
(H & E × 10,   MH 17729.)

The frequency of metastases in the basal ganglia, the thalamus and the hypothalamus was approximately in proportion to the size of these structures. Lesions
located in these structures may cause unusual symptoms (Sciarra and Sprofkin,
1953; Lewis and Johnson, 1968; Moolten, 1972).

Several metastatic lesions to the pineal gland were seen in the present series
(Fig. II-13). Other researchers reported involvement of the pineal gland in 1 to 4
per cent of patients with malignant tumors (Ortega et al., 1951; Halpert et al., 1960;
France, 1975).

Microscopic Findings (with Light and Electron Microscopes)

General Features

Sharp demarcation from the surrounding nervous tissue is a characteristic
microscopic feature of metastatic tumors (Figs. II-30C, p. 51 and 16A, p. 39).

Metastatic tumors usually form a solid mass of tumor cells, which may be
shown by electron microscopy to form various types of cell junctions. In general,
the mass compresses the surrounding tissues. Infiltration by loose tumor cells into
the neuropil is rarely observed. The exceptions to this rule are lymphomas (Fig.
II-14), leukemias, melanomas (Fig. II-36B, p. 56), and oat cell carcinomas of the
lung (Fig. II-39, p. 58). In the periphery of the metastatic tumor nodule, tongue-
like masses of tumor cells tend to grow around blood vessels (Fig. II-42C, p. 61).

In general, the histology of the metastatic tumors is affected by the structure
of the primary tumors and by the adequacy of the blood supply. Differentiated
carcinomas usually mimic the structure of the primary. In undifferentiated tumors,
the tumor cells grow and pile up around the blood vessels, and after reaching a thickness of about 200 to 300 μm, those cells beyond this limit become necrotic.

Fig. II-14 Intraparenchymal spread of lymphoma.

High-magnification micrograph illustrating the tumor spread along the white matter bundles. (H & E × 100, MH 78199.)

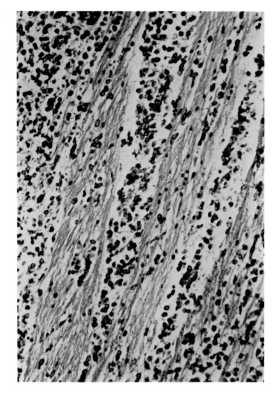

Histological Patterns

Adenocarcinoma with tall columnar epithelium

Glands lined by a single layer of tall columnar epithelium characterize metastatic adenocarcinomas of lung (Fig. II-15) and colon origin (Fig. II-16). Sometimes carcinoma from the ovary and other sites may have a similar histologic pattern. The basal aspect of the epithelium, resting on a basal lamina, always faces the stroma (Fig. II-17) or, at the edge of the nodule, the surrounding nervous tissue (Fig. II-15C).

The nucleus is located in the basal portion of the cell. The fine structures of these tumors have been described by some authors (Obiditsch-Mayer and Breitfellner, 1968; Kuhn, 1972; Bedrossian et al., 1975; Fenoglio et al., 1975). Well-developed rough endoplasmic reticulum, Golgi apparatus and secretory granules can be seen between the nucleus and the apical portion of the cell. Some of these tumors secrete mucin (Fig. II-18). Microvilli are present at the apical surface. Various types of cell junctions occur between cells.

Adenocarcinoma with low columnar epithelium

Glandular structures lined by this type of epithelium are often seen in metastatic carcinomas of the breast (Figs. II-19 and 20), gastrointestinal tracts other than the colon (Fig. II-21A), the prostate (Fig. II-21B) and the uterus (Figs. II-22 and 23). The tumor may form definite acini, but sometimes they grow as solid tumor masses without any distinct gland formation. Minute lumens surrounded by microvilli can be shown by the electron microscope (Figs. II-24 and 25).

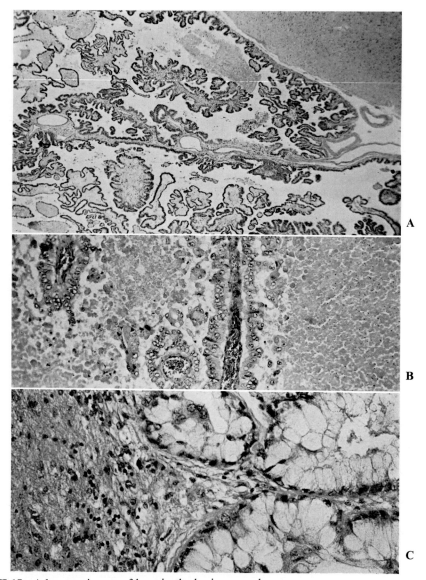

Fig. II-15 Adenocarcinoma of lung in the brain parenchyma.
A. Two of the three gyri of the cerebrum were replaced by metastatic papillary adenocarcinoma. Tumor cells extended along the pial and perivascular surfaces in a single layer abutting the connective tissue. (H & E × 34, MH 20548.)
B. A single layer of columnar epithelial cells along the blood vessels. The rest of the tumor was necrotic, especially in areas remote from the vessels. (H & E × 100, MH 21838.)
C. Higher magnification of the margin of a mucin-producing adenocarcinoma. The tumor is well demarcated from the surrounding brain (left). (H & E × 200, MH 22150.)

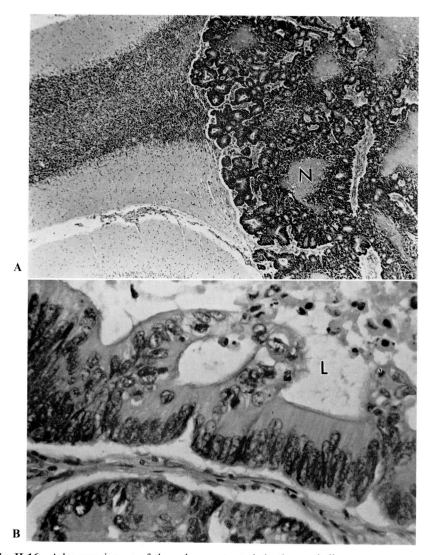

Fig. II-16   Adenocarcinoma of the colon, metastasis in the cerebellum.
A.   A tumor on the right side of the micrograph has a distinct margin separating it from the cerebellar tissue on the left.   A glandular arrangement is evident and necrotic foci are marked (N).   (H & E × 34, MH 19537.)
B.   Higher magnification of a similar tumor illustrated in A.   Tall, columnar epithelial cells lie between the lumen (L) and a connective tissue band.   Nuclei are located at the basal aspect and the apical portion is marked by a brush border.   (H & E × 310, MH 20214.)

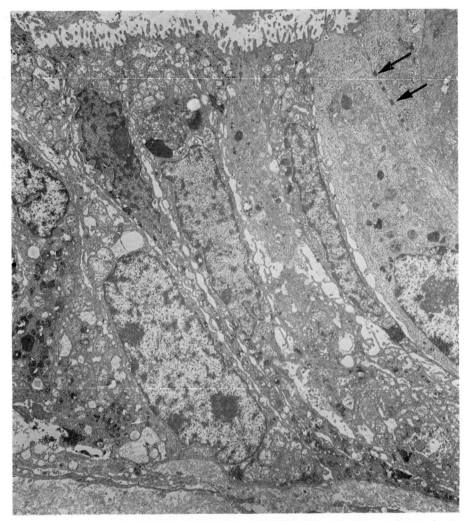

Fig. II-17 An electron micrograph of a metastatic differentiated adenocarcinoma in the brain of a 72-year-old man with progressive dementia. The lumen in the upper portion of the micrograph and the columnar arrangement of the tumor cells connected by well-developed desmosomes (arrows) are seen. The basal surfaces of the cells are covered by a basal lamella facing the connective tissue space. (× 3,200, NS 7659.)

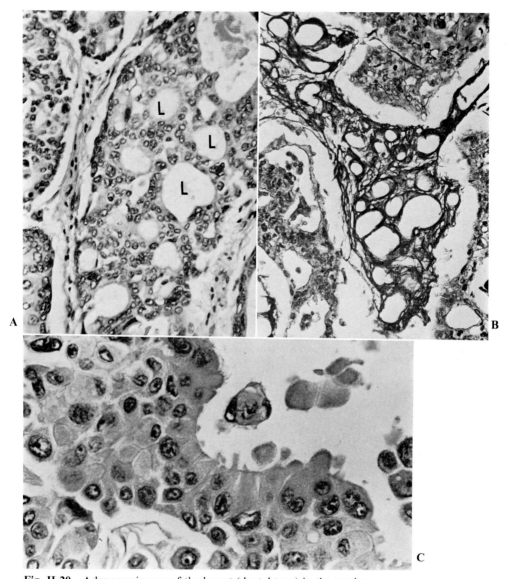

Fig. II-20 Adenocarcinoma of the breast (ductal type) in the cerebrum.
A. Lumens (L) of the glandular structures are evident. Tumor cells are separated by connective tissue septa. (H & E × 200, MH 22081.)
B. Reticulin stain of a tumor similar to that illustrated in A. The connective tissue septa contain strongly argentophilic fibers. Nests of epithelial tumor cells are seen in the upper, right and left sides of the illustration. (Wilder × 200, MH 20312.)
C. Higher magnification of the luminal aspect of the tumor. Tumor cells are compactly arranged. Cellular protrusions are seen. (H & E × 310, MH 21019.)

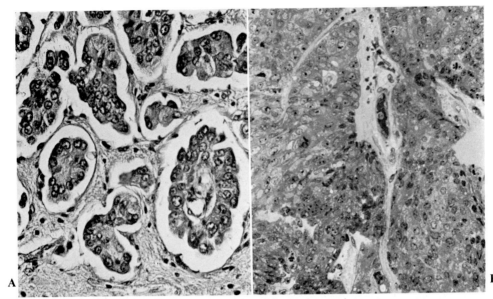

Fig. II-21   Metastatic adenocarcinomas from various primary sites.
A.   Higher magnification of nests of adenocarcinoma of the pancreas invading cerebral tissue.   (H & E × 200, MH 22203.)
B.   Adenocarcinoma of the prostate invading the dura.   (Epon embedding.   Toluidine blue × 100, NS 7768.)

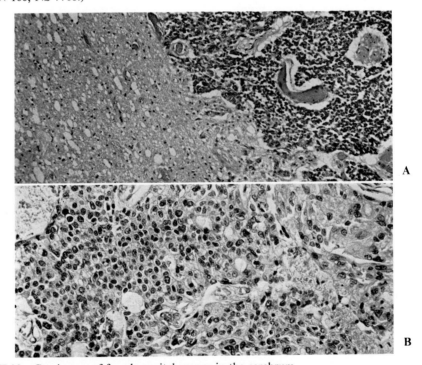

Fig. II-22   Carcinoma of female genital organs in the cerebrum.
A.   Endometrial adenocarcinoma (right) and edematous brain tissue (left) are sharply separated.   (H & E × 77, MH 19912.)
B.   Higher magnification of a tumor similar to that illustrated in A.   In this illustration, the epithelial nature of tumor is distinct, although the glandular structure is not apparent in this field.   (H & E × 100, MH 22176.)

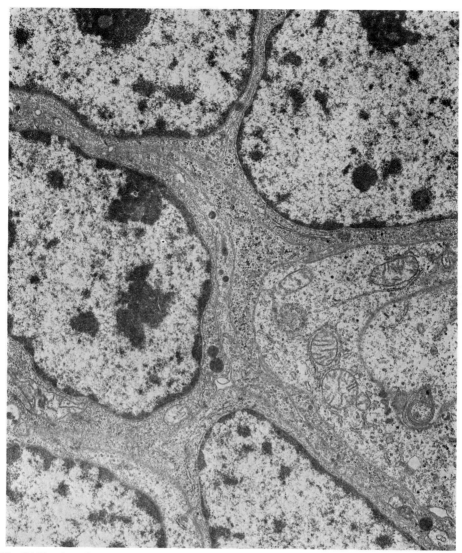

Fig. II-23 An electron micrograph of metastatic uterine adenocarcinoma in the brain. Tumor cells are compactly arranged with very narrow extracellular spaces. The cytoplasm is scanty and free ribosomes are evident. A few membrane-bounded dense bodies as well as mitochondria and other organelles are seen. Margination of the chromatin is evident in the nuclei. (× 10,000, NS 7742.)

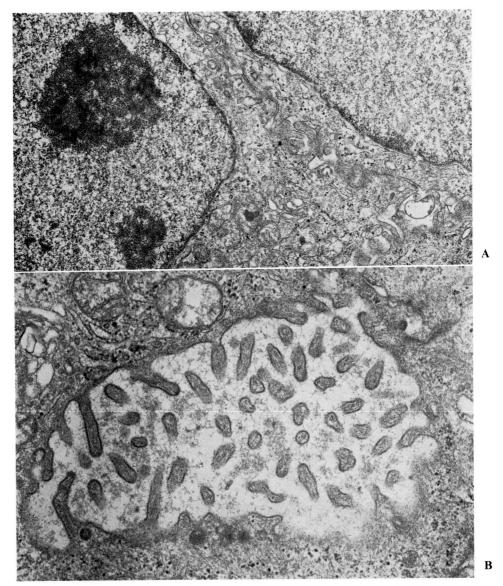

A

B

Fig. II-24 Electron micrographs of metastatic mammary carcinoma in the brain.
A. Tumor cells are intimately adherent to one another with narrow extracellular spaces.
The cytoplasm contains mitochondria, ribosomes, fibrils, Golgi apparatus and scattered
stacks of rough endoplasmic reticulum.   The nucleus contains a large nucleolus. ($\times$ 12,000,
NS 7767.)
B.   Many short microvilli project into a small lumen. ($\times$ 22,000, NS 7767.)

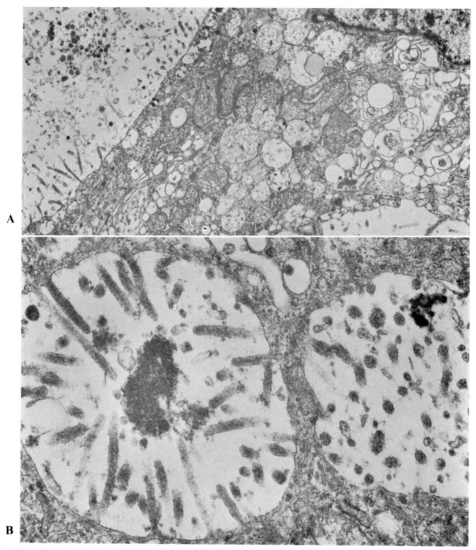

Fig. II-25 Electron micrographs of metastatic prostatic carcinoma in the brain.
A. A lumen of the gland is seen in the left upper portion. The apical surface is marked by long, slender microvilli projecting into the lumen. The cytoplasm on the right is crowded with well-developed membrane-bounded vacuoles, mitochondria, Golgi apparatus and other organelles. ($\times$ 5,600, NS 7768.)
B. Higher magnification of the microlumen of the tumor illustrated in A. Light microscopy showed many vacuolated areas within the tumor tissue. As seen in the electron micrograph, these actually represent small lumens. Slender microvilli project into the lumens. ($\times$ 25,000, NS 7768.)

Renal carcinoma

Cells of adenocarcinoma of the kidney (clear cell carcinoma) have characteristic, abundant, pale cytoplasm (Fig. II-26). Gland formation is rare. The electron microscope reveals abundant glycogen and lipid granules in the pale areas of the cytoplasm (Fig. II-27) (Hirano and Zimmerman, 1972).

Thyroid carcinoma

Metastatic thyroid carcinoma can be identified, if colloid-containing follicles are observed (Figs. II-28 and 29).

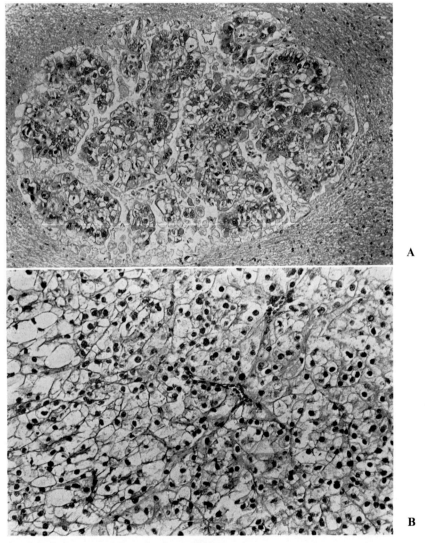

A

B

Fig. II-26   Renal adenocarcinoma in the cerebrum.
A.   A metastatic tumor nodule compresses the surrounding brain tissue. (H & E × 100, MH 21723.)
B.   Higher magnification of a tumor similar to that illustrated in A. Tumor cells have distinct, clear cytoplasm (clear cell carcinoma). (H & E × 280, NS 7933.)

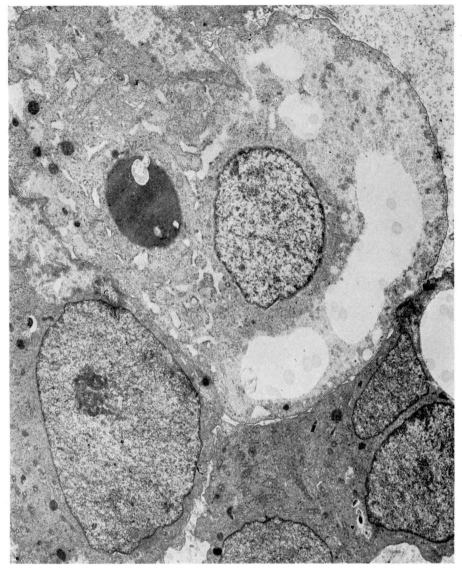

Fig. II-27 An electron micrograph of a renal adenocarcinoma in the brain. The tumor cells have markedly distended cytoplasms due to the accumulation of glycogen granules. (× 8,000, NS 5913.)

Squamous cell carcinoma

This tumor type is seen in metastatic carcinomas of the lung (Fig. II-30), esophagus (Fig. II-31A), uterine cervix, and other origins (Fig. II-31B). It is rare to see keratinization in metastases to the brain (Fig. II-32). The cells of the well-differentiated tumor have well-developed desmosomes, interdigitations and tonofilaments within the cytoplasm (Fig. II-33).

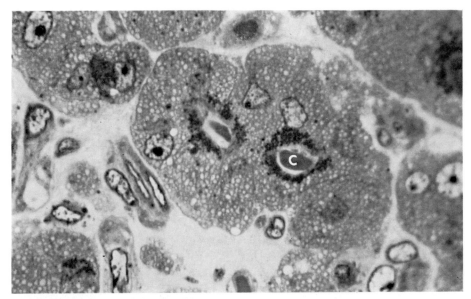

Fig. II-28   Carcinoma of the thyroid.
Carcinoma of the thyroid illustrating the characteristic follicles which contain colloid (C) surrounded by epithelial cells.   The apical portions of these cells contain a dark granular substance.   The rest of the cytoplasm contains numerous pale granular areas corresponding to mitochondria.   Vascular channels are seen in the connective tissue stroma.   (Epon embedding, Toluidine blue × 1,200, NS 77207.)

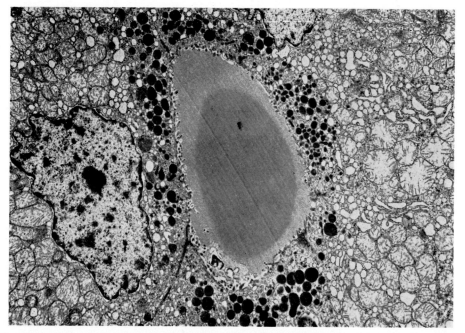

Fig. II-29   Electron micrograph of metastatic thyroid carcinoma.
A colloid substance fills a central lumen which is surrounded by several tumor cells.   The apical portion of the tumor cells are marked by membrane-bounded electron dense granules of variable size.   Most of the cytoplasm is filled with numerous mitochondria.   Well-developed junctional apparatuses are evident.   (× 4,000, NS 77207.)

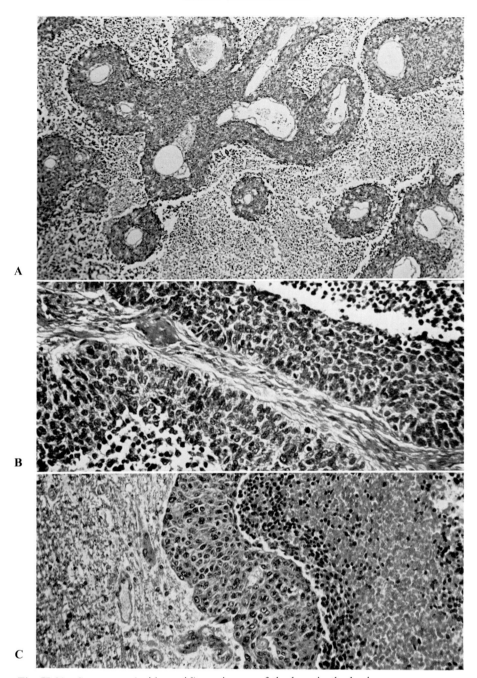

Fig. II-30 Squamous (epidermoid) carcinoma of the lung in the brain.
A. Nests of tumor cells around blood vessels. The nests are approximately 300μm thick
and are surrounded by necrotic tumor cells. (H & E × 50, MH 21126.)
B. Higher magnification of a tumor similar to that illustrated in A. The tumor cells are
seen around a vessel and the connective tissue stroma. The upper and lower portions of the
micrograph show necrosis. (H & E × 240, MH 757.)
C. The tumor is clearly demarcated from the compressed brain tissue (left), where endothelial proliferation is evident. Tumor cells at some distance from the edge of the boundary
of the tumor are necrotic (right). (H & E × 120, OS 1804.)

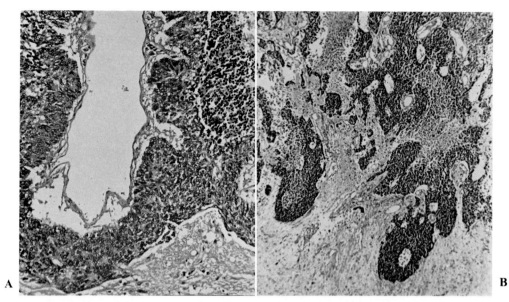

Fig. II-31 Metastatic squamous cell carcinoma from various primary sites.
A. Squamous cell (epidermoid) carcinoma of the esophagus in the pons. (H & E × 100,
MH 22462.)
B. Low magnification of an urotherial carcinoma of the bladder. (H & E × 100, MH
20186.)

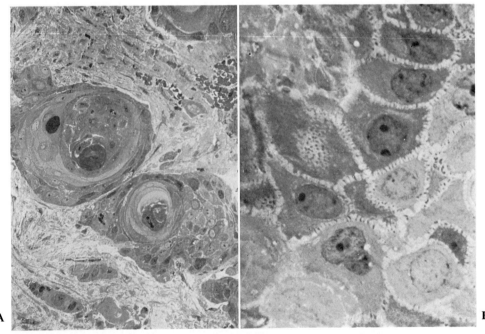

Fig. II-32 A keratinizing squamous cell carcinoma.
A. Nests of tumors containing centrally keratinized pearly structures. (Epon embedding,
Toluidine blue × 420, NS 77179.)
B. Higher magnification of an area of squamous epithelial cells similar to that illustrated in
A. The epithelial cells are connected by many intercellular bridges. (Epon embedding,
Toluidine blue × 1,000, NS 77179.)

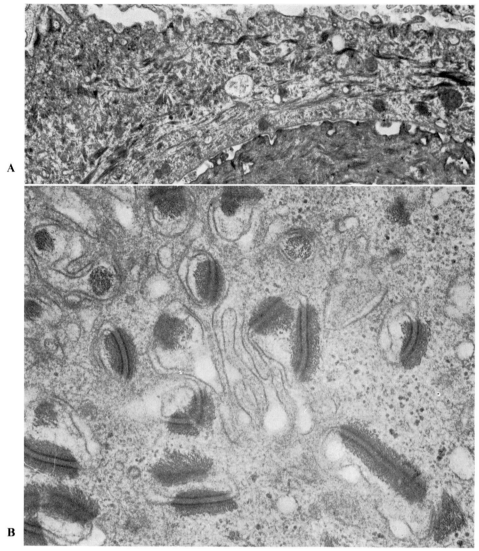

Fig. II-33 Electron micrographs of metastatic squamous cell carcinoma.
A. The tumor cells contain large numbers of tonofilaments. ($\times$ 8,800, NS 77179.)
B. Marked interdigitation of adjacent tumor cells and well-developed desmosomes.
($\times$ 30,000, NS 77179.)

Choriocarcinoma

Metastatic choriocarcinoma shows the same biphasic pattern as the primary lesion. Two groups of cells, syncytiotrophoblasts and cytotrophoblasts, are intermixed irregularly (Fig. II-34).

Melanomas

This group of metastatic tumors has a variety of histological patterns in the CNS. One pattern consists of compactly arranged polygonal cells which pile up around blood vessels in rosette formation (Fig. II-35). Tumors showing this pattern usually show a clear margin and do not infiltrate the adjacent tissues. In another pattern, spindle-shaped melanoma cells diffusely infiltrate the nervous

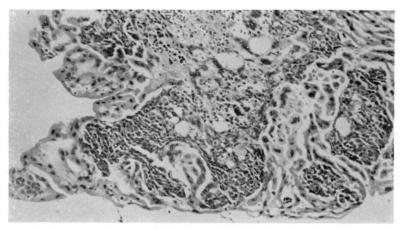

Fig. II-34 Carcinoma of female genital organs in the cerebrum.
A choriocarcinoma showing the characteristic Langhans and syncitial cells. (H & E
× 100, NS 6775.)

tissue (Fig. II-36). A third pattern consists of tumor cells invading the Virchow-
Robin spaces in multiple sites (Fig. II-56A and B, p. 76). This pattern is usually
seen in the gray matter without obvious leptomeningeal dissemination (see also
p. 77). Some tumor nodules are pigmented and some are not. Even within a
single tumor nodule, both melanotic and amelanotic areas may be seen. Melanosomes can be seen with the electron microscope (Figs. II-37 and 38). Immature
melanosomes have been identified even in amelanotic cells (Toshima et al., 1968; Fu
et al., 1975).

Oat cell carcinoma

Diffuse infiltration of the nervous tissue by spindle-shaped tumor cells is seen
in this tumor (Fig. II-39), which is similar to some cases of melanoma (Fig. II-36B).

Sarcomas

Nodules of metastatic soft part sarcomas are usually well-demarcated and
there is usually little tendency of tumor cell infiltration of the parenchyma (Fig.
II-40A and B). Vascular proliferation is not pronounced. Thin-walled, dilated
blood vessels in fibrosarcoma were characteristic features (Fig. II-41). In a case of
metastatic fibrosarcoma, however, the pseudopalisading of tumor cells around foci
of necrosis identical to that seen in glioblastoma multiforme was observed (Fig.
II-40C).

Lymphomas and leukemias

The tumor cells tend to grow along the perivascular space and in the surrounding neural tissue (Barnard and Scott, 1975). In the white matter, they infiltrate
nerve fibers (Fig. II-14). Pronounced proliferation of reticulin fibers is seen
around blood vessels.

Reaction of Surrounding Tissue

Vascular reaction

Proliferation of blood vessels occurs within the nervous tissue surrounding
the metastatic foci for a distance of approximately 1,000 μm. The intensity of

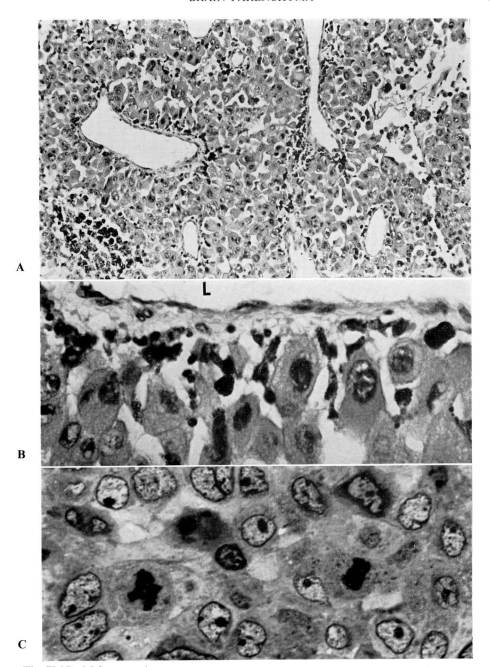

Fig. II-35   Melanoma. 1.

A.   Tumor cells are seen between vascular channels which have a thin walled sinusoidal pattern.   Coarse black pigment granules are seen around the perivascular areas and in the necrotic areas at the left lower corner of the micrograph.   (H & E × 100, MH 20305.)

B.   Higher magnification of A, illustrating pigment deposits in the tumor cells surrounding a blood vessel.   The lumen (L) of the vessel is seen.   (H & E × 490, MH 20305.)

C.   Higher magnification of a melanoma showing three distinct mitotic figures.   The tumor cells contain distinct nucleoli, but the melanin pigment is less apparent in this preparation. (Epon embedding, Toluidine blue × 1,200, NS 8040.)

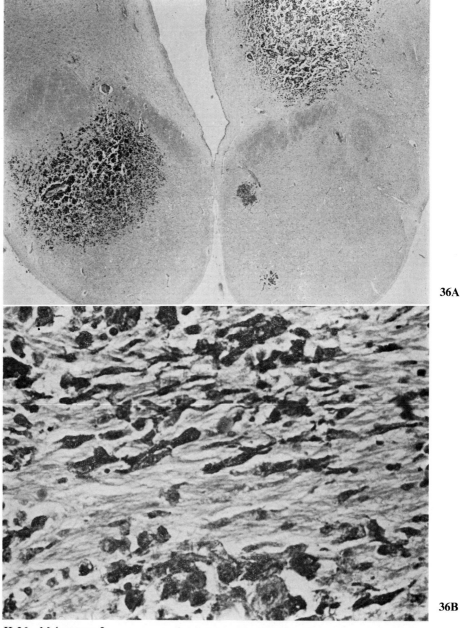

36A

36B

Fig. II-36 Melanoma. 2.
A. Several metastatic nodules of various sizes located in the hypothalamus. (H & E × 12, MH 19968.)
B. Spindle-shaped tumor cells infiltrate along the nerve fibers. (H & E × 240, MH 17764.)

Fig. II-37 An electron micrograph of metastatic melanoma in the brain (1).
The electron-dense melanin granules (melanosomes) are characteristic cytoplasmic features. Tumor cells show slender projections. (× 9,600, NS 7827.)

Fig. II-38 Electron micrograph of a metastatic melanoma in the brain (2).
Melanosomes and well-developed Golgi apparatus in a tumor cell. (× 17,000, NS 7827.)

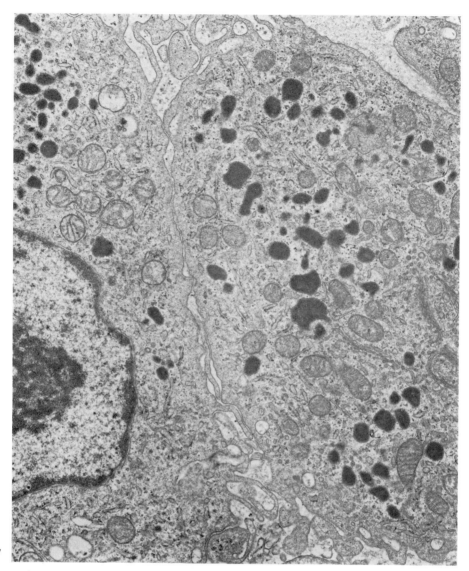

37

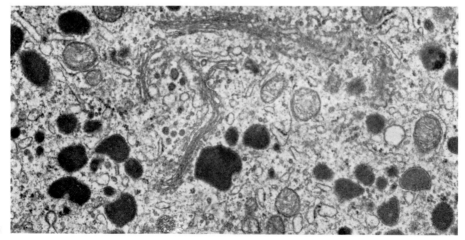

38

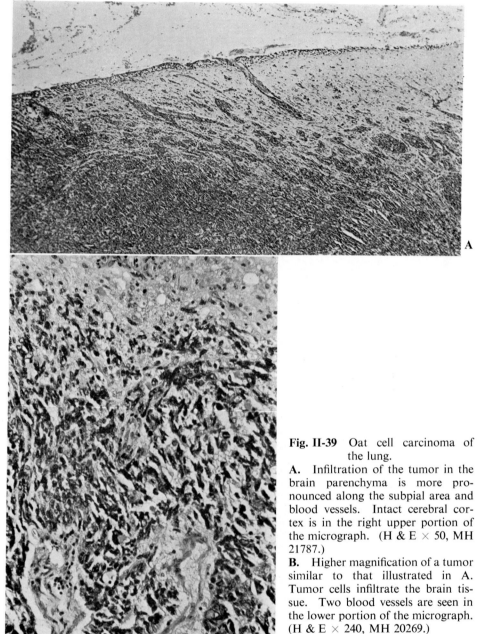

Fig. II-39 Oat cell carcinoma of the lung.
A. Infiltration of the tumor in the brain parenchyma is more pronounced along the subpial area and blood vessels. Intact cerebral cortex is in the right upper portion of the micrograph. (H & E × 50, MH 21787.)
B. Higher magnification of a tumor similar to that illustrated in A. Tumor cells infiltrate the brain tissue. Two blood vessels are seen in the lower portion of the micrograph. (H & E × 240, MH 20269.)

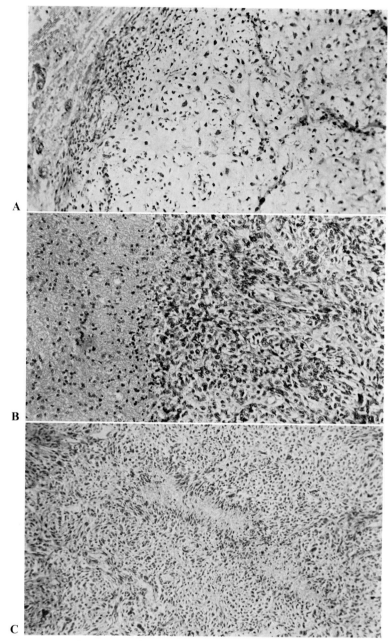

Fig. II-40   Metastatic sarcomas in the cerebrum.
A.   The margin of a chondrosarcoma in the brain. (H & E × 77, MH 13875.)
B.   The margin of a fibrosarcoma. As shown in A, the margin of the tumor is rather distinct although it is not encapsulated. The tumor cells and surrounding brain tissue are intermingled in a complex manner. (H & E stain × 100, MH 22068.)
C.   A fibrosarcoma showing pseudopalisading of nuclei around a necrotic zone. (H & E × 77, MH 22068.)

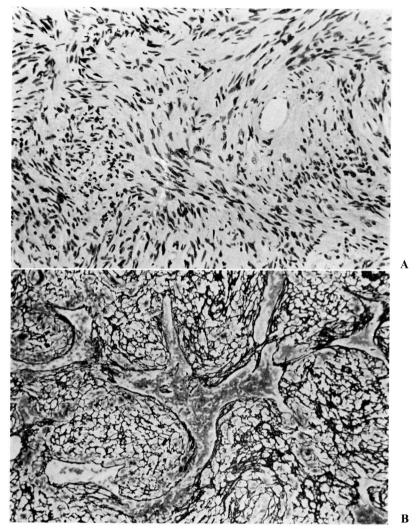

Fig. II-41 Metastatic fibrosarcoma in the cerebrum.
A. This is the histological appearance of a fibrosarcoma. Spindle-shaped cells are compactly arranged. A cross section of a blood vessel is seen. (H & E × 170, MH 17189.)
B. Reticulin stain of a tumor similar to that illustrated in A. A pronounced argentophilic network is a characteristic feature of fibrosarcoma. Fiber-free channels indicate vascular lumens. (Wilder × 100, MH 22068.)

vascular proliferation is maximal in the area adjacent to the tumor, where endothelial proliferation is conspicuous and the lumens of the blood vessel become narrow. Sometimes, the blood vessels are coiled in a manner reminiscent of renal glomeruli. However, endothelial proliferation is rarely as extensive as that seen in the gliomas. Aggregates of abnormally distended thin-walled vessels can be frequently seen at the periphery of the nodules (Fig. II-42A and B) (Gough, 1940; Hägerstrand, 1961).

In the center of the tumor nodule, the network of blood vessels becomes disperse and loose (Fig. II-19B), the lumens distended and the vessel walls thin. In areas of necrosis, there are almost no recognizable blood vessels.

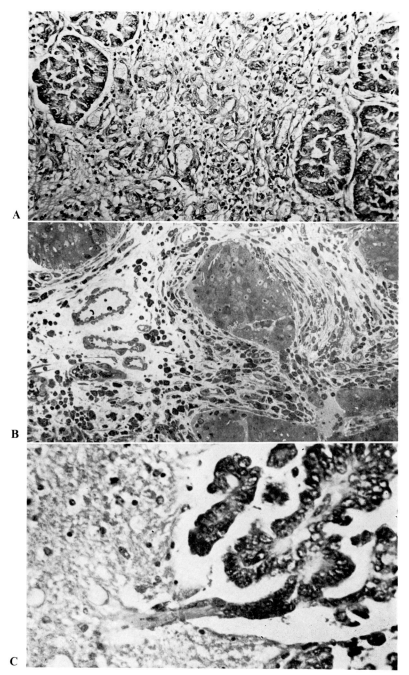

Fig. II-42 Vascular proliferation associated with metastatic tumor.
A. Nests of tumor cells from a lung carcinoma in brain tissue are surrounded by many small vascular channels. (H & E × 100, MH 20434.)
B. The center of a focus of metastatic breast carcinoma in the cerebrum. There is ample connective tissue between the nests of epithelial cells. Blood vessels show the marked endothelial proliferation. The surrounding edematous areas contain numerous cells as well as numerous fibroblasts. (Epon embedding, Toluidine blue × 200, NS 7663.)
C. Tumor cells extend into the perivascular space of the small vessel. Metastatic breast carcinoma in the cerebellum. (H & E × 200, MH 20843.)

It remains to be seen whether vascular proliferation is in fact induced by a tumor angiogenic factor as described by Folkman et al. (1971, 1976, 1977).

In depth structural studies of the endothelium reveal abnormalities which may vary depending upon the nature of the tumor (Nyström, 1960; Hirano and Zimmerman, 1972; Hirano et al., 1974; Hirano and Matsui, 1975; Hirano, 1976a). The cytoplasm of the endothelial cells may become irregular in shape, with some very

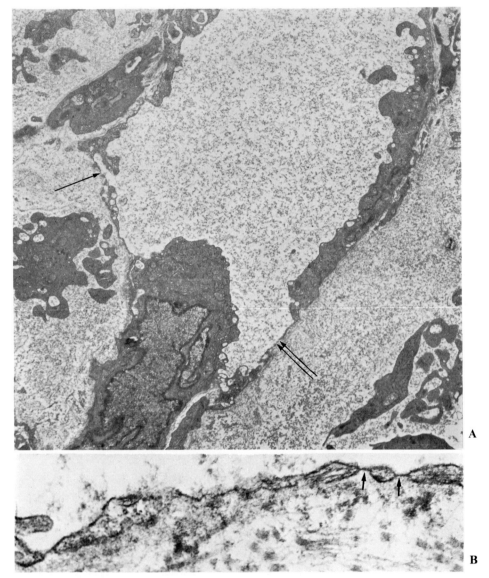

Fig. II-43 Electron micrographs of the blood vessels in metastatic brain tumors. 1.
A. Low magnification of a blood vessel within a focus of metastatic lung carcinoma in the cerebellum. The thickness of the endothelial cell is variable. The arrows indicate an area with numerous fenestrae. The blood vessel is surrounded by extracellular space filled with edema fluid and scattered collagen fibers. (× 4,000, NS 6619.)
B. Higher magnification of an abnormal blood vessel within a focus of metastatic renal carcinoma in the brain. Arrows indicate fenestrae. Collagen fibers are seen in the perivascular space. (× 58,000, NS 7907.)

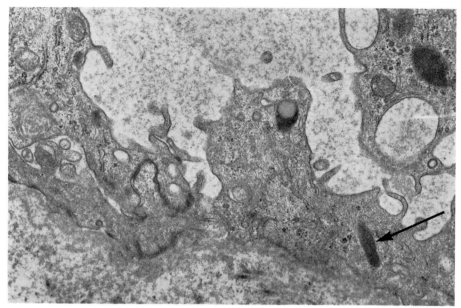

Fig. II-44 Electron micrograph of the blood vessel in metastatic brain tumor. 2. Metastatic breast carcinoma in the cerebrum. Marked infolding of the surface of the endothelial cells is seen. There are many fibrils in the cytoplasm. The arrow indicates a Weibel-Palade body. (× 15,000, NS 7663.)

thick portions and others which are quite thin, sometimes containing variable numbers of fenestrae (Fig. II-43). The thick areas contain a variety of organelles, some of which are unusually abundant, such as pinocytotic vesicles, Weibel-Palade bodies (Fig. II-44) (Weibel and Palade, 1964) and fibrils. Marked infolding of the luminal and basal surfaces may occur.

The lumen of the blood vessels in metastatic lesions may contain tumor cells. These are most often found in small veins or venules. Tumor cells usually do not penetrate the arterial wall but remain in the adventitia. Exceptions are melanomas and choriocarcinomas in which the cells may invade the media. The latter event may result in the formation of aneurysms and actual rupture. Tumor infiltration of the venous wall is often seen in the cases of lymphoma and leukemia (Leeds et al., 1971).

Connective tissue reaction

Connective tissue in the brain is confined to the perivascular regions. Some metastatic tumors, such as large cell carcinoma of the lung (Fig. II-45), are accompanied by pronounced connective tissue proliferation. Inflammatory cells, as well as fibroblasts, are seen in the layer of collagen-containing connective tissue. When the tumor reaches the leptomeninges and breaks through the pia, it may trigger a marked connective tissue proliferation in this area.

Radiation therapy may result in replacement of the tumor cells by fibrous connective tissue. The necrotic tumor tissue might be gradually surrounded by a fibrous capsule not usually seen in untreated patients (Plate II-2B, p. 33).

Calcifications in the stroma may occasionally occur (Potts and Svare, 1964).

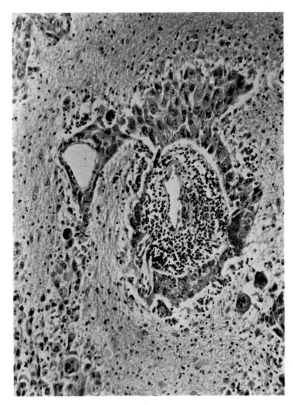

Fig. II-45 Undifferentiated large cell carcinoma of the lung.

Tumor cells in the brain tissue surrounding a blood vessel. The perivascular space is infiltrated by many lymphocytes. (H & E × 120, MH 20098.)

Infiltration of the metastatic tumor by lymphocytes and plasma cells is almost always seen, but the degree varies from case to case (Fig. II-46). Round cell infiltration may occur within the tumor itself, but this is more commonly seen at the periphery of the mass. The cells are most often seen in perivascular cuffs. Macrophages are most often found in groups in necrotic areas or in areas of accumulation of secretory products.

Reaction of the nervous tissue

Edema, especially of the white matter, is the most obvious change in the nervous tissue surrounding the metastatic lesion (Fig. II-47A, B and Plate II-2C, p. 33). The eosinophilic and PAS-positive edema fluid penetrates the white matter bundles. Electron microscopic study reveals the osmiophilic edema fluid in the extracellular spaces (Figs. II-48 and 49). Often the changes in the endothelium described above are associated with edema in adjacent tissues (Klatzo et al., 1962; Hirano et al., 1967; Hirano, 1969; Hirano and Matsui, 1978).

Neuronal cell bodies and their processes in the vicinity of the metastatic tumor may show a variety of changes. Vacuolation and swelling, especially of axons, are prominent features (Fig. II-50A). On the other hand, neurons, entrapped by the growing tumor, sometimes appear well preserved (Figs. II-47C and 50B).

A large number of reactive swollen astrocytes in the surrounding tissue are an invariable accompaniment of metastatic lesions (Fig. II-51). The cytoplasmic contents of the hypertrophic astrocytes vary depending on the stage of involvement.

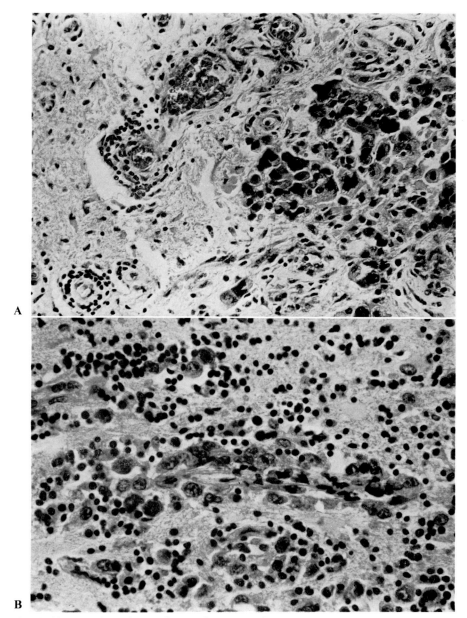

Fig. II-46 Lymphocytic reaction to the metastatic tumor.
A. The margin of a focus of metastatic carcinoma of the lung in the spinal cord. Lymphocytic cuffing around several blood vessels is evident in the neural tissue adjacent to the tumor. The hyperchromatic and bizarre nuclei of the tumor cells are seen. (H & E × 240, MH 22309.)
B. Diffuse lymphocytic infiltration is seen in the brain tissue in the presence of metastatic adenocarcinoma of the adrenal gland. (H & E × 370, MH 18004).

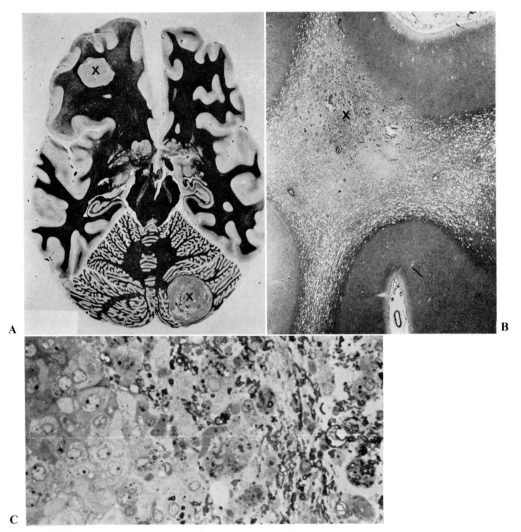

Fig. II-47 Involvement of white matter in metastatic tumors.
A. A horizontal section of the brain showing metastatic carcinoma (X) from the breast in the cerebellum and centrum semiovale. Swelling of the centrum semiovale and pallor of the white matter are obvious. (Myelin stain, MH 6434.)
B. Small nodules of metastatic breast carcinoma (X) are seen in the subcortical area. The adjacent white matter is severely vacuolated and distended. (Luxol fast blue-periodic acid Schiff × 10, MH 21077.)
C. Higher magnification of a metastatic squamous cell carcinoma from the lung. Tumor cells are seen on the left side of the field and darkly stained myelinated fibers are dispersed. Several macrophages are seen in the edematous area on the right. (Epon embedding, Toluidine blue stain × 390, NS 8025.)

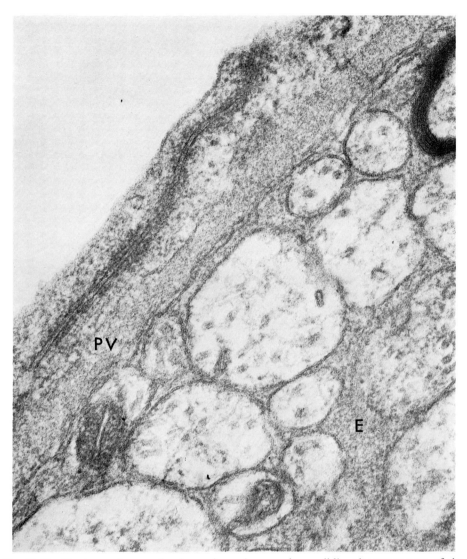

Fig. II-48 Electron micrograph of a perivascular area in a mildly edematous area of the brain of a rat subjected to a foreign body implantation in the forebrain. The extracellular space (E) between the cell processes, as well as the perivascular space (PV), are filled with electron-dense edema fluid. This is a common feature, also seen in vasogenic edema, due to a break in the blood-brain barrier in various pathological processes including metastatic tumors. An elongated endothelial cell junction is visible. (× 88,000.)

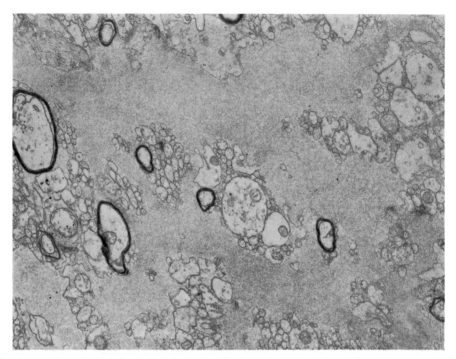

Fig. II-49   A region of the brain with marked edema in an experimental rat treated as described in Figure II-48.   ($\times$ 3,600.)

Watery swelling and an increase of glycogen granules may occur. More often there is pronounced accumulation of various organelles, especially filaments, resulting in an eosinophilic hypertrophied cytoplasm.

The pia mater may resist invasion by metastatic tumors. For example, cells of adenocarcinoma line up on the pia with their basal aspects facing the pial surface, and the secretory surface is directed towards the brain (Fig. II-15A, p. 38 and 60C, p. 81). When a metastatic tumor spreads from the subarachnoid space, the tumor cells again line up on the pial surface with their basal aspect on the pia, and the apical portion is directed towards the arachnoid (Fig. II-60A, p. 81).

Path of Dissemination

It is difficult to determine with certainty the dissemination route of each metastatic lesion by routine pathological examination (Nersesyants, 1951; Vorderwinkler, 1951). Occasionally, however, we recorded interesting findings which may suggest the route of the metastases. Many routes have been proposed as the pathways through which malignant tumors reach the CNS or its coverings. We will first describe two pathways which are generally accepted: blood-borne metastases through arteries, and direct invasion by the tumor from adjacent tissues.

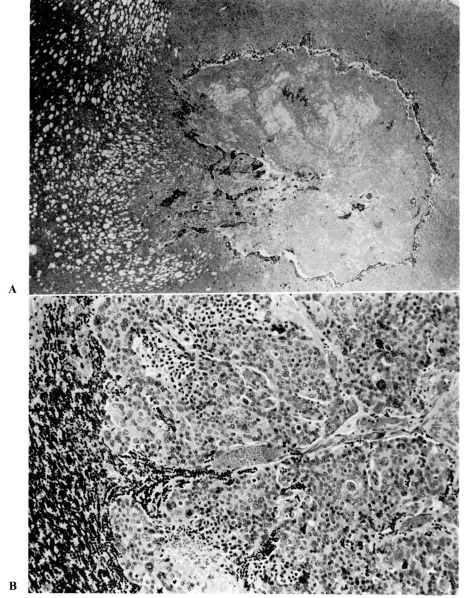

Fig. II-50 Neurons adjacent to a metastatic tumor.

A. A large zone of necrosis is surrounded by darkly stained metastatic tumor cells from the breast. On the left side of the field, numerous spongy, vacuolated areas are seen in the white matter. This corresponds to the axonal damage secondary to necrosis in the cerebral cortex, as well as to edema. (H & E × 16, MH 20042.)

B. A metastatic breast carcinoma in the granular cell layer of the cerebellum. The granular cells are entrapped between the tumor cells. (H & E × 120, MH 21367.)

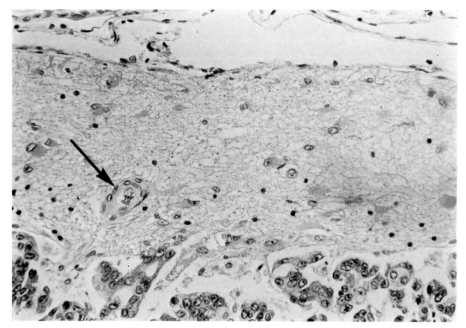

Fig. II-51   Glial reaction to the metastatic tumor.   The pial surface of the molecular layer of the cerebral cortex is seen in the upper portion of the illustration.   The metastatic tumor from the lung is seen at the bottom.   The astrocytes are markedly hypertrophic.   One blood vessel (arrow) shows endothelial proliferation.   The neuropil is pale and spongy, suggesting necrosis and edema.   (H & E × 240, MH 20560.)

Blood-borne Metastases Through Arteries

Nodular metastases in the brain parenchyma and other intracranial tissues are thought to be formed by blood-borne tumor cells.

Microscopic examination of the brain sometimes reveals emboli consisting of clumps of tumor cells in a fibrin network within the small vessels (Fig. II-52A and B).   The embolism is often accompanied by infarction of the surrounding nervous tissue (Fig. II-52C).   These emboli may be numerous throughout the brain (shower emboli).   Tumor embolism has been repeatedly described (Baker, 1942; Globus and Meltzer, 1942; Eason, 1950; France, 1975; Warren et al., 1977).   It is assumed that following intravascular proliferation, the tumor penetrates the vessel wall and produces metastatic nodules (Wood et al., 1961).   Two different arrangements of tumor nodules in the early stage may be observed.   A single nodule may be found at the center of the infarct (Fig. II-53A).   In other situations, numerous, small nodules arranged in a circle may be located at the periphery of the infarct (Fig. II-53B and C).   It is thought that these histologic findings represent early stages in the formation of blood-borne metastases.   On some occasions small metastatic foci are found without infarct of the surrounding tissue (Fig. II-54).

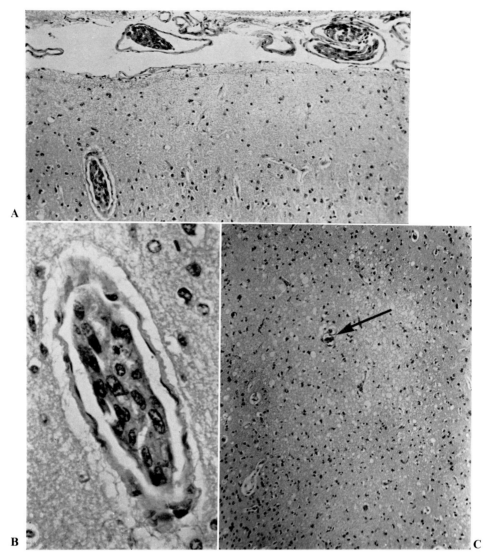

Fig. II-52 Tumor emboli.
A. Lumens of three vessels contain nests of tumor cells of breast cancer. There are no apparent infarcts in the adjacent cerebral cortex in this picture. (H & E × 100, MH 20519.)
B. Higher magnification of one of the tumor emboli shown in A. (H & E × 420, MH 20519.)
C. Low magnification of an infarct in the cerebral cortex. Marked sponginess and a pale background of the tissue are evident. A blood vessel containing tumor cells is seen in the center of the fresh infarct (arrow). (H & E × 77, MH 19376.)

Direct Invasion from the Adjacent Tissues

The CNS may be invaded by primary or secondary tumors of the neighboring tissues. As in the former example, cancers of the nasal sinuses and of the pharynx may invade the base of the skull and reach the intracranial tissues, destroying the bony structures or penetrating the bony canals.

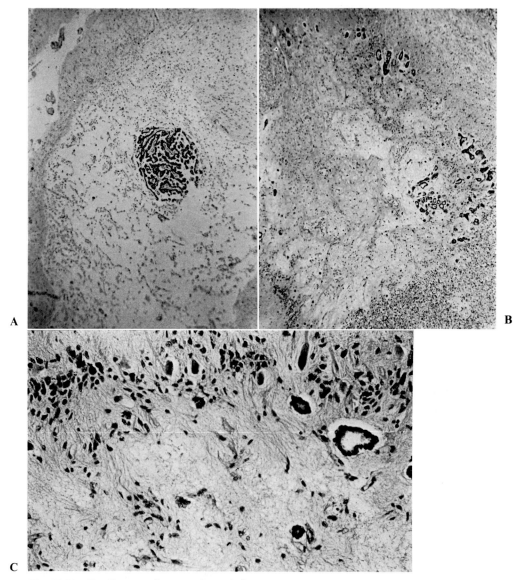

Fig. II-53 Small nests of tumors in an infarct.
A. A small metastatic nodule of lung cancer is seen in the center of the infarct in the cerebral cortex. In this case multiple foci of infarcts were seen in the brain. They were often associated with tumor deposits as illustrated in this picture. This may indicate tumor emboli and possible early stages of metastatic tumor growth. (H & E × 34, MH 17337.)
B. Multiple foci of metastatic mammary carcinoma at the margin of an infarct in the cerebellum. (H & E × 43, MH 76190.)
C. Higher magnification of B. Loss of granule cells, ischemic changes of Purkinje cells and gliosis are due to the infarction. Minute nests of metastatic tumor cells are evident. (H & E × 200, MH 76190.)

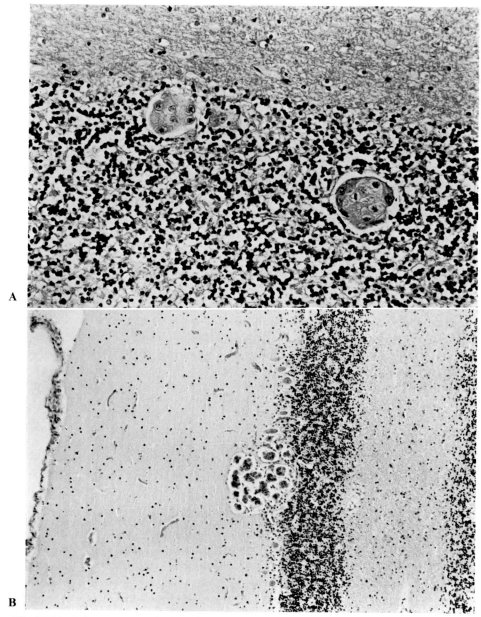

Fig. II-54 Minute metastatic deposits of lung cancer in the cerebellar cortex.
A. Two nodules of metastatic tumor cells are evident in the granular cell layer of the cerebellum. (H & E × 240, MH 21409.)
B. A group of tumor cells form a minute nodule in the Purkinje cell layer extending into the molecular layer of cerebellum. (H & E × 90, MH 20843.)

Tumor metastases to the skull and the dura may also invade the CNS. This process is often observed in cases of metastatic breast carcinoma (Fig. II-65C, p. 86). A similar sequence of events may be observed when the spinal epidural tissue is invaded directly by tumors from the vertebrae, as in multiple myeloma, or from the paravertebral lymph nodes with metastases.

These two mechanisms of formation of CNS metastases do not seem to account for all metastases. Various other mechanisms may be proposed.

Blood-borne Metastases Through the Vertebral Venous Plexus

The venous system known as Batson's plexus is named after the author who described its role in tumor metastases (Batson, 1940 and 1942). This system, which has been studied by many authors (Herlihy, 1947; Anderson, 1951; Coman and De-Long, 1951; Abrams, 1957; Henriques, 1962; Crock et al., 1973; Dommisse, 1975), is composed of three major interconnected parts: the epidural plexus, the plexus in the vertebral body, and the paravertebral plexus. This system gets the drainage from the vessels of the spinal cord and has main connections with the sacral venous plexus, the azygos system and the cranial dural sinuses. These valveless veins function as blood reservoirs, and any subtle change of venous pressure alters the direction of blood flow.

The Batson's plexus is thought by some authors to be the route of metastases of tumors arising in the pelvic or abdominal organs and proceeding to the spine (Viadana et al., 1976; Vider et al., 1977). It seems appropriate to acknowledge the role of this system in the metastases to the spine or to the spinal epidural tissues. There is no direct evidence, however, that this system is a route for intracranial metastases (Willis, 1973).

Lymph-borne Metastases

The lymphatic channels enter the cranial cavity or the vertebral canal along the blood vessels and are distributed in the dura and the spinal epidural tissues. The role of the lymphatics in the formation of metastases in the CNS is not clear, but the possibility that at least some CNS metastases are lymph-borne cannot be ruled out. In some old reports, the connection between the subarachnoid space and the lymphatic system and its role in diffuse leptomeningeal carcinomatosis was emphasized, but this hypothesis has not been widely accepted (Field and Brierley, 1948; Bowsher, 1957).

Metastases via the Peripheral Nerves

This hypothetical route has been applied mainly to explain diffuse leptomeningeal involvement. The tumor emboli are thought to be carried in the lymphatics in the peripheral nerve (Knierim, 1908; Alpers and Smith, 1938; Grain and Karr, 1955; Heathfield and Williams, 1956; Gonzales-Vitale and Garcia-Bunuel, 1976), but the doubt of the existence of a lymphatic system in the peripheral nerves contradicts its possible role in the tumor diffusion (Friedell and Parsons, 1961; Larson et al., 1966;

Rhodin et al., 1967).

According to our observations, tumors which enter the endoneurium show some tendency to extend continuously along the nerve fiber. Therefore, this route is probably not a mechanism of "distant" metastasis but may serve for local extension of the tumor (Fig. II-64, p. 85 and Fig. II-72, p. 94).

Leptomeningeal Involvement

In the following section, we describe pathologic characteristics of diffuse leptomeningeal involvement by metastatic neoplasms. This type of involvement of the CNS was observed in 2.7 per cent of the patients with carcinoma or sarcoma (Table II-2). Other authors reported a rate of 0.8 per cent and 1.5 per cent (Chason et al., 1963; Gonzalez-Vitale and Garcia-Bunuel, 1976). The most common primary tumors produced were breast carcinoma, lung carcinoma and melanoma, which accounted for 33, 28 and 17 per cent of the leptomeningeal carcinomatoses respectively (Table II-6 and Fig. II-3). Olson et al. (1971) reported similar results. It has also

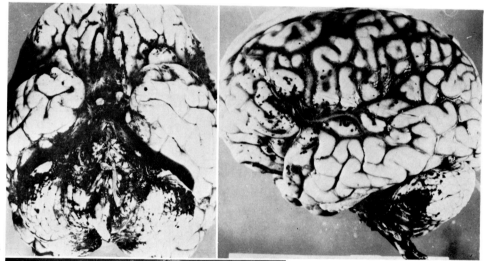

A   B

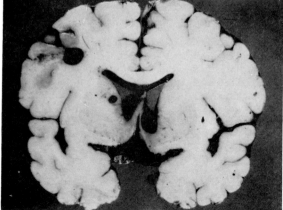

C

Fig. II-55 Meningeal and metastatic spread of melanoma. The subarachnoid space is well delineated by dark plaques of melanoma. Tumor deposits and large fissures are seen in the basal cistern. **A, B** and **C.** (A 48-year-old man developed sudden loss of consciousness. Subarachnoid hemorrhage was found. Autopsy did not reveal a definite primary site, but there were metastases in the lungs and many other organs. In the central nervous system, the tumor invaded the leptomeninges. There were several metastatic nodules in the brain parenchyma. MH 17764.)

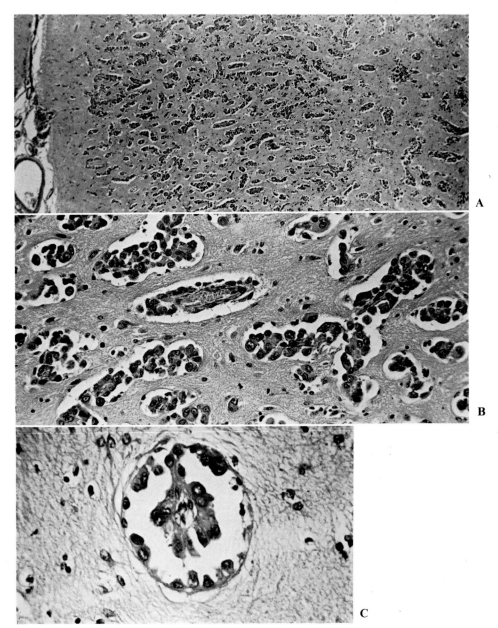

Fig. II-56 "Encephalitic" type of metastases.
A. Infiltrations of the cerebral cortex with a characteristic pattern of the spread of the tumor along blood vessels. This feature may be regarded as a marked exaggeration of the vascular pattern in the cerebral cortex. Metastatic melanoma. (H & E × 40, MH 12890.)
B. Higher magnification of A, showing the spread of the tumor cells virtually confined to the perivascular spaces. (H & E × 190, MH 12890.)
C. Micrograph similar to B. In this instance, the primary origin was breast carcinoma. In contrast to the extensive connective tissue proliferation in the leptomeninges, little connective tissue is seen in this tumor invading the Virchow-Robin space. Fibrillary astrocytes are seen in the brain tissue. (H & E × 230, MH 78183.)

been reported that gastric carcinoma may frequently form metastases of this type (Meissner, 1953; Meyer and Reah, 1953; Grain and Karr, 1955; Toyokura et al., 1957; Tokoro, 1959; Little et al., 1974; Gonzales-Vitale and Garcia-Bunuel, 1976).

The CNS lesions of lymphoma and leukemia frequently consist of this type of lesion. Leukemia affects the leptomeninges more frequently (22%) than lymphoma (11%) (Table II-3). Acute leukemia, especially in young patients, affects the lepto-meninges more frequently.

The leptomeningeal lesion is usually diffuse, but sometimes it consists of multiple, disseminated discrete plaques (Fig. II-55A and B). Lymphomas and leukemias affect the leptomeninges diffusely (Plate II-1C, p. 32), while carcinomas may show both patterns. Another uncommon pattern is the so-called "encephalitic" type of lesion (Madow and Alpers, 1951), where numerous inconspicuous plaques are formed almost exclusively in the gray matter. Microscopic examination of lesions of this type disclosed neoplastic cells mainly in the perivascular spaces of smaller vessels, so-called Virchow-Robin spaces, while only a small number of the cells were seen in the subarachnoid space of the brain surface (Fig. II-56).

Grossly, the affected brain usually shows moderate swelling. The leptomeninges affected by metastatic tumors usually appear thickened and opaque. Although pigmented melanoma may be recognized grossly, it is difficult to identify metastatic leptomeningeal carcinoma when tumor cells form thin sheets only. Leptomeningeal involvement is mainly observed in areas of the CNS with larger subarachnoid spaces, probably reflecting the flow of CSF. The basal cistern and its connecting cisterns, the ventral surface and the cerebellopontine angle of the brain stem and the Sylvian fissure are the sites of predilection (Fig. II-55A and B). In the vertebral canal, the dorsal surface of the cord (Fig. II-77A, p. 99), the cauda equina (Fig. II-59C, p. 80) and the nerve roots within the dural sleeves are frequently involved (Alpers and Smith, 1938; Olson et al., 1971, 1974).

On microscopic examination, tumor cells are found in all the spaces containing cerebrospinal fluid and in the delineate areas such as the Virchow-Robin spaces, which are rather obscure in the normal condition (Figs. II-57 and 58). Neoplastic cells usually lodge and grow on the inner surface of the arachnoid, arachnoid trabeculae, pia, adventitia of vessels and the sheath of the nerve root (Figs. II-59 and 60). However, cells of lymphoma and leukemia and cells of mucin-producing adenocarcinoma (signet ring cells) may occasionally be observed floating in the CSF.

Cytologic examination of CSF has been applied to diagnosing metastases to the CNS, and is important especially in leukemia and malignant lymphoma. This procedure is an essential step towards treatment, confirming the clinical diagnosis of leptomeningeal involvement (Koss, 1979).

A variety of carcinomas may show the histologic characteristics of the primary lesion. The arrangement of the cancer cells forms a single layer or a stratified plaque with occasional central necrosis (El-Batata, 1968; Little et al., 1974). Our series includes several examples of squamous cell carcinomas (Fig. II-59A).

The pia mater and glial membrane beneath it usually prevent tumor infiltration into the brain parenchyma, but in advanced stages, the tumor may break through the surface and invade the brain.

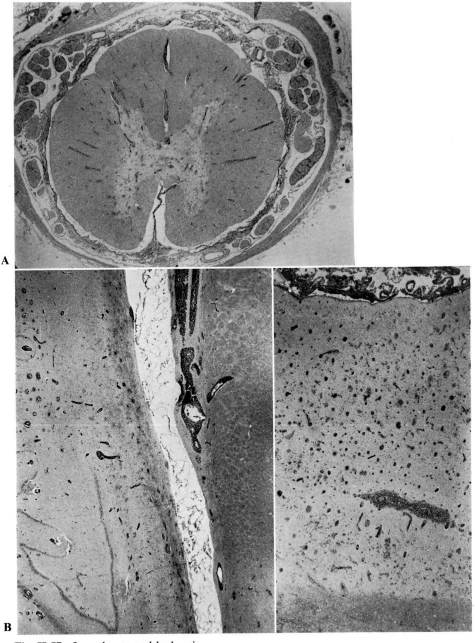

Fig. II-57 Lymphoma and leukemia.

A. Leptomeningeal spread of acute lymphocytic leukemia. The vascular pattern of the spinal cord is clearly visualized due to perivascular cuffing of tumor cells. (H & E × 11, MH 22552.)

B. Perivascular cuffing by the tumor cells of a lymphocytic lymphoma in the paraventricular area of the temporal horn. This case also has leptomeningeal lymphomatosis, which is not illustrated in this picture. The choroid plexus in the ventricle is entirely free of tumor cells in spite of its rich vascular network. (H & E × 11, MH 21978.)

C. The subarachnoid and Virchow-Robin spaces are marked by tumor cells. Extensions of tumor cells into adjacent brain tissue from the perivascular spaces are present although they are not clearly seen at this low magnification. (H & E × 11, MH 22552.)

Fig. II-58 Intraparenchymal spread of lymphoma. Extension of the tumor cells from the subarachnoid space into the Virchow-Robin space of the optic nerve.
(H & E × 43, MH 21978.)

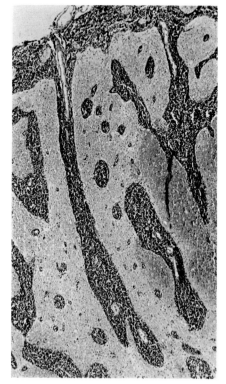

Nodular metastases in the brain parenchyma adjacent to the ventricular system may rupture into the ventricles and develop many nodules on the ventricular wall, as well as in the subarachnoid space (Fig. II-55C) (Miller and Constans, 1950; Wilkins and Wu, 1971; Olson et al., 1974). The choroid plexus is less frequently affected than expected because of its rich vasculature and net-like structure (Fig. II-61). When it is affected, the tumor cells usually accumulate in the tela chorioidea, which is connected to the subarachnoid space. On rare occasions, the choroid plexus is the only structure involved (Globus and Meltzer, 1942; Gonzales-Vitale and Garcia-Bunuel, 1976). We have not observed selective involvement of the arachnoid villi by metastases, in keeping with the observations by Olson et al. (1974).

Cranial nerve roots (including olfactory and optic nerves) and spinal nerve roots are frequently infiltrated by tumor cells (Altrocchi et al., 1972; Bramlet et al., 1976; Ushio et al., 1977a). The segment of the root affected by metastatic carcinoma often appears as a localized spindle-shaped mass (Figs. II-59C and 62A). On the other hand, leukemias and lymphomas usually cause diffuse swelling of the roots (Figs. II-62B and 63) (Hunt et al., 1960; Van Allen and Rahme, 1962; Jacobsen and Lester, 1970). The tumor cells lodge on the arachnoid, wrap around the root and extend to the root sheath in each fascicle. Then the tumor cells in the subarachnoid spaces may infiltrate the endoneurium (Plate II-3A and B, p. 92) and proliferate along the nerve fiber in both directions (Figs. II-63 and 64), but they rarely extend beyond the level of the spinal ganglia distally, or the junction with the CNS proximally (Fig. II-63C) (Alpers and Smith, 1938; Clausen et al., 1956; Urich, 1974; Inoue, 1978).

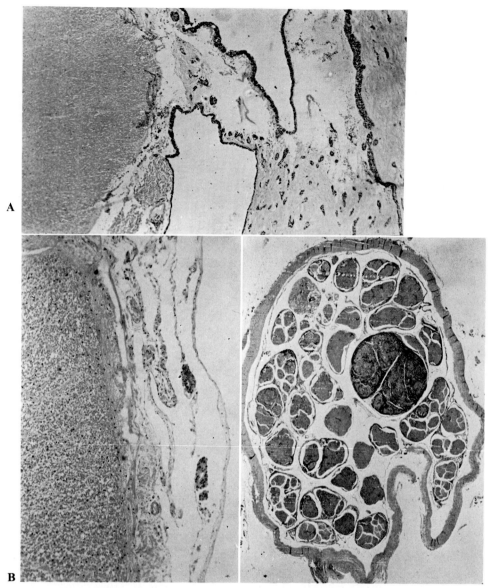

Fig. II-59 Metastatic tumor in the leptomeninges of the spinal cord.
A. Layers of tumor cells extend in the subarachnoid space along the surface of the septa of the posterior aspect of the cord. The lining of tumor cells on the right side of the picture corresponds to the inner surface of the arachnoid membrane. In addition, many small tumor nodules are disseminated in the subarachnoid space, where proliferation of the connective tissue is seen. A few tumor nodules are also seen in the dura mater. This is squamous cell carcinoma from the cervix. (H & E × 43, MH 21285.)
B. Two small isolated tumor nodules are seen in the subarachnoid space. Metastasis from prostatic carcinoma. (H & E × 77, MH 15424.)
C. Cross section of the cauda equina surrounded by dura mater. A markedly enlarged root is due to the massive infiltration by melanoma. In addition, tumor infiltration is seen as a dark deposit in the leptomeninges. (H & E × 8, MH 21084.)

60C. A normal (left) and necrotic (right) gyri of the cerebral cortex. A layer of papillary →
adenocarcinoma cells surrounds a blood vessel on the right with their basal aspects abutting the vessel wall. Another layer of tumor cells covers the necrotic gyrus. Their basal aspect of the cells faces the pia mater, while the apex is directed inward. (H & E × 120, MH 22073.)

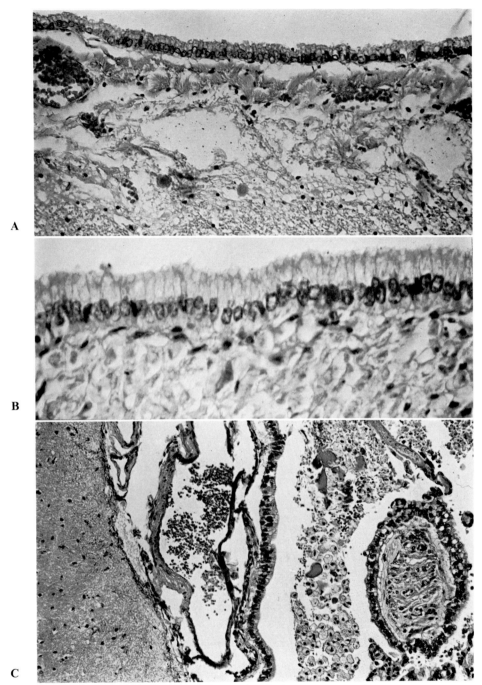

Fig. II-60 Arrangement of adenocarcinoma in relation to nervous tissue.
A. A single layer of columnar epithelial cells extend along the pial surface of the spinal cord. Between the spinal cord (below) and the tumor, a thick band of collagenous tissue containing blood vessels is evident. The pial border is not clear but corresponds roughly to the area where corpora amylacea are seen. Note that the basal aspect of the tumor faces the pial surface. (H & E × 240, MH 77195.)
B. A single layer of adenocarcinoma abuts on the surface of the spinal nerve root. The basal aspect of the tumor cells runs along the outer surface of the root sheath. (H & E × 490, MH 77195.)

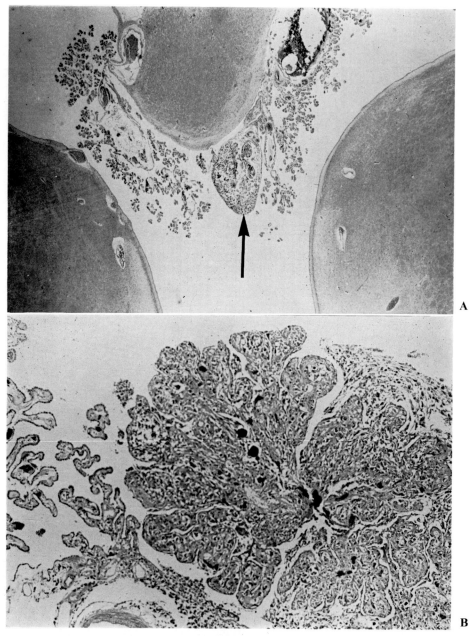

Fig. II-61 Metastatic tumors in the choroid plexus.
A. The arrow indicates a single tumor nodule in the choroid plexus at the foramen of Monro. Metastatic melanoma. (H & E × 12, MH 19968.)
B. Tumor nodules in the choroid plexus of the fourth ventricle. Marked proliferation of the stroma, associated with the tumor cells is evident. Intact choroid plexus is seen on the left side. Dense spherical deposits are calcospherites which have no pathological significance. Tumor cells are also seen in the ventricle (right upper corner). Invasion into the tela chorioidea is seen. Metastasis of lung cancer. (H & E × 50, MH 22356.)

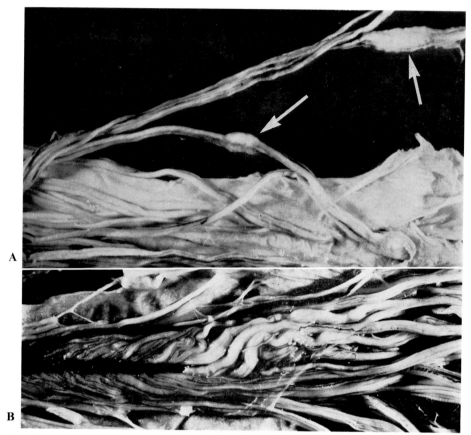

Fig. II-62 Metastatic tumor nodules in the spinal nerve roots.
A. Focal spindle-shaped enlargements (arrows) of the roots are due to tumor growth. (A 62-year-old woman, who had swollen lymph nodes one year earlier, developed motor weakness, which started in the left upper extremity. Autopsy, performed six months later, revealed squamous cell carcinoma of the lung that metastasized to the liver, vertebrae and other organs, including the brain parenchyma and leptomeninges. MH 18324.)
B. Diffuse thickening of the spinal nerve roots. (Malignant lymphoma, the same case as in Fig. II-7B MH 78191.)

The manner of infiltration to the roots varies according to the structural differences between the sheath and stroma of the root, compared to the architecture of the CNS and the distal peripheral nerves. There are abundant narrow subarachnoid spaces between rootlets. Tumor propagation towards the CNS through the endoneurium is impeded by the glial membrane at the junction of the CNS (Shantha and Bourne, 1968; McCabe and Low, 1969; Gamble, 1976; Low, 1976).

The vessels in the subarachnoid space, usually the veins or adventitia of the arteries, may also be invaded by metastatic tumors.

Stromal proliferation differs in various primary neoplasms. Breast carcinoma and reticulum cell sarcoma are often associated with dense fibrous stroma (Fig. II-77, p. 99). Inflammatory cells are seen around the vessels in some cases. Hydrocephalus of a mild or moderate degree may be present in cases of leptomeningeal involvement.

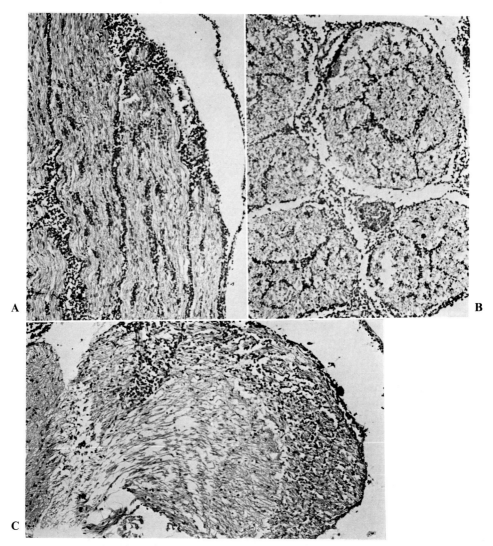

Fig. II-63   Acute lymphocytic leukemia involving the roots.
A.   Longitudinal section of a spinal root.   Due to the subarachnoid spread of tumor cells, the patterns of the perineurium and nerve bundles are clearly outlined.   Invasion of tumor cells into the endoneurium is also evident in some areas.   (H & E × 96, MH 22552.)
B.   Cross section of a spinal nerve root of the same case as that illustrated in A.   (H & E × 96, MH 22552.)
C.   The entrance zone of a posterior root into the spinal cord of the same case as that illustrated in A.   The marginal zone of the posterior root is marked by diffuse infiltration of tumor cells.   On the other hand, the central zone of the root, as well as the spinal cord on the left, are free of tumor cells.   (H & E × 96, MH 22552.)

Paths of Dissemination

There are many hypotheses to account for leptomeningeal spread of metastases (Willis, 1973).   Two paths are proposed for arterial-borne metastases: the choroid plexus (Moberg and Reis, 1961) and the leptomeningeal vessels (Price and Johnson, 1973).   Our findings support the conclusion that dissemination from the choroid plexus is relatively rare.

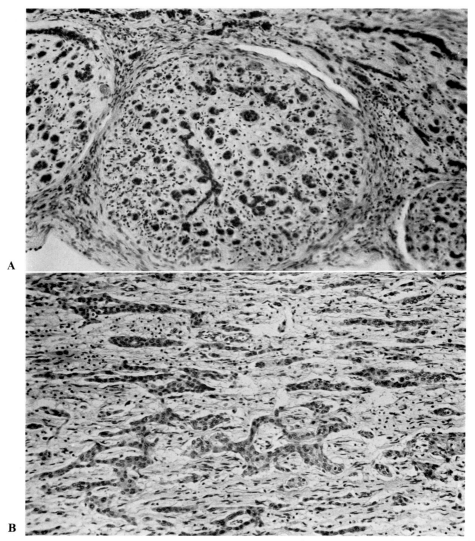

Fig. II-64   Adenocarcinoma of the breast involving the spinal nerve roots. The tumor extends along the nerve fibers.   Cross section (A) and longitudinal section (B) of the spinal nerve roots.   (H & E × 90, MH 17429.)

Contiguous growth of primary or secondary lesions of adjacent tissues (such as the dura, the brain parenchyma, the eyes or the nose) is an important source of dissemination.   Chason et al. (1963) reported frequent association of nodular metastasis of the brain parenchyma with leptomeningeal dissemination.

Other hypothetical paths, mainly the route through the peripheral nerves, are discussed elsewhere (p. 74).

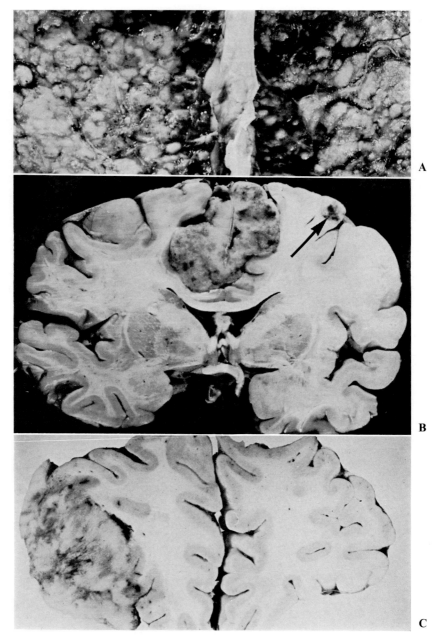

Fig. II-65 Dural metastasis from breast carcinoma.
A. Characteristic multiple dural metastases, which lined inner surface of the dura. (A 62-year-old woman, who was operated on for breast carcinoma nine years earlier, developed generalized seizures. Autopsy, performed four months later, revealed metastases to the lung, lymph nodes and many other organs including the cerebrum, dura mater and the pituitary gland. MH 14269.)
B. A large metastatic tumor in the falx compressing the adjacent brain tissue. An additional small intracerebral tumor (arrow) is also seen. (A 78-year-old woman, who was operated on for breast carcinoma 35 years previously developed bilateral weakness of the lower extremities. Autopsy revealed metastatic breast carcinoma in the lungs, vertebrae, dural falx and cerebrum. MH 15627.)
C. Dural metastasis invading the leptomeninges and extending into the brain tissue. (A →

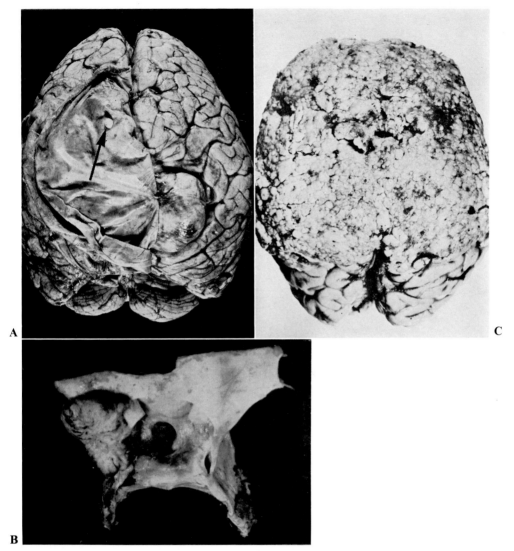

Fig. II-66 Dural metastases of various tumors.
A. Sarcoma. Large and small (arrow) dural metastases resembling meningioma. (A 51-year-old woman, who was operated on for sarcoma that probably originated in the uterus, developed back pain and then motor and sensory disturbance of the left lower extremity. Autopsy revealed undifferentiated sarcoma that metastasized to the kidney, bones and other organs. Metastases were also observed in the dura, both lobes of the pituitary gland and the spinal epidural space at the mid-thoracic level. MH 19215.) (From Hirano et al., 1980)
B. A metastatic nodule in the sphenoidal region from carcinoma of the colon, resembling meningioma in this location. (A 58-year-old man who was operated on for carcinoma of the colon one year prior to admission. No neurological deficits were noted. The brain parenchyma, as well as the base of the skull and adjacent dura contained a tumor. MH 18639.)
C. Multiple myeloma involving the skull that spread to the entire epidural surface of the dura mater. (A 59-year-old woman who had had back pain for one year. Autopsy revealed severe bony involvement including the skull. Metastases invaded the dural leaflets and protruded into the subdural surface in one area. MH 11706.)

→ 52-year-old woman who was operated on for breast carcinoma three years previously. No neurological deficit was noted. Autopsy revealed metastases to the skull, dura mater, pituitary gland and cerebrum. MH 11762.)

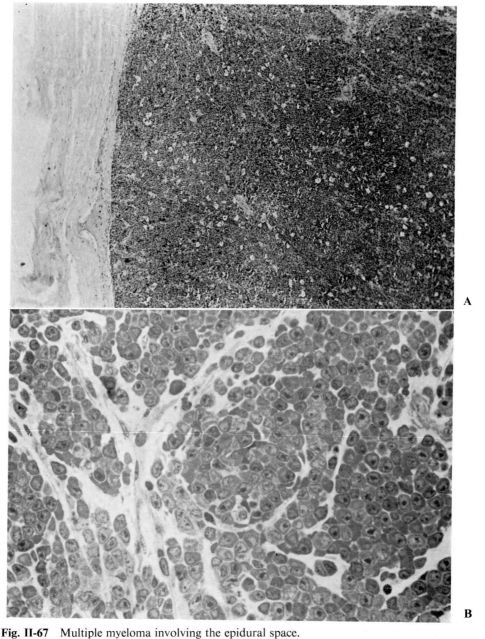

Fig. II-67 Multiple myeloma involving the epidural space.
A. Tumor growth in the skull compressing the dura mater on the left. Infiltration of some tumor cells into the dural layer is visible. (H & E × 50, MH 21405.)
B. Higher magnification of the multiple myeloma in the epidural space of the spinal cord. (Epon embedding, Toluidine blue × 490, NS 77192.)

Dural Metastases

Dural metastases have not been studied as extensively as those to the brain or the leptomeninges. In our autopsy series dural metastases were observed in 10 per cent of the patients with carcinoma and sarcoma (Table II-2).

Mammary carcinoma accounted for 51 per cent of the dural metastases. Lung carcinoma, melanoma and carcinoma of the gastrointestinal tract were next in frequency (Table II-6 and Fig. II-3). Reports on the frequency of dural metastases are quite varied. Willis found a relatively low rate, three per cent of the patients with cancer (Willis, 1973). In breast carcinoma alone, the frequency was as high as 31 per cent in our series (Table II-2), 33 per cent in the study by Abrams et al. (1950), and 50 per cent in that of France (1975).

Dural involvement was observed in 13 per cent of our cases of lymphomas, leukemias and multiple myelomas (Table II-3). Some other authors have reported a higher rate of dural involvement of 65 per cent in lymphoma patients (Janota, 1966), and 66 per cent in acute lymphocytic leukemia patients (Moore et al., 1960).

Macroscopic findings

Dural metastases of carcinoma and sarcoma are usually multifocal (Fig. II-65A) and the nodules protrude into the subdural space. They often have adhesions to the arachnoid and invade the arachnoid and the brain (Fig. II-65B and C). Sometimes they mimic meningioma clinically and on gross inspection (Fig. II-66A and B, Schaerer and Whitney, 1953). Lymphomas may occasionally form nodules similar to those seen in carcinomas. In contrast, multiple myeloma involves the skull first, extends to the epidural space and then infiltrates the dura itself (Figs. II-66C, 67 and 68). It rarely reaches the subdural surface. In some metastatic

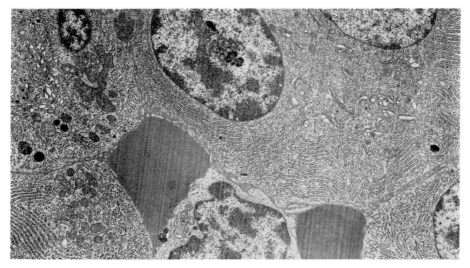

Fig. II-68 Metastatic multiple myeloma. Portions of several tumor cells and erythrocytes are seen. The tumor cells show the characteristic pattern of well-developed rough endoplasmic reticulum. ($\times$ 4,800, NS 7006.)

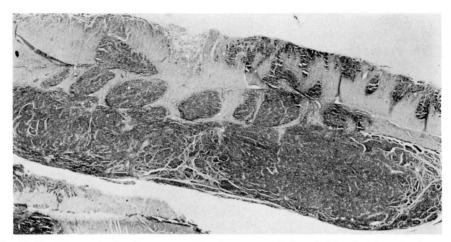

Fig. II-69 Metastatic dural tumors. The dura mater is invaded by darkly stained tumor nodules. The subdural space forms large tumor masses. Tumor nodules in the epidural surface suggests bony involvement. Prostatic carcinoma. (H & E × 16, MH 20097.)

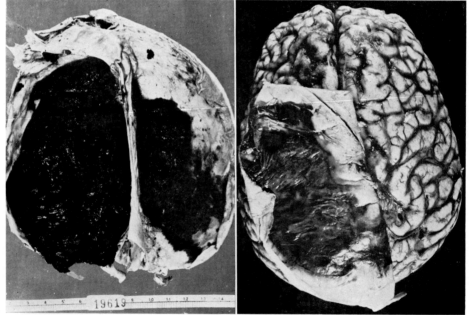

A   B

Fig. II-70 Subdural hemorrhage.
A. A bilateral, fresh subdural hematoma in a case of leukemia. (An 86-year-old woman who was found to have monoblastic leukemia one month previously. Autopsy revealed recent hemorrhages in the brain as well as a subdural hemorrhage. MH 19619.)
B. Chronic subdural hematoma in a case of prostatic carcinoma. Tumor cells were not seen in the hematoma in this case. Yet chronic subdural hematoma with dural metastasis was occasionally observed. (A 64-year-old man, who was operated on for prostatic carcinoma two years previously, developed pain. Autopsy showed metastases to the lungs, liver, bones and spinal epidural space at the mid-thoracic level. MH 19173.) (From Hirano et al., 1980.)

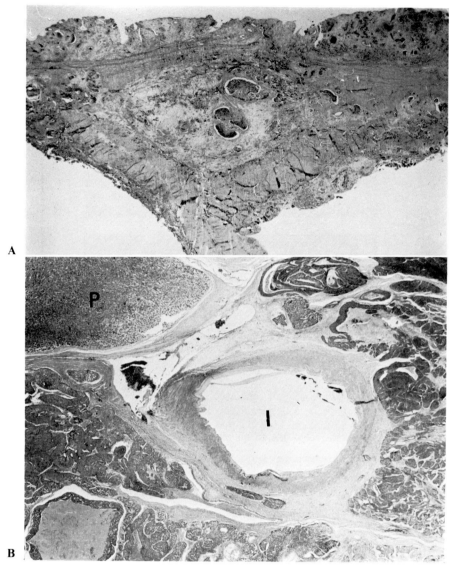

Fig. II-71 Invasion of dural sinuses by metastatic tumors.
A. The dura mater and superior sagittal sinus involved by breast carcinoma. The sinus is occluded and small vascular channels are filled by tumor cells. (H & E × 12, MH 20468.)
B. Portion of the cavernous sinus, pituitary gland (P) and internal carotid artery (I). Extension of a nasopharyngeal squamous cell carcinoma is seen in the region of the cavernous sinus including the dura mater. (H & E × 12, MH 18266.)

carcinomas, dural masses may also be contiguous with metastases to the skull (Fig. II-69).

Dural involvement by leukemia is usually microscopic and no obvious abnormalities are discernible on macroscopic examination. However, subdural membranes may be frequently observed as a consequence of small hemorrhages (McDonald, and Burton, 1966; Pochedly, 1977c), and sometimes massive subdural hematoma is noted (Fig. II-70A) (Pitner and Johnson, 1973).

In metastatic carcinoma and sarcoma, we occasionally found subdural hema-

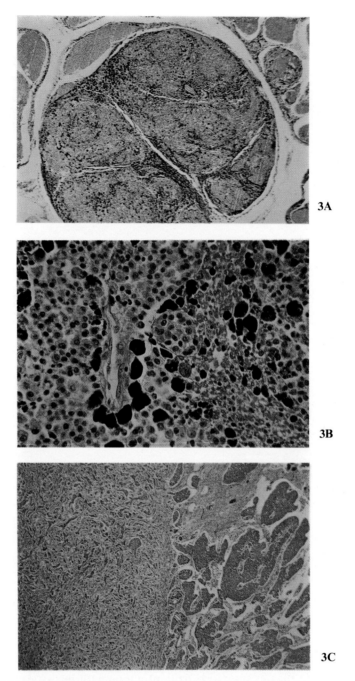

3A

3B

3C

Plate II-3A Melanoma cells infiltrating one of the spinal nerve roots in a case of diffuse leptomeningeal involvement. (H & E × 33, MH 21084.)

Plate II-3B Higher magnification of Plate 3A. Tumor cells infiltrate the endoneurium and encircle the remaining nerve fibers (red stained). Some tumor cells have abundant melanosomes, whereas others have only a small amount of pigment. (H & E × 330.)

Plate II-3C Dural metastasis (left) from a breast carcinoma invading the cerebral cortex. The subdural tumor is divided into small clusters by proliferated connective tissue stroma, a feature that is not prominent in the tumor within the brain parenchyma. (H & E × 33, MH 21823)

tomas: a few were large enough to produce symptoms (Fig. II-70B) (Westenhöffer, 1904; Purckhauer, 1929; Russel and Cairns, 1934; Baker, 1938; Meyer and Reah, 1953; Braun et al., 1973; Leech et al., 1974; Ambiavagar and Sher, 1978).

Venous sinuses are occasionally occluded as a complication of dural involvement. We observed 15 such cases with superior sagittal sinus obstruction and eight cases with cavernous sinus obstruction. In six of the 15 cases with superior sagittal sinus obstruction, breast cancer was the causative factor (Fig. II-71A).

Carcinomas of the nasal sinuses and the pharynx were the most frequent source of cavernous sinus obstruction: four out of eight cases (Fig. II-71B). Similar cases were reported by others (Mones, 1965; Korenman and Mones, 1970; Willis, 1973).

The proxymal portion of the cranial nerves and spinal nerves may be invaded in the dural sleeves by metastatic dural tumors. Unsöld et al. (1980) reported a case with metastatic lung cancer in the cavernous sinus which involved cranial nerves. By this route, a metastatic tumor may reach the leptomeninges and result in diffuse leptomeningeal involvement (Figs. II-71B and 72).

Microscopic findings

The histology of metastatic carcinoma to the dura usually mimics the primary lesion (Fig. II-73A). These lesions are often associated with marked proliferation of the fibrous connective tissue (Fig. II-74), contrary to the brain metastases (Fig. II-73B and Plate II-3C, p. 92).

Leukemic cells are usually located around the venous plexus between the two dural leaflets. Tumor cell clusters are also seen in the superficial layers of the subdural or epidural surfaces. The subdural membrane contains hemosiderin-laden macrophages and neoplastic cells (Pochedly, 1977c).

In obstructed dural sinuses, subendothelial and intraluminal tumor growth are observed. Neoplastic growth in the lumen of small veins is frequently observed (Fig. II-73C).

Path of Dissemination

Dural involvement may be contiguous with tumor growth in the skull. Naheedy et al. (1980) found that 15 per cent of the cases with skull metastasis on radiological examination had contiguous dural invasion. It is questionable whether dissemination along the path of the meningeal arteries accounts for most dural metastases. Various other hypotheses which have been proposed to explain dural metastases are mentioned in another section (p. 74). Small nodules of metastatic carcinomas lodged between the two leaflets of the dura are probably derived via the venous pathway. Leukemic infiltration to the dura also appears to be derived from the venous plexus. Frequent tumor growth in the lumens of the veins suggests that the role of the venous route may be important, at least in tumor propagation within the dura.

Metastatic Tumors in the Vertebral Canal

Malignant tumors may affect various tissues in the vertebral canal. The most common form of involvement is spinal epidural metastasis. The spinal leptomeninges and the spinal nerve roots may also be affected as a part of diffuse leptomeningeal involvement. The third and least common form is intramedullary metastasis to the cord. These three types of lesions are described below.

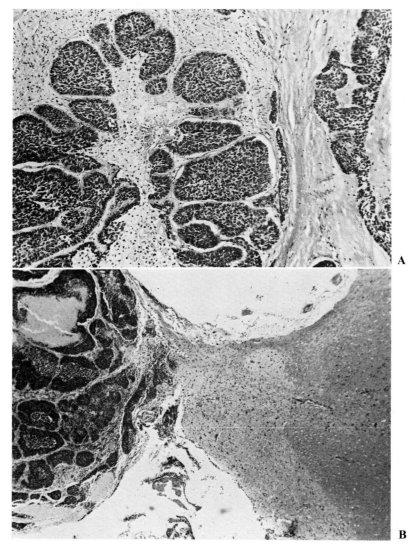

Fig. II-72 Direct invasion of cranial nerves by a squamous cell carcinoma of the nasopharynx (A) and the base of the tongue (B).
A. Cross section of a cranial nerve in the dural sleeve. (H & E × 170, MH 18266.)
B. Extension of the oral carcinoma in the facial nerve which stops abruptly at the exit from
the pons on the right. (H & E × 34, MH 19276.)

Fig. II-73 Metastatic breast carcinoma in the dura mater.
A. High magnification of metastatic deposits in the falx. (H & E × 200, MH 21791.)
B. Subdural extension and infiltration of the brain tissue are seen. Aggregates of tumor
cells are present in the brain (right) in contrast to prominent connective tissue proliferation in
the leptomeninges (left). (H & E × 100, MH 21823.)
C. Distended vascular channels in the dura mater filled with tumor cells. (H & E × 100,
MH 20408.)

Fig. II-74 Metastatic dural tumors. High magnification of an adenocarcinoma of the
lung that metastasized to the dura mater. The tumor forms acini surrounded by prominent
connective tissue stroma. (H & E × 120, MH 76198.)

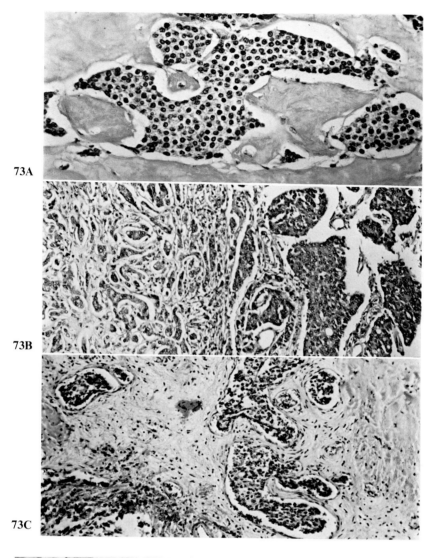

73A

73B

73C

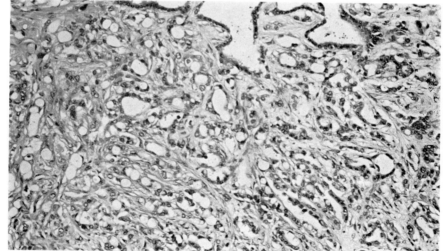

74

Spinal Epidural Tissue

The frequency of spinal epidural metastases of carcinomas and sarcomas was 4.2 per cent in our series and eight per cent in another (Abrams et al., 1950). Primary tumors most frequently observed in this type of metastasis were carcinomas of the lung and breast, followed by carcinomas of the gastrointestinal tract, prostate, and the urinary tract (Table II-6 and Fig. II-75). Similar observations were reported by Neustaedter (1944), Chandler et al. (1954), Perese (1958), Barron et al. (1959), Wright (1963), Vieth and Odom (1965b) and Gilbert, R. W. et al. (1978).

Five per cent of the patients with lymphoma and leukemia showed involvement of the spinal epidural tissue. Multiple myeloma frequently produces such lesions. Clarke (1956) reported involvement of the spinal epidural tissue by multiple myeloma in 20 per cent of the patients. Among various types of lymphomas, Hodgkin's desease may affect the spinal epidural tissue (Chandler et al., 1954; Williams et al., 1959; Bhagwati and McKissock, 1961; Vieth and Odom, 1965b; Verity, 1968; Mullins et al., 1971).

In general, the epidural tissue at the thoracic level is the most frequently involved (Barron et al., 1959; Gilbert, R. W. et al., 1978). However, some primary tumors, such as prostatic carcinoma, colonic carcinoma and renal carcinoma, have a predilection for lower levels.

In some instances, the symptoms caused by the spinal epidural tumor were the initial signs of cancer (Barron et al., 1959). This has been recorded for lung carcinoma, prostatic carcinoma and lymphoma (Bhagwati and McKissock, 1961; Wright, 1963; Vieth and Odom, 1965b).

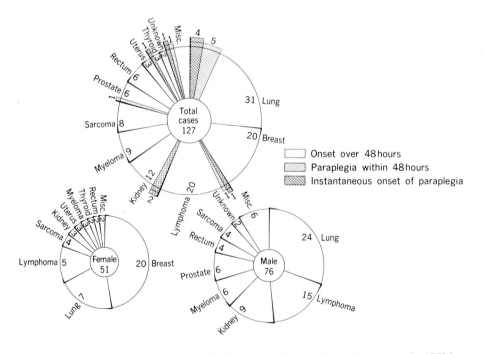

Fig. II-75　Primary sites for spinal epidural metastases. (From Barron et al., 1959.)

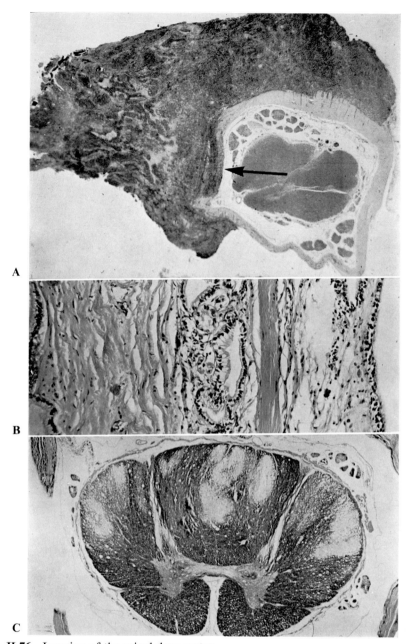

Fig. II-76 Invasion of the spinal dura mater.
A. A large epidural metastasis of adenocarcinoma of the kidney which is seen invading the dura mater at the arrow. (H & E × 5, MH 20528.)
B. Epidural (right), intradural (center) and subdural (left) regions are all infiltrated by a papillary carcinoma. (H & E × 100, MH 77195.)
C. The spinal cord of the mid-thoracic segment shows necrosis of irregular shape, which was caused by an epidural deposit of Hodgkin's disease. (Woelke × 8, MH 21282.)

Macroscopic findings

Epidural tumors are usually contiguous growths of tumors in the vertebrae attached to the dura mater and extended vertically for the length of a few vertebrae. The tumors are often anterior or lateral to the cord (McAlhany and Netsky, 1955; Bhagwati and McKissock, 1961), but in some instances the tumor may encircle the dural tube entirely. Sometimes the epidural tumor is associated with vertebral collapse.

Microscopic findings

Metastatic tumor is found in the epidural fatty tissue, spinal dura, and sometimes in the subdural layer (Fig. II-76A and B). However, an obvious subdural tumor is rarely associated with the epidural lesion (Chandler et al., 1954). On rare occasions, the tumor grows almost exclusively on the subdural surface (Rogers and Heard, 1958; Beehler, 1960; Feiring and Hubbard, Jr., 1965).

The compressed spinal cord may show irregular foci of complete necrosis or less severe lesions, consisting of vacuolation in the neuropil and demyelination (Fig. II-76C). The white matter is more severely affected. The ganglion cells, adjacent to the necrotic foci, do not usually show ischemic changes. These features are different from ordinary arterial occlusion. McAlhany and Netsky (1955) also reported similar findings and showed that the necrotic foci often appeared just beneath the tumor or on the opposite side. They also described relative sparing of the anterior column. In some experimental studies, the epidural mass caused a disturbance in the local blood flow, which resulted in vasogenic edema and necrosis (Doppman et al., 1973; Ushio et al., 1977d). The spinal cord, with its long-standing cord compression, shows Wallerian degeneration of both the ascending and descending tracts.

Path of Dissemination

Spinal epidural growth usually follows vertebral metastases of carcinomas or multiple myeloma. Gilbert, R. W. et al. (1978) reported frequent co-existence (85%) of vertebral and epidural lesions at the same level.

Lymphomas usually involve the spinal epidural tissue by direct extension through the intervertebral foramen from the affected paravertebral lymphatic tissue (Williams et al., 1959; Bhagwati and McKissock, 1961). Some of these metastatic tumors may spread by other routes, such as the veins and lymphatics, as mentioned in another section (p. 74).

Spinal Leptomeninges and Nerve Roots

These tissues are involved with metastatic tumors as a part of diffuse leptomeningeal involvement (Fig. II-77). The cauda equina is frequently infiltrated by tumor cells and may cause the initial symptoms in diffuse leptomeningeal involvement and is therefore of importance in symptomatological or neuroradiological evaluation (see also p. 285) (Van Allen and Rahme, 1962; Guyer and Westbury, 1968; Jacobsen and Lester, 1970). On rare occasions, leptomeningeal involvement is confined to the vertebral canal (Parsons, 1972; Olson et al., 1974).

Leptomeningeal involvement may lead to infiltration of the spinal cord by tumor cells. In some cases, tumor cells fill the entire subarachnoid space around the spinal cord.

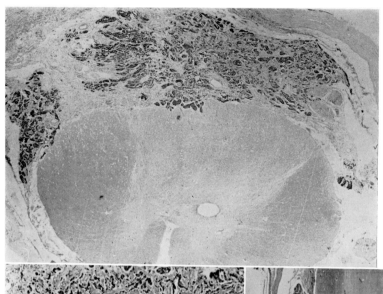

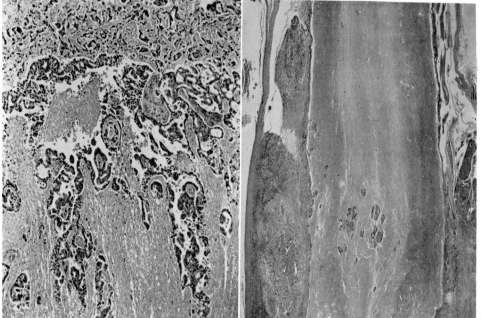

Fig. II-77 Metastatic tumor in the leptomeninges of the spinal cord.
A. A metastatic tumor is evident in the dorsal aspect of the spinal cord. Although tumor cells, in general, spread diffusely in the subarachnoid space, they may form tumor masses in certain areas as shown in this case. A few tumor nodules have invaded the posterior aspect of the spinal cord. Adenocarcinoma from the parotid gland. (H & E × 10, MH 17486.)
B. Invasion of tumor cells from the leptomeninges into the spinal cord. Metastatic breast carcinoma. (H & E × 43, MH 21077.)
C. Low power view of a longitudinal section of the spinal cord showing the leptomeningeal tumor mass and small deposits of tumor nodules in the spinal cord. The spinal cord is surrounded by a mass of tissue that contains not only tumor cells but also extensive proliferation of connective tissue and meningeal cells. (H & E × 4, MH 20827.)

Intramedullary Lesions (Fig. II-78)

Nine cases of intramedullary metastases in the spinal cord were observed among 180 cases of metastatic tumors involving the vertebral canal. Barron et al. (1959) reported two such cases out of 127 cases with metastases in the vetebral canal. Our nine cases reflect 0.3 per cent of all patients with carcinoma or sarcoma. Chason et al. (1963) reported a rate of 1 per cent for spinal intramedullary metastases among patients with carcinoma. Most of the intramedullary metastases were accompanied by brain metastases.

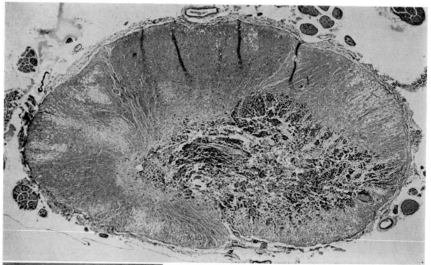

A

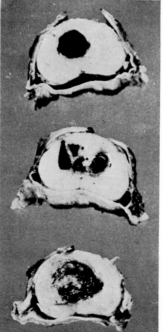

Fig. II-78 Intramedullary metastasis in the spinal cord.

A. A metastatic carcinoma from the lung. (H & E × 12, MH 16877.)

B. (A 59-year-old woman who developed motor weakness of the left upper extremity which progressed to left hemiparesis. Autopsy revealed anaplastic carcinoma of the lung that metastasized to the lymph nodes and adrenal gland. The cerebrum, cerebellum, pons and spinal cord contained metastatic nodules. MH 20269.) (From Hirano et al., 1980.)

B

Of the total number of cases of metastatic tumors in the parenchyma of the CNS, 1.6 per cent were located in the spinal cord in our series, and 5 per cent and 2.5 per cent in other series respectively (Chason et al., 1963; Burger and Vogel, 1976).

The sources of metastases to the spinal cord are almost identical with those for parenchymal brain metastases. They consisted of six cases of lung carcinoma, two cases of breast carcinoma and one case of melanoma. Hughes (1978) reviewed 40 cases in four series and reported similar findings (Benson, 1960; Chason et al., 1963; Sherbourne et al., 1964; Willis, 1973).

The tumors in the spinal cord often extend vertically for the length of a few vertebrae. The microscopic appearance is identical to that in the brain parenchyma. Some of the more recent reports on this subject were published by Mastalgia and Kakulas (1970), Edelson et al. (1972), Cashion and Young (1973) and Morariu and Serban (1974).

Pituitary Gland

The pituitary gland is a common target organ of metastatic tumors despite its small volume (0.5–0.6 grams in weight). Metastases to the pituitary gland or its capsule were observed in six per cent of the patients with carcinomas and sarcomas in our series (Table II-2). Others recorded this event in 1.8, 3.8, 8.3 and 1.0 per cent of their cases (Abrams et al., 1950; Hägerstrand and Schonebeck, 1969; Rossemann et al., 1970; Kovacs, 1973). Lymphomas, leukemias and multiple myelomas affected the pituitary gland and its capsule in 16 per cent of our cases.

Breast carcinoma was the most frequent source of metastases in the pituitary gland (50% of 205 cases with pituitary metastases), followed by the lung (22%), the gastrointestinal tract, the nasal sinuses, and the pharynx (Table II-6 and Fig. II-3). In 526 cases of breast carcinoma, we found pituitary gland involvement in 103 cases (20%). Other authors reported the frequency of pituitary gland involvement to be 9 to 28 per cent (Gurling et al., 1957; Sumulder and Smets, 1969; Duchen, 1966; Hägerstrand and Schonebeck, 1969; Kistler and Pribram, 1975; Oi et al., 1978).

The high rate of metastases recorded for the pituitary gland may be partially explained by the more thorough routine examination of this region as compared with other parts of the CNS.

The majority of metastatic tumors in the pituitary gland were asymptomatic. Diabetes insipidus, the only symptom of pituitary dysfunction in our series, was observed in six patients among 103 cases of pituitary meatastases from breast cancer. All patients had lesions on the posterior lobe of the pituitary gland and five cases had extensive lesions which invaded the infundibulum or the hypothalamus. Duchen (1966) also described four cases of diabetes insipidus in 161 cases of pituitary gland metastases from the breast. Teears and Silverman (1975) also reported six cases of diabetes insipidus among 88 cases of pituitary gland metastases. The ratio of 2.4 to 20 per cent for diabetes insipidus has been reported for metastatic pituitary tumors (Jones, 1944; Blotner, 1958; Houck et al., 1970).

Other hormonal disturbances were not detected during the clinical course of our patients. Houck et al. (1970) reported similar observations.

Table II-23 Pituitary involvement by metastatic malignant neoplasms.

Location of metastases	Carcinoma & sarcoma	Lymphoma & leukemia*	Total
Anterior lobe	43	5	48
Posterior lobe	102	13	115
Capsule	43	84	127
Pituitary gland total**	**205**	**96**	**301**

  *   Including multiple myeloma.
 **   Includes some cases, for which location in the pituitary gland was not available.

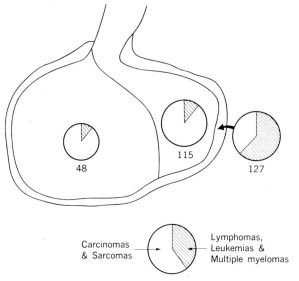

Fig. II-79 Secondary tumors in the pituitary gland. Graphic
presentation of Table II-23.

Data showing involvement of the component regions of the pituitary gland, namely the anterior lobe, the posterior lobe and the capsule is shown in Table II-23 and Figure II-79. Carcinoma has an obvious predilection for the posterior lobe, while lymphomas and leukemias tend to involve the capsule.

Three paths for pituitary gland involvement by metastatic tumors may be considered: blood-borne metastases, direct invasion by the tumor from neighborning tissues, and infiltration by leukemic or lymphoma cells.

In the first type of involvement, tumor cells metastasize presumably into the pituitary gland, especially into the posterior lobe, through the arteries. Most of the cases with metastases in the anterior lobe also have lesions in the posterior lobe.   In some cases, the tumor was considered to be first established in the posterior lobe with secondary invasion to the anterior lobe across the pars intermedia. In other instances, nodules in the anterior lobe were independent of those in the posterior lobe (Fig. II-80A and B).

The unique vascular architecture of the pituitary gland probably explains why carcinomas metastasize more frequently into the posterior lobe rather than the anterior lobe. The anterior lobe has a very limited primary arterial supply, and it is supplied by the portal system which enters through the posterior lobe of the pituitary gland (Green, 1951; Page and Bergland, 1977).

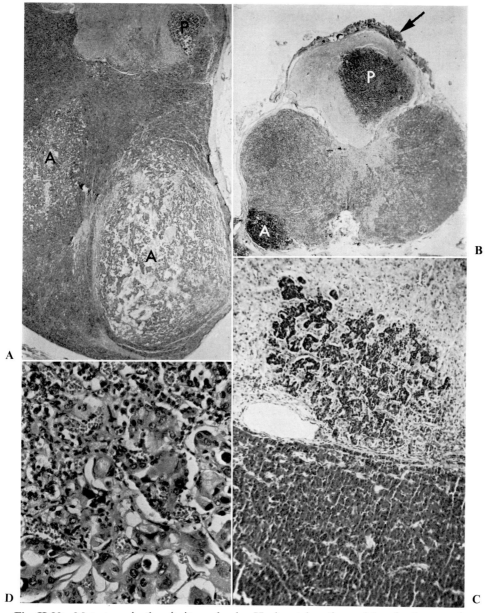

Fig. II-80 Metastases in the pituitary gland. Horizontal sections of the gland.
A. Two large metastatic nodules are seen on the anterior lobe (A) and one in the posterior lobe (P). Carcinoma of the lung. (H & E × 9, MH 19534.)
B. Metastatic deposits in the anterior lobe (A), posterior lobe (P) and capsule (arrow). Carcinoma of the lung. (H & E × 4, MH 20653.)
C. Metastatic carcinoma of the lung in the posterior lobe. (H & E × 80, MH 18093.)
D. Higher magnification of metastatic breast carcinoma in the anterior lobe. Large tumor cells infiltrate the small pituitary cells. (H & E × 150, MH 20042.)

The appearance of metastatic foci in the posterior lobe is almost identical to those in the brain parenchyma. The slight differences are due to the preexisting nerve fiber bundles, pituicytes and the rich vascular network of the pituitary gland. The tumor nodules sometimes have an irregular margin (Fig. II-80C). Tumor cells grow among the preexisting, fine vascular network. We observed that endothelial proliferation and glial responses are often inconspicuous in this region.

In the anterior lobe, metastatic tumors usually invade the glandular structures, growing along the rich vascular networks of small vessels (Fig. II-80D and Plate II-4A, p. 110). Some metastatic nodules have large necrotic centers.

Willis (1973) reviewed 16 reports of blood-borne metastatic lesions to the pituitary gland, most having originated from breast carcinoma. Other papers with comments on this subject were contributed by Meyer and Reah (1953), Das Gupta and Brasfield (1964), Koyama and Takakura (1969) and Epstein et al. (1973).

The second type of involvement of the pituitary gland was via direct invasion from a tumor in the base of the skull by tumors of the head and neck region. We observed 11 such cases in 155 cases of these primaries; most of them were carcinomas of the pharynx and nasal sinuses (7 cases). Teoh (1957) reported an incidence of 23 per cent (7 of 31 cases) of pituitary gland invasion by nasopharyngeal carcinomas. It is also possible that some metastases to the pituitary gland represent a direct extension from metastatic tumors in the base of the skull.

Infiltration of the pituitary gland by leukemic cells was more frequent than in malignant lymphomas. We observed infiltration in the pituitary gland in 28 per cent of the patients with leukemias. Masse et al. (1973) reported 46 per cent of pituitary gland metastases in leukemic patients, most of which were limited to the capsule. The severe infiltration is usually limited to the outer layer of the capsule. This infiltration was contiguous with bone marrow involvement of the sella turcica, as observed in several large microscopic sections that included the decalcified bony structures. Although the capsule of the pituitary gland is the only site of involvement in many cases, infiltration into the pituitary gland was observed in about one fifth of lymphomas and leukemias with pituitary involvement. Leukemia may also cause diabetes insipidus when the lesions are located in the posterior lobe or in the hypothalamus (Joseph and Levin, 1956; Rosenzweig and Kendell, 1968; Roy and Johnson, 1970).

Skull and Vertebrae

The bone is one of the most frequent sites of metastatic tumor growth. Metastases to the bone occurred in 34 per cent of the cases of carcinoma and sarcoma in our series. The vertebrae are affected most frequently among the whole skeletal system (Willis, 1973). The incidence of vertebral metastases was 15 per cent in our series and over 30 per cent in some other series (Drury et al., 1964; Fornasier and Horne, 1975). Skull involvement occurred in five per cent of the cases of carcinoma, including those due to direct invasion from pharyngeal or nasal tumors. Courville and Abbott (1945) estimated the real rate of skull metastases between 15 and 20 per cent based on several reports.

The primary tumors which most frequently caused generalized bone metastases were carcinomas of the breast, lung, thyroid, prostate, kidney, melanoma and sarcoma. Among those tumors, breast carcinoma, sarcoma and thyroid carcinoma frequently affected both the vertebrae and the skull, while prostatic and lung carcinoma frequently metastasized to the vertebrae alone. On the other hand, carcinomas of the nasal sinuses and the pharynx frequently invaded the skull. Neuroblastoma, which is a relatively rare tumor, showed frequent bony metastases.

The most frequent tumors with skull involvement, excluding the hematogenous neoplasms, were breast carcinoma, which accounted for 48 per cent of the skull involvement, lung carcinoma (14%) and carcinoma of the head and neck region (12%) (Table II-6). This list of the primary origin for skull metastasis was similar to other reports (Courville and Abbott, 1945; Perese, 1959). According to Willis (1973), the calvarium is more frequently involved than the base of the skull.

The most common primary sources of vertebral metastases in our series were breast carcinoma (33%) and lung carcinoma (28%), followed by carcinoma of the gastrointestinal tract and prostatic carcinoma (Table II-6). Similar results, but with more involvement by uterine carcinoma, are reported by other authors (Arseni et al., 1959; Drury et al., 1964). In some other series, lymphoma and multiple myeloma were important sources of metastases (Chandler et al., 1954; Fornasier and Horne, 1975) (see also Table II-3, p. 8 and p. 281).

The thoracic spine is most frequently affected by metastatic tumors (Arseni et al., 1959, Fig. II-81). However, if individual vertebrae are examined, the fifth lumbar vertebra is reported to be most often involved (Drury et al., 1964). The site of vertebral metastases differs for various primary tumors. Carcinomas of the pelvic organs frequently involve the lower spine.

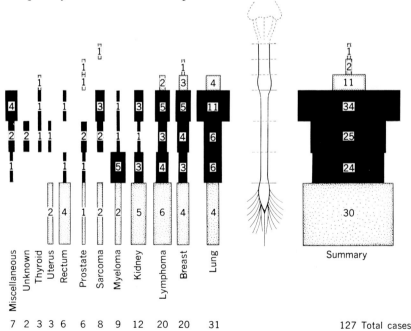

Fig. II-81 Level of vertebral metastases and primary sites, a radiologic analysis. (From Barron et al., 1959.)

Macroscopic findings

Metastases in the skull are usually multiple and consist of distinct nodules (Fig. II-82A and B). Sometimes, however, diffuse involvement with irregular margins is also observed (Fig. II-82C). The outer surface is often smooth on pathological examination and shows no tumor invasion into the adjacent tissue. On the other hand, the inner surface often shows adhesion or contiguous growth in the dura mater.

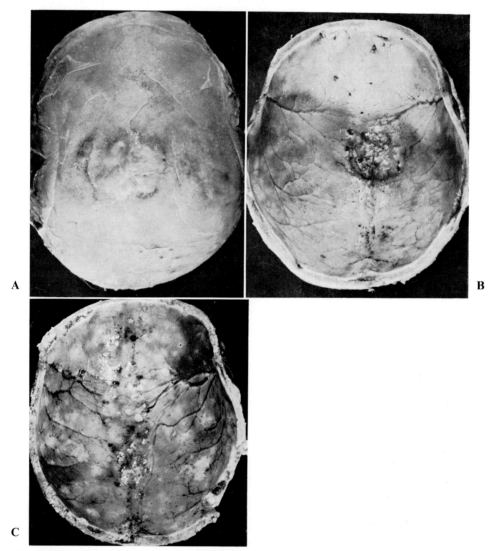

Fig. II-82 Metastatic tumors in the skull.
A and **B.** The outer surface of the tumor (Fig. A) is smooth compared to the inner surface (Fig. B) because the former is covered with the periosteum. (A 59-year-old woman who was operated on for breast carcinoma five years previously. No neurological deficits were noted. Autopsy revealed metastases in the lung, liver and other organs including the dura, cerebrum, cerebellum and posterior lobe of the pituitary. MH 19790.) (A: From Hirano et al., 1980.)
C. (A 62-year-old woman with metastatic squamous cell carcinoma involving the calvarium and other organs. MH 17952.)

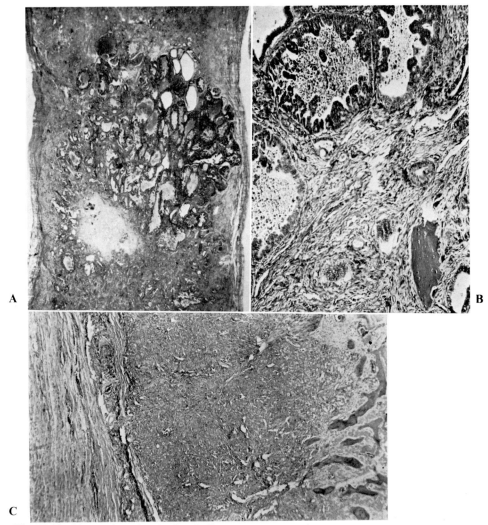

Fig. II-83 Tumor invasion in the skull.
A. Metastatic adenocarcinoma from the lung. (H & E × 10, MH 20242.)
B. Higher magnification of a tumor similar to that illustrated in A. (H & E × 72, MH 20434.)
C. A metastatic prostatic carcinoma in the skull extending into the dura mater on the left in the illustration. (H & E × 32, MH 19567.)

There are two types of metastatic bony lesions; osteolytic and osteoblastic (Fig. II-83). The most notable example of tumors with osteoblastic lesions is the prostatic carcinoma. In these situations, the affected bone becomes thick and sclerotic and may sometimes show spicules. Other primary tumors also occasionally produce osteoblastic lesions. Usually, bone metastases have a mixture of both osteoblastic and osteolytic lesions (Sharpe and McDonald, 1942; Schaerer and Whitney, 1953; Shapiro and Janzen, 1959; Potter, 1970; Burger and Vogel, 1976).

The vertebrae are often affected at multiple levels. The lesion usually begins in the vertebral body and extends into the lamina. This is an important path of invasion of the spinal epidural tissue. It may result in vertebral collapse causing compression of the spinal cord.

Path of Dissemination

In addition to direct invasion and arterial-borne metastases, the vertebral venous plexus (Batson's plexus) may provide a route for local metastasis (see also p. 74). Other authors have proposed direct invasion of the vertebrae from affected paravertebral lymph nodes (Blythe et al., 1975).

Some Unusual Metastases

Metastases into Primary Brain Tumors

We found 42 cases of primary brain tumors coexisting in patients with secondary tumors in the CNS and its coverings. These were 18 meningiomas, 11 pituitary adenomas, four gliomas, four epidermoids, two schwannomas, two lipomas and one colloid cyst. Clinically, these lesions were not diagnosed as primary brain tumors during life, and most of them were asymptomatic.

We found three cases of metastases to meningiomas. The primary sources were carcinomas of the breast (Fig. II-84A and Plate II-4B, p.110), kidney, and malignant lymphoma. In addition to these three cases, two more such cases were observed after the completion of this survey. In one case, a glioma contained metastatic melanoma, and in the other case, choristoma of the infundibulum was infiltrated by lymphoma cells (Fig. II-84B and Plate II-4C, p.110).

There are many reports of meningioma as fertile soil for secondary tumor growth. Wu and Hiszczynskyj (1977) reviewed 17 such cases reported by others and added one case of their own. Two additional cases which were not included in Wu's report (Hockley, 1975; Gyori, 1976), and three cases of our own, brings the total number of meningiomas containing metastases to 23 cases. In these 23 cases, the primary tumors included seven lung carcinomas, six breast carcinomas, four renal carcinomas and six of other origins, including two cases of unknown primary sites.

Metastases to gliomas are extremely uncommon and we found only two such reports (Posnikoff and Stratford, 1960; Rubinstein, 1972). As for other kinds of brain tumors, schwannoma and ependymoma were reported to contain metastatic tumors (Wallach and Edberg, 1959; Rubinstein, 1972). No choristoma has ever been reported to contain the metastases.

Coexistence of Cerebral Metastases of Two Different Origins

Our series included 104 patients with malignant tumors that originated from two or more different organs. Among them, we found a single case in which two different kinds of secondary growth were seen in the cranial cavity. In this case the brain parenchyma contained metastatic nodules from lung carcinoma, and the capsule of the pituitary gland was infiltrated by lymphoma cells.

In another peculiar case, both the epithelial and mesodermal elements of a carcinosarcoma, which originated in the lung, produced two different histologic types of metastases in the brain parenchyma and in the posterior lobe of the pituitary gland.

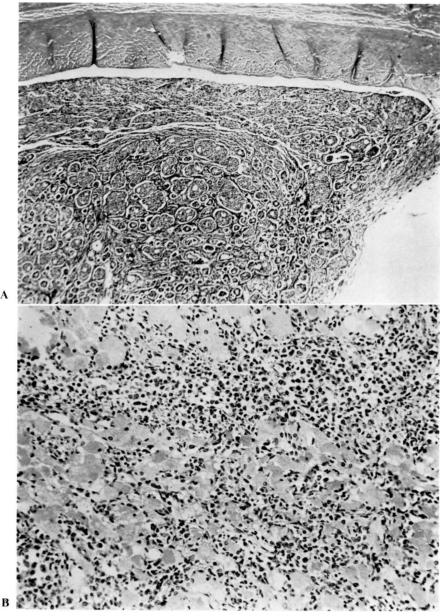

Fig. II-84 Metastatic tumor in the primary intracranial neoplasm.
A. Metastatic breast carcinoma in meningioma. Numerous small nodules of metastatic deposits are seen in a background of meningioma. (H & E × 120, MH 13277.)
B. A choristoma (large pale cells) is infiltrated by cells of lymphocytic lymphoma (small dark cells). (H & E × 190, MH 7824.)

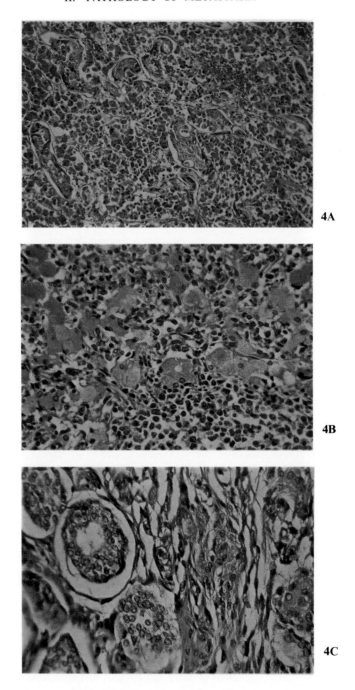

4A

4B

4C

Plate II-4A   Metastatic adenocarcinoma of the colon in the anterior lobe of the pituitary
gland.   (H & E × 50, MH 22274.)
Plate II-4B   Adenocarcinoma of the breast which metastasized into meningioma.   (H & E
× 330, MH 13277.)
Plate II-4C   Malignant lymphoma (lymphocytic type) invading a choristoma (large pink
cells) in the infundibulum.   In this case, the entire brain and the leptomeninges are involved.
(H & E × 330, MH 7824.)

Similar situations in extracranial metastases were reviewed by Minckler et al. (1970) and Willis (1973).

CONCLUSION

The body of statistical data compiled in this review of a large autopsy series provided information about numerous parameters regarding the involvement of the central nervous system at the terminal stages of metastatic neoplasms. It confirmed and emphasized the features of metastatic tumors in the central nervous system documented in the literature. It also contributed additional data about metastases to the dura mater and pituitary gland.

On morphological analysis, a clearer delineation of the histopathology of the metastatic tumor was facilitated by the markedly contrasting background provided by the nervous tissue. In addition, the unique anatomy of the central nervous system was accentuated by the presence of the metastases.

III. CLINICAL FEATURES OF INTRACRANIAL METASTATIC TUMORS

GENERAL STATISTICAL DATA

Primary Tumor

The results of the survey to be reported in this chapter are based on two sources of clinical information: patients treated at our clinic (Department of Neurosurgery of the National Cancer Center Hospital and the University of Tokyo Hospital) from 1959 through 1978, a period of 20 years, and those reported in the All Japan Brain Tumor Registry (1981). During this period, 616 cases of metastatic brain tumors were treated at our clinic. The frequency of primary sites for these metastatic brain tumors is shown in Table III-1. Lung cancer is the most frequent source (45.1%) and breast cancer is the second (16.2%). Gastrointestinal and urogenital cancers

Table III-1 Primary sources of intracranial metastatic tumors.

Site of primary neoplasm	Clinical cases		Autopsy cases	
	Univ. of Tokyo & N.C.C.*	All Japan Registry (1981)	Montefiore**	N.C.C.
Lung	278 (45.1%)	563 (41.1%)	349 (29.9%)	144 (42.2%)
Breast	100 (16.2)	154 (11.2)	278 (23.8)	44 (12.9)
Gastrointestinal	42 (6.8)	131 (9.5)	98 (8.4)	36 (10.6)
Genitourinary	42 (6.8)	137 (10.1)	110 (9.4)	29 (8.5)
Melanoma & Skin	6 (1.0)	13 (0.9)	47 (4.0)	5 (1.5)
Head & Neck	19 (3.1)	61 (4.5)	29 (2.5)	10 (2.9)
Thyroid	12 (1.9)	17 (1.2)	15 (1.3)	4 (1.2)
Leukemia	26 (4.2)	6 (0.4)	92 (7.9)	27 (7.9)
Lymphoma	8 (1.3)	13 (0.9)	112 (9.6)	17 (5.0)
Sarcoma	21 (3.4)	33 (2.4)	20 (1.7)	14 (4.1)
Others	62 (10.1)	67 (4.9)	17 (1.5)	8 (2.3)
Unknown	0 (0.0)	174 (12.7)	0 (0.0)	3 (0.9)
Total	**616 (100.0)**	**1,369 (100.0)**	**1,167 (100.0)**	**341 (100.0)**

* National Cancer Center Hospital, Tokyo.	Total No. of autopsies	3,849	4,191
** Montefiore Hospital and Medical Center, New York. These cases are including metastasis to the spinal canal (see Table II-1).	Ratio of intracranial involvement	30.6%	8.2%
	Ratio of brain examination	99.4%	34.1%

Table III-2 Primary origin of intracranial metastatic tumors

Authors		No. of cases	Primary tumors							
			Lung	Breast	Digestive tract	Genitourinary organs	Skin including melanoma	Endocrine organs	Leukemia lymphoma sarcoma	Others & unknown
Krasting*	1906	139	20.9%	28.8%		25.6%				50.4%
Grant	1926	49	12.2	30.6	4.1	18.4	14.3			20.4
Dunlap	1932	77	11.7	15.6	13.0	22.1	6.5	5.2	3.9	15.6
Baker	1942	114	21.1	21.1	15.8	18.4	7.9	6.1		9.6
Globus	1942	33	57.6	—	18.2	6.1		15.2		3.0
Neustaedter	1944	52	15.4	26.9	5.8	7.7	3.8			40.4
Tom	1946	82	22.0	15.9	15.9	11.0	8.5	3.7	3.7	19.5
Kiefer	1947	100	35	10	10	25				
Rupp	1948	42	50.0	7.1	4.8	4.8		4.8		28.6
Elvidge & Baldwin	1949	88	22.7	15.9	4.5	13.6		2.4	2.3	35.2
Earle**	1954	167	57.5	0.6	10.5	12.6	7.1	2.3	2.9	5.1
Chao et al.	1954	38	60.5	18.4	2.6	2.6	2.6	—	5.3	5.3
Lesse & Netsky	1954	207	24	34	5.8	6.2	1.4	2.9	11.1	14.6
Störtebecker	1954	158	15.8	7.0	9.5	24.7	7.6	1.3		34.2
Ask-Upmark	1956	14	35.7	21.4	14.3	21.4				7.1
Labet	1956	154	36.4	9.6	5.1	3.2				35.0
Petit-Dutailis et al.	1956	107	47.7	10.3	8.4	13.1	3.7	0.9	1.9	14.0
Garde et al.	1958		22.6	23.8	11	3.6				39
Perese	1959	162	21.6	24.1	8.0	11.1	9.3	3.1	9.9	12.9
Simionescu	1960	195	38.1	22.6	3.6	12.5	6.2	2.7	1.1	13.3
Chu & Hilaris	1961	218	33.9	39.0	2.8	7.8	4.6		5.0	6.9
Blatt & Højgaard	1963	69	50.7	10.1	13.0	7.2	5.8	1.4	1.4	10.1
Chason et al.	1963	63	54.4	15.9	9.5	6.4	4.8			11.0
Richards & McKissock	1963	389	64.8	5.9	4.9	4.6	1.5	0.3	0.5	17.5
Aronson et al.	1964	397	46	13	9	7	3	4	10	8
Støier	1965	124	29.0	5.6	7.3	18.5	13.7	0.8		25.0
Vieth & Odom	1965a	313	27.5	16.3	5.1	7.0	20.2		2.6	21.3
Order et al.	1968	108	63.0	13.9	9.3	5.6			2.8	13.9
Penzholz	1968		32.4	19.3	4.8	11.3	8.0			24.2
Koyama & Takakura	1969	101	42	18	10	1	3	1	15	10
Nisce et al.	1971	560	25	39		8				28
Raskind et al.	1971	51	51.0	17.6	5.9	5.9	5.9		3.9	9.8
Takeuchi	1971	90	41	10	12.2	6.6		4.4	7.8	18
Castaigne	1972	222	43	10	6	7	3			31
Haar & Patterson, Jr.	1972	167	30	11	7	3	16		8	25
Constans et al.	1973b	167	15.6	36.5	10.2	9.0		4.2	1.2	16.2
Deutsch et al.	1974	88	35.2	23.9	4.5	10.2	5.7	1.1	2.3	13.6
Paillas et al.	1974b	172	31.9	22.6	10.9	13.2	5.1	1.6	0.5	13.3
Young et al.	1974	162	46.3	26.2		8.0	6.8			11.7
Takakura	1976	325	40.0	12.0	9.5	2.7	2.4			33.4
Tomita et al.	1977	88	61.4	8.0	8.0	2.3	1.1	6.8		4.5
All Japan Registry	1981	1,369	41.1	11.2	9.5	10.1	0.9	1.2	4.1	21.7
Current study										
New York (Autopsied cases)	1981	1,177	29.7	23.6	8.3	8.5	4.0	1.3	13.9	1.4
Tokyo (Clinical cases)	1981	616	45.1	16.2	6.8	6.8	1.0	1.9	8.9	13.2

* Krasting's material cited by Grant (1926)
** All male cases (Male Veteran's Hospital)

are the third most common sources of brain metastasis. Since gastric cancer is the most frequent malignant tumor in Japan, brain metastasis from gastrointestinal cancers is not so rare. The All Japan Brain Tumor Registry has revealed the same tendency of primary sites, in which lung cancer is the most predominant primary tumor for brain metastasis (41.1% of all metastatic brain tumors). Since the incidence of melanoma in Japan is lower than in European countries or the United States, the lower ratio of brain metastasis is generally noted. Statistical analysis of the primary sites of intracranial metastases has demonstrated a higher incidence of leukemia or lymphoma in autopsied cases compared to clinical ones. This tendency is accepted based on the data of clinical cases which were collected in neurosurgical clinics.

Primary sources of intracranial metastasis of malignant tumors have been reported by many investigators (Table III-2). The ratio of primary tumors is quite different depending on the background of each clinic. Recently, the increase of lung cancer as the primary source for metastatic tumors of the central nervous system is generally noted.

Age

There are two peaks in the age distribution of intracranial metastases of malignant neoplasms. The highest frequency in our clinical series was found between the ages of 55 and 59 years. This frequency in our series completely agrees with the data of the All Japan Brain Tumor Registry (Figs. III-1 and 2). Another peak was observed in children. Primary tumors of intracranial metastases in children are mainly leukemia, neuroblastoma, retinoblastoma, some sarcomas (rhabdomyosarcoma, etc.) and malignant lymphoma (Bailey et al., 1939). Our series demonstrated a higher incidence of metastatic tumors in children than the All Japan Brain Tumor Registry, since pediatric clinics at the National Cancer Center Hospital are actively working and more patients were consulted there for neurosurgical management than the average neurosurgical clinic. The age distribution of all patients with primary brain tumors is demonstrated in Figure III-3. The peak incidence was found in patients between the ages of 40 and 49, which is slightly lower than those with metastatic tumors. The peak incidence of primary brain tumors in children was found between the ages of 5 and 14 years, but that of metastatic tumors was found in ages under 9 years. The ages between 15 to 19 years are the most dormant for both primary and metastatic brain tumors. No patients over the age of 80 having metastatic brain tumors were encountered clinically.

The average ages at the onset of neurological symptoms due to intracranial metastatic tumors are summarized in Table III-3. The average age of onset was 56 years for lung cancer and 49 years for breast cancer patients. Intracranial metastases appear at relatively younger ages for patients with choriocarcinoma, thyroid cancer and various sarcomas.

The overall incidence of intracranial metastatic tumors was higher in men than in women, but this sex difference depends on the cancer types of the patients. If lung cancer is the major source, the incidence in men is higher than in women [Globus

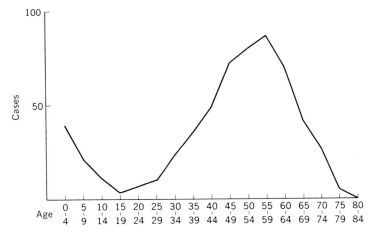

Fig. III-1 Age distribution of intracranial metastases of malignant neoplasms (616 cases).

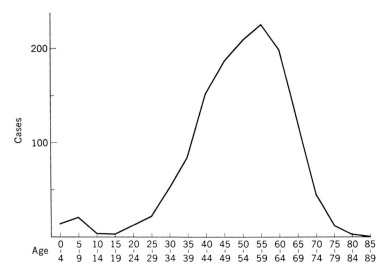

Fig. III-2 Age distribution of intracranial metastases of malignant neoplasms (All Japan Brain Tumor Registry 1981, 1,360 cases).

and Meltzer (1942), Elvidge and Baldwin (1949), Knights, Jr. (1954a, b), Simionescu (1960), Nisce et al. (1971) and Haar and Patterson, (1972)]. Richards and McKissock (1963) examined only cases of lung cancer and the ratio of incidence in men and women was 213:39. When the major source of the primary tumor was breast cancer, the ratio is naturally reversed. Strang and Ajmone-Marsan (1961) reported that the incidence of their cases was higher in women than men.

Sex

The sex and age distribution of intracranial metastatic tumors is shown in Figure III-4. According to the All Japan Brain Tumor Registry, 55.9 per cent of 1,369 patients

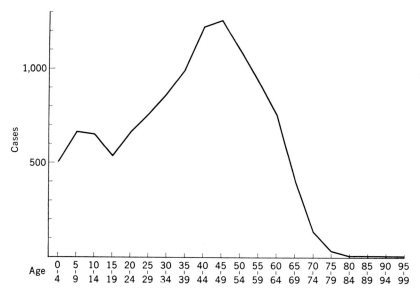

Fig. III-3 Age distribution of all brain tumors (All Japan Brain Tumor
Registry 1981, 11,584 cases).

Table III-3 Incidence of intracranial metastatic tumors*. Average
age at onset of neurological symptoms and sex distribution.

Primary tumor	No. of cases	Average age of onset (years)	Sex ratio M : F
Lung	289	56 ± 10	3.4 : 1
Breast	100	49 ± 10	0 : 100
Gastrointestinal tract	42	52 ± 11	2 : 1
Esophagus	6	53 ± 11	5 : 1
Stomach	26	49 ± 13	1.5 : 1
Rectum	7	53 ± 8	6 : 1
Liver, Pancreas	3	58 ± 10	
Genitourinary organs	42		
Uterus	18	51 ± 7	
Choriocarcinoma	4	30 ± 7	
Testis	3	43 ± 16	
Kidney	15	54 ± 6	2 : 1
Bladder	2	Adult	
Head & Neck	19	52 ± 12	3 : 1
Parotid	6	41 ± 11	5 : 1
Thyroid	12	43 ± 12	1 : 3
Sarcoma**	21	40 ± 17	6 : 1

 * Including some new data.
** Excluding cases of children.

were male.   In our clinical series, 56.6 per cent were male and 43.4 per cent were
female.   Of 289 lung cancer patients, 223 (77.2%) were male and 66 (22.8%) were
female.   Therefore, the number of male patients was 3.4 times more than that of
female patients.   The age distribution of lung cancer metastasized to the brain ranged
from 25 to 78 years, and its peak incidence was between the ages of 55 and 59 years
in male patients and 45 to 49 years in female patients (Fig. III-4).

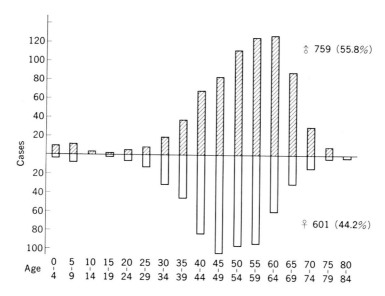

Fig. III-4 Sex and age distribution of intracranial metastatic tumors
(All Japan Brain Tumor Registry 1981, 1,360 cases).

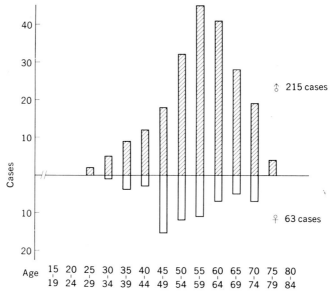

Fig. III-5 Sex and age distribution of intracranial metastatic tumors from
lung cancer (278 cases).

According to our clinical data, there were no significant differences in age or
sex distribution for any histological type of lung cancer (Table III-4). Our data from
autopsies, however, showed different rates of incidence of various types of lung cancer
for each sex. And the frequency of brain metastasis also differed among histological
types (see p. 16). It is controversial whether the brain is susceptible to tumor cells of

Table III-4 Distribution of each histological type, sex and the average age at onset of neurological symptoms of intracranial metastatic tumors from lung cancer.

Histological type	Male		Female	
	No. of cases	Average age of onset	No. of cases	Average age of onset
Adenoca.	107	56 ± 10	38	54 ± 11
Squamous cell ca.	34	56 ± 10	11	58 ± 11
Large cell ca.	16	57 ± 8	3	51 ± 9
Small cell ca.	31	55 ± 10	4	61 ± 7
Unknown	35		10	
Subtotal	223	56.3 ± 10.3 (25–78 years)	66	54.6 ± 10.0 (33–73 years)
Total		**289 cases***	**55.9 ± 10.3**	

* Including recent data.

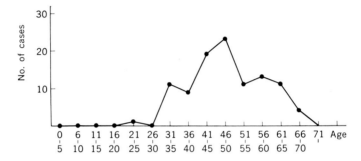

Fig. III-6 Age distribution of intracranial metastatic tumors from breast cancer (102 cases).

certain histological types. Koletsky (1938), Bryson and Spencer (1951), and Hazra et al. (1972) stressed that adenocarcinoma and small cell carcinoma metastasized more easily to brain than squamous cell carcinoma. Knights, Jr. (1954b) and Halpert et al. (1960) opposed this view. The age distribution of breast cancer patients is shown in Figure III-6.

The total rate of other primary neoplasms was approximately the same for both men and women. The number of male patients was, however, more than female for gastrointestinal, head and neck cancers and various sarcomas. Especially for gastric cancer, the number of male patients was more than twice that of female patients. On the contrary, the number of female patients was three times more than that of males for thyroid cancer.

Location

Many investigators admitted that intracranial metastatic tumors appear in every part of the brain. Kindt (1964) reported that the area of the middle cerebral artery is the predominant site for metastasis, since the blood flow is maximal because of the anatomical and physical situation. It was also commonly noted that tumors are situated mostly in the subcortical or cortical regions (Willis, 1952; Toyokura, et al., 1957). Ask-Upmark (1956) calculated the ratio of the weights of the cerebrum to cerebellum to be 9 to 1. In 45 cases of brain metastases collected from the literature and his own materials, he found that metastases to the cerebrum were only three times as frequent as metastases to the cerebellum. He postulated the histological affinity of the cerebellum for metastasis. There were several other reports that the frequency of cerebellar metastasis is higher than the cerebrum per unit weight (Meyer and Reah, 1953; Onuigbo, 1958; Chason et al., 1963). There is, however, no definite evidence to support the hypothesis by Ask-Upmark.

Table III-5 Number of intracranial metastatic tumors in supra- and infra-tentorial space*.

Location	No. of tumors
Supratentorial	992 (78.8%)
Infratentorial	133 (10.6)
Supra-and infra-tentorial	134 (10.6)
Total	**1,259 (100.0)**

* All Japan Brain Tumor Registry (1981).

Recent statistical analysis of the location of intracranial metastatic tumors has demonstrated the actual incidence more clearly. Among 1,259 intracranial metastases accumulated by the All Japan Brain Tumor Registry, 992 cases (78.8%) were supratentorial, 133 cases (10.6%) infratentorial, and the remaining 134 cases (10.6%) were located both in the supra- and infra-tentorial spaces (Table III-5). The ratio of the number of tumors in the supratentorial space to that in the infratentorial space is 7.5 to 1; this is almost equivalent to the weight ratio of the cerebrum to the cerebellum.

The locations of intracranial tumors in various anatomical sites have been reported by many investigators. Some of the data is summarized in Table III-6.

Table III-6 Location of intracranial metastatic tumor.

Author	Simionescu* 1960	Lang & Slater 1964	Støier 1965	Vieth* (1) & Odom 1965a	Vieth** (2) & Odom 1965a	Olivecrona 1967	Haar & Patterson 1972	Constans et al. 1973b
Total no. of cases	109	284	171	133	78	195	167	163
Location								
Frontal	50%	21%	11%	27%	21%	21%	22%	16%
Temporal	11	14	12	14	11	14	13	26
Parietal	17	18	43	30***	22	19	26	18***
Occipital	4	8	8	14	12	5	8	5
Cerebellum	15	12	14	8	14	12	19	15
Brain stem	1	3	4	2	4	1	1	6
Meninges	1	1	1		6		2	
Calvarium		5				1		
Pituitary gl.	2					2		
Others		16	6		11	1	10	
Multiple						24		15

*   In cases of single metastasis.
** In cases of multiple metastases.
*** Including parieto-temporal, parieto-frontal and parieto-occipital tumors.

Table III-7   Location of intracranial metastatic tumors*.

Frontal lobe	182 (19.7%)
Temporal lobe	92 (10.0)
Parietal lobe	249 (27.0)
Occipital lobe	68 (7.4)
Diffuse	7 (0.8)
Chiasmal region	16 (1.7)
Third ventricle	1 (0.1)
Lateral ventricle (ant. horn-body)	4 (0.4)
Lat. ventricle (trigonum)	2 (0.2)
Lat. ventricle (temp. horn)	13 (1.4)
Corpus callosum and septum pellucidum	12 (1.3)
Rostral brain stem and basal ganglia	31 (3.4)
Pineal region	7 (0.8)
Aqueduct	2 (0.2)
Cerebellar vermis	9 (1.0)
Cerebellar hemisphere	62 (6.7)
Fourth ventricle	4 (0.4)
Cerebello-pontine angle	5 (0.5)
Caudal brain stem (pons and medulla)	4 (0.4)
Optic nerve	3 (0.3)
Calvarum	38 (4.1)
Skull-base, medial	32 (3.5)
Skull-base, paramedial	44 (4.8)
Tentorium	3 (0.3)
Sagittal sinus	2 (0.2)
Sphenoid ridge	1 (0.1)
Olfactory groove	15 (1.6)
Tuberculum sellae	14 (1.5)
Total	**922 (100.0)**

*   All Japan Brain Tumor Registry (1981).

The frontal and parietal lobes are the most common sites of metastatic tumors.   The details of location of intracranial metastatic tumors reported by the All Japan Brain Tumor Registry (1981) are shown in Table III-7.   In this table, it should be noted that some locations such as the chiasmal region and tuberculum sellae might be better categorized as one site, but all sites are classified according to the technical coding system of the registration.   The parietal lobe, where 27.0 per cent of all metastatic tumors are located, is the most predominant site for metastases.   The second most predominant site is the frontal lobe, where 19.7 per cent are located.

There is no difference in laterality.   Støier (1965) reported that the number of

Table III-8   Laterality of intracranial metastatic tumors*.

Right	505 (36.9%)
Left	463 (33.8)
Bilateral	182 (13.3)
Central	82 (6.1)
Non specified	62 (4.5)
Unknown	74 (5.4)
Total	**1,369 (100.0)**

*   All Japan Brain Tumor Registry (1981).

tumors situated on right and left side were 63 and 65 respectively. Laterality of tumors reported by the All Japan Brain Tumor Registry (1981) is summarized in Table III-8. On the right side, there were 505 (36.9%) tumors, and on left side, 463 (33.8%). One hundred eighty-two cases (13.3%) had tumors bilaterally, and in 82 cases (6.1%) the tumors were located centrally. Non-specified cases in the table included those with meningeal carcinomatosis.

Number of Tumors

Problems regarding the number of metastatic tumor nodules are important for establishing therapeutic schedules including surgery, and have been reported in many papers (Table III-9). In autopsied materials, more than 80 per cent of the patients had multiple metastatic tumor nodules. Galluzzi and Payne (1956) reviewed previously published papers and examined their own cases, and concluded that a single metastatic tumor was found only in 13.9 per cent of all 741 cases. From a clinical point of view, the decision for surgical removal of the metastatic brain tumor is generally made under the consideration of whether the number of tumors is single or multiple. Since there was technical difficulty in finding small metastatic tumor nodules in the brain by angiography or RI scintigram, they were often not clinically detected. In reports based on surgical information, the ratio of single tumors was especially

Table III-9 Number of metastases in brain (Ratio of single metastatic tumor).

Author		Total no. of cases	Ratio of single metastasis
Krasting	1906	145	33%
Grant	1926	26	50
Globus & Meltzer	1942	52	42*
Rupp	1948	42	40
Walther	1948	103	40
Flavell	1949	85	2
Baker et al.	1951	100	30
Meyer & Reah	1953	106	30
Earle	1954	161	45
Lesse & Netzky	1954	121	20
Störtebecker	1954	82**	82
Ask-Upmark	1956	151	40
		696***	35
Galluzzi & Payne	1956	741***	14
Toyokura et al.	1957	39	36
Simionescu	1960	137**	69
Richards & McKissock	1963	147	27
Chason et al.	1963	200	15
Lang & Slater	1964	284**	66
Vieth & Odom	1965a	211	56
Koyama & Takakura	1969	63	30
Nisce et al.	1971	91	40
Takakura (Current study)	1981	246**	54

*   The original report cited 57 cases including 5 cases of meningeal carcinomatosis.
**   All surgical cases.
*** Review.

high, since the patients were preselected by surgical indications.   Störtebecker (1954) reported that 82 per cent of 82 surgical patients had asingle metastases.   Simionescu (1960) and Lang and Slater (1964) also reported similar statistic figures that 69 per cent of 137, and 66 per cent of 284 operated patients had single metastases respectively.   Our 246 surgical cases were analyzed, and single metastases was found in 54 per cent, multiple metastases in 33 per cent, meningeal carcinomatosis in eight per cent and diffuse infiltration in five per cent of all cases.   If meningeal carcinomatosis and diffuse infiltration are excluded, the ratio of cases with single metastases becomes 62.0 per cent (134/216).   According to the data of the All Japan Brain Tumor Registry, single metastases was found in 63.6 per cent, multiple metastases in 29.3 per cent and meningeal carcinomatosis in 7.1 per cent among a total of 1,295 intracranial metastatic tumor patients.   These patients were accumulated solely from neurosurgical clinics.

Recent examinations by CT have, however, solved most of the technical problems for detecting the presence of small metastatic tumor nodules.   It is possible to detect a tiny nodule with a diameter as small as 3 mm.   The number of metastatic tumors clinically found has, therefore, approached the real figures analyzed by autopsy.   Actually, multiple metastatic tumors are found in more than 80 per cent of patients today.   It has for a long time been considered that there is no surgical indication for multiple intracranial metastatic tumors.   Some patients with multiple metastases were, however, successfully treated by surgical removal of a major nodule and chemoradiotherapy for remaining small tumors.   Tiny tumors, with diameters of only a few millimeters each, were eradicated later by continuous maintenance of chemotherapy, and those patients have been in good condition for more than one year.   Considering these cases, it might be necessary to redraw a classical standard therapeutic schedule and establish new approaches of treatment using multidisciplinary concepts in surgery, radiation, chemotherapy and immunotherapy.

The actual number of metastatic nodules counted in 211 autopsied cases by Vieth and Odom (1965a) were: single, 56.4%; two nodules, 17.1%; three nodules, 10.9%; four to five nodules, 9.5%; six to eight nodules, 3.3%; more than eight nodules, 1.9%.

Metastatic Leptomeningeal Tumors

Leptomeningeal involvement by carcinoma cells was first described by Eberth in 1870 under the name of "endothelioma of the pia," but its metastatic nature was not clarified.   Case reports of such pathological changes without any associated parenchymal metastasis were also reported by Oppenheim (1888), and Saenger (1900) under the name of "carcinomatose" and Lilienfeld and Benda (1901) as "Metastatischer Karzinose."   Siefert (1902) described the clinical signs and the histological observations of multiple carcinomatosis of the central nervous system.   The term "meningeal carcinomatosis" was first adopted by Beerman in 1912 for diffuse leptomeningeal involvement by carcinoma cells.   Various other nomenclatures were used by different authors: metastatic carcinoma to the leptomeninges (Strange, 1952), carcinomatosis of the meninges (Fischer-Williams et al., 1955; Heathfield and Williams, 1956), leptomeningeal carcinomatosis (Grain and Karr, 1955), carcinosis meningum (Moberg and Reis, 1961); meningitis due to carcinomatosis (McMillan, 1962), etc.

Since preoperative or antemortem diagnosis was difficult especially in the early stages of dissemination due to technical difficulties in the cytological examination of cancer cells in the cerebrospinal fluid, the metastatic leptomeningeal tumor was thought to be a rare form of metastatic intracranial tumors. Spriggs (1954) collected from the literature only 66 cases in which malignant cells were found in the cerebrospinal fluid. Techniques to detect cancer cells in the cerebrospinal fluid have, however, been much improved in the past decade, and metastatic leptomeningeal tumors have been found to be a relatively common complication of systemic cancer (Olson et al., 1974).

Table III-10 Metastatic leptomeningeal tumors.

Primary tumor	Total No. of cases	Age	Duration from primary tumor detection to the onset of neurological symptoms
Stomach cancer	6	30–58 yrs.	Pre-exist—27 months
Breast cancer	4	31–42	5–26
Uterine cancer	4	41–66	Co-exist—22
Lung cancer	3	38–71	Pre-exist—3
Malig. lymphoma	4	children—17	Pre-exist—24
Rhabdomyosarcoma	1	child	15m
Retinoblastoma	6	children	Average 18.2 months
Subtotal	**28**	**children—71**	**Pre-exist—27**
Leukemia	26	children—31	Average 11.8 months
AML	20		
ALL	4		
CML	2		
Total	**54**	**children—71**	**Pre-exist—27**

The rate of metastatic leptomeningeal tumors is about 7.1 per cent (92/1,295 cases) of all metastatic intracranial tumors collected by the All Japan Brain Tumor Registry. In our clinical 616 intracranial metastatic tumors, 52 cases (8.4%) of leptomeningeal involvement were encountered, 26 of which were leukemia. Primary tumors other than leukemia were stomach cancer (6 cases), breast cancer (4), uterine cancer (4), lung cancer (3), malignant lymphoma (4), rhabdomyosarcoma (1) and retinoblastoma (6) (Table III-10). Since melanoma is relatively rare in Japan, only one patient was treated, but no definite evidence of leptomeningeal involvement was obtained clinically. CT has, however, demonstrated clearly leptomeningeal carcinomatosis in recent cases. On the other hand, stomach cancer is the most common malignancy, and it metastasizes often in the form of meningeal involvement. The six cases listed in Table III-10 were verified to have leptomeningeal tumors by autopsy or clinical evidence. The age distribution was from 30 to 58 years (five women and one man). Since the overall incidence of intracranial metastasis of stomach cancer in men is three times more than that in women, men seem to be more susceptible to leptomeningeal involvement than women. But it is not conclusive, because the number of patients was limited. Breast cancers also metastasize frequently in leptomeningeal form. The predominant age distribution of intracranial metastatic tumors is from 31 to 42 years for breast cancer.   Only three patients with lung cancer showed definite clinical evidence of leptomeningeal involvement.   Leptomeningeal involvement of malignant lymphoma, rhabdomyosarcoma and retinoblastoma were all observed in children.   Only one case of malignant lymphoma was detected at the age of 17.   Out of 26 leukemia patients, 22 were children, since co-operative treatment by neurosurgeons and pediatritians was carried out in the National Cancer Center Hospital, and most adult patients with leptomeningeal involvement of leukemia had escaped from the current study.   The rate in our series of leptomeningeal involvement of acute myelocytic leukemia (AML) is higher than that of acute lymphocytic leukemia (ALL), which is the more common type in children in Europe and the United States (Hardisty and Norman, 1967; Price and Johnson, 1973).   Recent statistical data in Japan has, however, shown a similar tendency since the number of ALL patients is increasing.

Primary tumors for leptomeningeal metastasis in the United States are different. According to Olson and others (1974) of the Memorial Sloan-Kettering Cancer Center in New York, carcinoma of the breast and lymphomas accounted for 36 per cent and 28 per cent of all 50 cases respectively.   Of the remainder, 16 per cent were caused by lung cancer, 10 per cent by malignant melanoma, 4 per cent by adenocarcinoma of the pancreas, and a single case was due to sarcoma.   In two cases, the primary tumor could not be determined.   There were no patients with stomach cancer.   Leukemia was not included in their study.

In 29 cases of leptomeningeal tumors studied by Little and others (1974) at the Mayo Clinic in Rochester, Minnesota, carcinoma of the breast and lung accounted for 31 per cent and 24 per cent respectively.   Of the remainder, 14 per cent were caused by stomach cancer, and 10 per cent by malignant melanoma.   There was only one case each of carcinoma of the pancreas, uterus, gastrointestinal tract (not verified) and skin.   In two cases, the primary tumors could not be determined. Leukemia was also not included.

SYMPTOMS AND SIGNS

Onset of Neurological Symptoms

Background regarding types of patients differs largely in each hospital.   In the National Cancer Center Hospital, a majority of the patients have a history of treatment for malignancies and the metastatic tumors of the central nervous system are generally detected after or at the same time as establishment of diagnosis for primary tumors. They are categorized as "post-found" and "coexisting" types of metastatic tumors.   On the other hand, they are often found before detecting primary tumors (pre-existing types) in general neurosurgical clinics, since the patients, whose neurological symptoms appear earlier than those of primary site, are referred to as having primary tumors of the central nervous system.

The duration between the discovery of the primary tumor and the appearance

Table III-11 Duration from establishment of diagnosis for primary cancer to that for intracranial metastasis*.

Duration	No. of patients
Pre-existing and co-existing type	176 (19.0%)
1– 6 months	286 (30.8)
7–12	139 (15.0)
1– 2 years	132 (14.2)
2– 3	67 (7.2)
3– 4	32 (3.4)
4– 5	32 (3.4)
5– 6	18 (1.9)
6– 7	15 (1.6)
7– 8	3 (0.3)
8–	30 (3.0)
Total	**928 (100.0)**

* All Japan Brain Tumor Registry (1981)

of neurological symptoms of intracranial metastasis, as reported by the All Japan Brain Tumor Registry (1981), is summarized in Table III-11. In one hundred seventy-six out of 928 cases (19.0%) verified metastatic intracranial tumors were found before, or almost at the same time as the primary tumors. Thirty per cent of the intracranial tumors were found one to six months after the primary tumor diagnosis. The duration is, however, significantly different for each primary tumor (Table III-12). In cases of lung cancer in our series, 24.7 per cent of all intracranial metastases are of the pre-existing type. The coexisting type is found in 10.0 per cent and the post-found type is in 65.3 per cent. With regard to metastatic tumors of the pre-existing type, the differential diagnosis from glioma was not easy, but it has become more accurate with the aid of computed tomography. Since multiplicity of tumors is one of the characteristics of metastatic tumors and those tumors can be easily demonstrated by CT, it is quite reasonable to suspect metastatic tumors before surgery when they are detected. Details of CT findings of metastatic tumors will be described in the following chapter. Chest x-ray examination will also offer suggestions as to the presence of primary or secondary lung tumors. In cases of metastatic tumors of the coexisting type, it is usually not difficult to diagnose. Every chest surgeon is always cautious about the presence of intracranial metastasis.

The neurological symptoms of intracranial metastasis appear most rapidly in cases of lung cancer because of the direct anatomical channel of the vascular system. The average duration between the establishment of primary lung cancer diagnosis

Table III-12 Duration between the detection of primary cancer and the development of neurological symptoms due to intracranial metastasis.

Type	Lung cancer		Breast cancer	
Pre-existing	64 cases (24.7%)		0 cases (0.0%)	
Co-existing	26	(10.0)	1	(1.4)
Post-found	169	(65.3)	70	(98.6)
(Average duration)	7.2 months (1–90 months)		42.4 months (1–15 y 6 months)	
Total	**259**	**(100.0)**	**71**	**(100.0)**

and the appearance of neurological symptoms due to intracranial metastasis was 7.2 months. The longest duration in our 259 cases was seven years and six months, but in 76 per cent of our cases, the initial neurological symptoms due to intracranial metastasis appear during six months after the detection of primary lung cancer. Constans et al. (1974) reported also that in 25 out of 37 (68%) intracranial metastatic tumors due to lung cancer, the neurological symptoms appeared in the initial six months after the detection of primary cancer. In their cases no intracranial metastasis developed after two years from the detection of primary lung cancer. On the contrary, in the cases of breast cancer, the average duration was 42.4 months and much longer than that of lung cancer. The longest duration in our series of breast cancer was 15 years and six months. In cases of Constans et al. (1974), the longest duration was 23 years after mastectomy, and 67 per cent of all intracranial metastases appeared three years after diagnosis of the primary tumor. In our series, in only one in 71 cases of breast cancer was brain metastasis detected at the same time the primary tumor was detected. No intracranial metastatic tumor of the pre-existing type was present in breast cancer. The average duration was longer in cases of cancers of the gastrointestinal organs, kidney and melanoma than for lung cancer. The initial neurological symptoms due to intracranial metastasis appear most frequently during one to five years after the detection of primary cancer in these cases.

There are two forms of onset of neurological symptoms due to intracranial metastasis: the acute type and the progressive type.

Acute Type

Neurological symptoms of the acute type develop by epileptic seizures or the sudden onset of headaches or conscious disturbances due to intracranial hemorrhage. Seizures, such as initial symptoms of intracranial metastatic tumors, were noted in 19.1 per cent of our cases. In most cases, seizures were of the Jacksonian type. The severity of post-ictal unilateral motor weakness was varied. In some patients, the symptoms disappeared a few hours after the seizure; in other cases, they persisted permanently. Grandmal seizures developed in some cases.

Intracranial hemorrhages appear in two forms: intraparenchymal hemorrhage adjacent to the tumor and subarachnoid hemorrhage. Subarachnoid hemorrhage accompanied with metastatic brain tumors was reported already half a century ago by Gate and Boyer (1932), Garin et al. (1932) and Huguenin (1935). Constans et al. (1974) found 52 cases of metastatic tumors in 188 brain tumor cases accompanied by subarachnoid hemorrhage. Melanoma and choriocarcinoma are the most common causes of such subarachnoid hemorrhages. The search for the etiology of intracranial hemorrhage is especially important in planning the therapeutic schedule, since the incidence of intracranial hemorrhage is considerably high in cancer patients, mainly due to coagulation crises induced by extensive chemotherapy. It is quite rare to detect aneurysms by angiography in cases of subarachnoid hemorrhage accompanied by metastatic brain tumors. The sudden onset of headaches, loss of consciousness and seizures are common symptoms of such subarachnoid hemorrhage as seen in cases of general vascular accidents. The level of consciousness depends on the severity of the hemorrhage and the induced brain edema.

In the fulminant type, the level of consciousness deteriorates rapidly. The patients do not generally respond to glucocorticoid therapy. Massive hemorrhage or irreversible destruction of the brain stem due to extensive brain edema triggered by epileptic seizures is the main cause for the rapid course of deterioration.

Progressive Type

This is a common type for the development of metastatic tumors in the central nervous system. Tumor cells metastasized through blood vessels or cerebrospinal fluid lodge in the parenchyma of the brain or the leptomeninges. As the tumor grows gradually, it induces brain edema around the tumor. Increased intracranial pressure by both tumor and brain edema produces symptoms such as headache and nausea. Various symptoms and signs of neurological deficit gradually appear before attacks of epileptic seizures. Constans et al. (1974) reported that the acute type of onset of neurological symptoms was found in 49 per cent and the progressive type in 51 per cent of their cases. In our series, more than 60 per cent of the cases were of the progressive type.

Neurological Symptoms and Signs

Metastatic Parenchymal Tumor

Neurological symptoms and signs appearing in the initial or early stage of intracranial (parenchymal) metastatic tumors are summarized in Table III-13 and 14. Headache is the earliest and most frequent symptom and it was complained of by 57.4 per cent of the patients. It starts generally as a mild headache, a feeling of nuchal stiffness or so-called "morning headache" as seen in primary brain tumors, and it gradually intensifies in severity. In the literature, the headache is the complaint most frequently recorded as a primary symptom: Hare and Schwarz (1939), 83%; Lang and Slater (1964), 32%; Penzholz (1968), 55%; Posner (1971), 33%; and Paillas et al. (1974b), 69%.

The headache does not, however, always reflect the intensity of increased intracranial pressure. Early meningeal involvement by the tumor intensifies the headache. On the contrary, it is often recognized that a headache subsides partially or completely even though the intracranial mass grows. It may be due to disturbances of consciousness or depression of mechanisms of pain perception. Nausea is also a common symptom accompanied by headache and was experienced by 40.2 per cent of the patients. Vomiting was observed in 31.4 per cent of them. It was noted that about 12 per cent of the patients complained of nausea without headache.

Unilateral motor weakness and sensory disturbances are the major neurological symptoms. In the early stages, they were experienced by 38.7 per cent of the patients, but they develop later in a greater number of patients. Actually, Posner (1971) reported that one third of the patients complained of unilateral weakness, but he noticed unilateral weakness in 63 per cent and unilateral sensory loss in 42 per cent of the patients presenting neurological signs.

Table III-13   Neurological symptoms and signs in 204 cases of parenchymal metastasis.

Symptoms and signs	No. of cases
Headache	117 (57.4%)
Nausea	82 (40.2)
Vomiting	64 (31.4)
Unilateral motor weakness	79 (38.7)
Mental and behavioral changes	44 (21.6)
Seizure	39 (19.1)
Visual disturbance	24 (11.8)
Diplopia	16 (7.8)
Aphasia	20 (9.8)
Dizziness (including vertigo)	11 (5.4)
Ataxia	10 (4.9)
Visual field loss	4 (2.0)
Impairment of cranial nerves	
I	1 (0.5)
III	9 (4.4)
IV	5 (2.5)
V	10 (4.9)
VI	15 (7.4)
VII	9 (4.4)
VIII	7 (3.4)
IX	2 (1.0)
X	1 (0.5)
XI	1 (0.5)
XII	3 (1.5)
Choked disc	63 (30.9)

Table III-14   Symptoms and signs of intracranial metastatic tumors.

	Størtebecker (1954) 154 cases			Lang & Slater (1964) 208 cases		Nisce et al. (1971)	Salerno et al. (1978)
	First Symptoms	Early Symptoms	Total	First Symptoms	Secondary Symptoms	560 cases	23 cases
Headache	43.7%	44.3%	88.0%	43.8%	51.0%	168 (33%)	9.1%
Nausea & vomiting	0.6	21.4	22.2	4.3	7.2	99 (17)	
Motor weakness	8.2	26.6	34.8	21.6	10.1	417 (75)	47.8
Sensory deficit						159 (28)	21.7
Seizure	22.1	17.8	39.9	14.4	8.7	101 (18)	34.8
Mental & behavioral changes	7.6	29.1	36.7	12.0	12.5	208 (41)	34.8
Impaired consciousness				6.7	9.6		
Failing vision	5.1	22.2	27.3	12.0	7.2	84 (15)	13.0
Visual field involvement							
Speech disturbance	5.1	12.0	17.1			81 (14)	
Dizziness, vertigo	7.6	16.4	24.0	2.4	5.8	74 (13)	56.5
Nystagmus						120 (21)	26.1
Diplopia						43 (8)	
Choked disc						101 (18)	

Epileptic seizures are often the initial symptoms, as stated earlier. They were found in 19.1 per cent of our patients. In the literature, seizures were recorded as early symptoms by many reporters: Lesse and Netsky (1954), 17%; Størtebecker (1954), 39%; Garde et al. (1958), 37%; Penzholz (1968), 22%; Posner (1971), 28%; and Paillas et al. (1974b), 39%. Simionescu (1960) reported that epileptic seizures were recorded in 29 per cent of the patients at the time of admission, and that such seizures were the initial symptoms in 25 per cent of all cases. He stated also that seizures in patients with cerebral metastasis demonstrate certain particular characteristics which might help to differentiate it from epilepsy associated with primary tumors of the brain or from genuine epilepsy. He found Jacksonian seizures without loss of consciousness in 37 per cent, Jacksonian seizures followed by loss of consciousness in 32 per cent, a state of continuous Jacksonian seizures in 14 per cent, and grand mal seizures in 17 per cent of the patients. Focal seizures, especially Jacksonian seizures, are characteristic in patients with metastatic brain tumors. Since metastatic tumors develop frequently in sites near the central sulcus, seizures often initiate into sensory or motor abnormalities in unilateral extremities or the face. Jacksonian-type seizures were noted in about 80 per cent of our cases at sometime during the entire course of the illness.

Seizures in cancer patients is a serious warning sign suggesting the presence of intracranial metastasis. Postictal unilateral weakness usually subsides in a few hours or a few days after the seizure. But when seizures reappear or continue, motor and sensory deficits may persist. It might be introduced by focal damage of the brain due to severe cerebral edema, ischemia or focal hemorrhage adjacent to the tumor. Any minor seizures should be promptly treated by administering anticonvulsants and glucocorticoids. Glucocorticoids are especially important in reducing brain edema and preventing further seizures. It was noted that grand mal seizures indicated the presence of multiple metastases (Simionescu, 1960). Paillas and associates (1974b) found grand mal seizures in 11 per cent of their cases. In our series, grand mal seizures were noted in nine of 39 patients (23.1%) having seizures, in which five patients had multiple metastases, two had meningeal involvement, one patient had a large single tumor in the frontal lobe and another had a infratentorial tumor. No single metastasis situated near the central sulcus was found in patients with grand mal seizures. On the contrary, even small tumors situated near the central sulcus may produce Jacksonian seizures. In Jacksonian-type seizures detected before the CT age, approximately 60 per cent of our patients had single metastasis.

Mental and behavioral changes are also major symptoms of metastatic intracranial tumors, recognized in 44 patients (21.6%). The most common symptoms were memory disturbance (14/44, 31.8%), mental deterioration (11/44, 25.0%) and disorientation (8/44, 18.2%). Character changes, euphorism, and hallucinations were also noted. Patients with mental or behavioral changes generally had tumors in the left frontal or temporal regions. The left frontal lobe was involved in 60 per cent of our cases having mental or behavioral changes, and 24 per cent of the patients had multiple metastases in the left hemisphere. One patient with meningeal carcinomatosis and one with a metastatic tumor in the paraseller region showed mental deterioration. A patient presenting extremely abnormal behavior had a large tumor in his left frontal lobe. Such mental or behavioral changes are not only influenced by the location of the metastatic tumor, but also largely by accompaning extensive brain edema; therefore, those psychiatric symptoms are often subsided by the administration of glucocorticoids. The frequency of mental or behavioral changes was varied: Hare and Schwarz (1939), 9%; Globus and Meltzer (1942), 40%; Garde et al. (1958), 14%; Simionescu (1960), 18%; Penzholz (1968), 10%; Posner (1971), 36%; and Paillas et al. (1974b), 14%.

Disturbance of visual acuity as an early symptom was experienced by 11.8 per

cent of our patients. Optic nerve atrophy following papilledema is the most responsible pathogenesis. In rare cases, cancer cells are disseminated surrounding the optic
nerve. Loss of visual field was experienced by only five patients (2.5%), but the
frequency might increase when it is carefully examined. Posner (1971) reported that
visual field loss was found in 35 per cent of his patients. Diplopia was also a common
complaint (7.8%), but the frequency did not differ from that observed in primary
tumors. The type of involvement of cranial nerves in our series is summarized in
Table III-13. Direct involvement of the trigeminal nerve causes severe neuralgia.
Loss of auditory acuity was noted in 3.4 per cent of the patients. Aphasia is a common symptom. One tenth of the patients complained of speech difficulties. Diabetes
insipidus was noted in one patient, whose posterior lobe of the pituitary gland was
invaded by the tumor.

As a common neurological sign, a choked disc was observed in 30.9 per cent of
the patients at the time of admission. The frequency of choked discs varies with
reporters, since the source of the patients differed in each hospital. In cancer
hospitals, patients in the early stage without choked discs are often referred to neurosurgeons, whereas in general neurosurgical clinics, patients already having choked
discs are generally referred to the treatment. The frequency of choked disc appearing
in the literature was: Hare and Schwarz (1939), 49%; Störtebecker (1954), 76%;
Labet (1956), 53%; Simionescu (1960), 45%; D'Andréa and de Divitiis (1966),
67%; Penzholz (1968), 68%; and Posner (1971), 39%.

A choked disc is not a reliable sign indicating increased intracranial pressure,
and it might be absent even when the intracranial pressure is greatly increased.
Simionescu (1960) reported that the number of metastases has no significant influence
on its frequency. Paillas and co-workers (1974b), however, noted that the presence
of choked disc indicated the presence of multiple metastases. Two thirds of their
patients having a choked disc had multiple metastases. The grade of the choked disc
does not indicate the size of the tumor. It is noted that the frequency of retinal
hemorrhage is higher in patients having metastatic brain tumors than those having
primary tumors. Simionescu (1960) reported that 45 per cent of the patients with
choked discs had extensive hemorrhages both in and around the papilla. This hemorrhage resembles that observed in patients with thrombosis of the central vein of the
retina, and this finding is rarely observed in cases of primary tumors.

Intracranial metastases of the pre-existing type are often encountered in neurosurgical clinics. In 94 verified cases reported by Støier (1965), 55 cases (58.5%)
were of the pre-existing type. The ratios of pre-existing type appearing in the literature
were: Störtebecker (1954), 32%; Simionescu (1960), 12%; Richards and McKissock
(1963), 11%; Lang and Slater (1964), 17%; Nisce et al. (1971), 8%; Steimle et al.
(1975), 51.3%. After surgical removal of the intracranial metastasis, the primary
source of the tumor could sometimes not be found. According to reports by Elvidge
and Baldwin (1949), Wagner (1955), and Simionescu (1960), the primary sources of
12 to 33 per cent of the cases remained unknown. In rare cases, the duration of the
pre-existing time was quite long. Russell and Rubinstein (1959) reported a duration
of four years in a case of lung cancer.

Metastatic Leptomeningeal Tumor

Symptoms arising from leptomeningeal involvement by metastatic tumors usually appear as late manifestations of systemic cancer, but some patients develop neurological symptoms prior to the detection of the primary tumor (pre-existing type). In our series, six out of 28 patients (21.4%) had neurological symptoms prior to the detection of the primary tumor. In the literature, neurological symptoms of lepto-meningeal infiltration appeared before the detection of the primary cancer in four out of 50 patients (Olson et al., 1974) and in 14 out of 29 patients (Little et al., 1974). The pre-existing type of leptomeningeal tumors were often found in cases of gastric cancer (3/6), but not in cases of breast cancer.

In the natural course of spreading and proliferation of tumor cells on the leptomeninges, the initial symptoms and signs generally appeared as minor troubles such as mild headaches or slight cranial nerve dysfunction. Since the growth of the tumor cells is, however, quite rapid, the symptoms and signs intensify day by day. The characteristics of the symptoms and signs of leptomeningeal involvement by cancer cells are well summarized by Olson and associates (1974) as follows: (1) the patient usually had symptoms and signs of structural disease involving the neuraxis at more than one anatomical site; (2) neurological signs indicated much more prominent and wide spread dysfunction than did the patient's symptoms.

The common initial symptoms and signs are summarized in Tables III-15 and 16.

Table III-15 Neurological symptoms of leptomeningeal metastatic tumor.

Symptoms	No. of cases			
	Olson et al. (1974) 50		Little et al. (1974) 29	Our series 28
	Initial complaint	Entire course		
Headache	19	25	17	19
Nausea and vomiting	6	18	10	10
Neck pain or stiffness			7	
Mental and behavioral changes	12	26	14	9
Seizures	4	13	4	2
Loss of consciousness	3	3		2
Lightheadedness	6	11		
Dizziness	1	4		1
Unsteady gait	5	12	5	6
Cranial nerve symptoms			19	
Loss of vision	4	11	3	3
Diplopia	4	11	12	9
Decreased auditory acuity	3	6		1
Tinnitus	0	4	2	1
Dysarthria	1	6	5	1
Dysphagia	1	5		1
Spinal root symptoms				
Pain	12	32	5*, 13**	6
Numbness			6, 6	4
Weakness	11	36	4, 4	5
Paresthesia	5	29		2
Bladder and bowel dysfunction	1	12		

* Upper extremity symptoms. ** Lower extremity symptoms.

Table III-16 Neurological signs of leptomeningeal metastatic tumor.

Signs	Olson et al. (1974) 50		Little et al. (1974) 29	Our series 28
	Initial exam.	All exam.		
Disturbed mental status	26	41	13	14
Abnormal extensor plantar responses	25	33		
Cranial nerve	39	47	21	20
I	0	2	3	1
II	7	18		
Papilledema	6	9	6	11
Loss of vision	1	8	4	3
Optic atrophy	0	2		2
III, IV, VI	23	35	7*, 6**	10
V	6	15	8	6
VII	21	22	12	7
VIII	15	19	6	6
IX, X	8	10	5	5
XI	2	2	1	2
XII	4	10	4	2
Spinal root				
Nuchal rigidity	8	17		15
Neck pain on manipulation	3	2		
Pain on straight leg raising	6	10		
Sensory deficit	25	31	3†, 7‡	7
Weakness	39	47	6, 13	7
Hyporeflexia	30	43	11, 13	8
Dysarthria	6	11		3
Gait disturbance	16	22		11

* Third nerve.   ** Sixth nerve.   † Upper extremity.   ‡ Lower extremity.

The most common initial symptom is headache. It is caused either by general increased intracranial pressure or focal irritation by tumor cell infiltration on the meninges. In about two thirds of our 28 patients, headache was an initial symptom. It was often very severe and accompanied by nausea and vomiting (10 cases). Since the tumor cells involve the cranial and spinal leptomeninges generally at the same time, pain in the extremities or lumbago is also a frequent initial symptom. Mental deterioration was not a common initial complaint, but it was generally seen in patients in more advanced stages. Changes of mental state included confusion, lethargy, memory disturbance and disorientation. In later stages, neurological signs of mental and behavioral changes were naturally seen in almost all patients. They were dementia, lethargy, confusion, irritability and anxiety. Seizure was seen in two patients but it was a less common initial symptom for patients having leptomeningeal metastasis compared with those having parenchymal solid metastasis.

For cranial nerve involvement, diplopia was the most common complaint. The involvement of the third, forth or sixth cranial nerves was found in ten patients. Loss of visual acuity was experienced by three patients. Papilledema was noted in one third of the patients (two thirds of the adult cases), and two patients had optic nerve atrophy. Cranial nerves V, VII and VIII were also commonly affected by tumor infiltration.

One fourth of the patients complained of pain or weakness of extremities due to infiltration of the tumor to the spinal root. Nuchal stiffness or rigidity was found in about half of the patients. According to Olson and associates (1974), 25 per cent of the patients had only spinal root symptoms initially, and an additional 15 per cent of them had spinal root symptoms combined with symptoms of other areas. However, 39 patients had signs referable to the spinal roots, usually lower motor weakness (39 cases), dermatomal or stocking type of sensory loss (25 cases), or absent deep tendon reflexes (30 cases). Pain due either to nerve root infiltration or spinal meningeal irritation was a prominent symptom. It should be noted that more symptoms and signs appear and intensify during the course of illness, as might be expected from the diffuse and infiltrative nature of leptomeningeal involvement by malignant tumor cells.

The lumbar puncture was not routinely performed, since it is hazardous for patients with high intracranial pressure. When CT suggests the presence of leptomeningeal infiltration of the tumor without masses in parenchyma, CSF examination might be worthwhile to perform. In our cases, CSF pressure was generally high and its maximum pressure was 800 mm H_2O. One case of lung cancer demonstrated the normal range of CSF pressure (110 to 75 mm H_2O after removal of 5 ml of CSF), but the cell count of the CSF was 1,850/3, including abundant tumor cells. The tumor cells in the CSF were examined either by the smear or cell culture technique. The presence of the tumor cells was demonstrated in all 16 cases tested. The other characteristics of the CSF findings were a higher concentration of protein and a low glucose content.

According to Olson and co-workers (1974), CSF was obtained from 47 out of their 50 cases. The pressures of CSF ranged 90 to 550 mm H_2O; white blood cell counts were from 0 to 500/mm³, with 0 to 95 per cent of polymorphonuclear cells. The protein concentration ranged from 24 to 1,200 mg/100 ml, and the glucose content from 0 to 225 mg/100 ml. Tumor cells were found in 21 cases in the initial examination, but only two patients showed normal cells after successive examinations. A low CSF glucose content always raises the suspicion of carcinomatous infiltration of the meninges. The glucose concentration decreased in 72 per cent of the patients and the protein content increased in 70 per cent of them.

According to Little and co-workers (1974), the CSF was examined in 21 out of 29 patients. Carcinoma cells were identified in the CSF of 17 patients. A decreased glucose content was found in 76 per cent, and the increased protein content was noted in 76 per cent of the patients. A pleocytosis, consisting of lymphocyte and polymorphonuclear leukocytes was not an uncommon finding.

The following cases are typical patterns of onset of the metastatic meningeal tumors.

Case 1 42-year-old woman. TU 670360. Breast cancer.
In March 1967, left mastectomy was performed for breast cancer. The patient received local radiotherapy (40 Gy.) and chemotherapy with Endoxan, since local lymph node metastases were noted. Five months later, she began to complain of headache, nausea and vomiting at the same time. Pain in both lower extremities, back pain and lumbago appeared. At the time of admission, marked nuchal rigidity was detected. Kernig's sign was positive. Mental states gradually deteriorated. Poor memory, delayed response for instructions, dementia and confusion were noticed. Marked papilledemas were seen on both sides. CSF pressure was 340 mm H_2O (70 mm H_2O after

removal of 7 ml of CSF). The total cell count was 480/3. Abundant atypical cells were detected. The protein content of CSF was elevated. The low glucose content of CSF was noted. No definite nodular metastases were detected in the parenchyma by RI scintigram and angiography. She was treated by ventricular drainage and hypophysectomy. She gained temporary palliation for three months.

Case 2   56-year-old woman. TU 660285. Gastric cancer.

The patient complained of headache in April 1966. She noticed her ataxic gait. Her mental state gradually deteriorated. Two months later, generalized convulsive seizures suddenly attacked her. Her visual acuity decreased gradually and she became almost blind. Nuchal rigidity was present at the time of admission. Right hyperreflexia was noticed. Marked papilledemas were seen bilaterally and optic nerve atrophy was later revealed. CSF pressure was 310 mm H_2O. The CSF contained innumerable atypical cells. Her symptoms and signs disappeared promptly after the drainage of the CSF. The neurological signs, however, appeared again and intensified very rapidly. She died three months later. Autopsy revealed the presence of gastric cancer as the primary tumor (Borrman III). Other metastases were found in bone marrow, the retroperitoneal tissue, para-aortic area, and pancreas. There were extensive disseminated matastatic tumors in the leptomenings. There were also three small nodular metastases in the cerebrum (both sides) and a nodule in the cerebellum.

There were 26 cases of leptomeningeal involvement by leukemia, in which 20 cases were children and six cases were adults (Table III-10). There were 19 cases of acute myelocytic leukemia (AML), three cases of acute lymphocytic leukemia (ALL) and two cases of chronic myelocytic leukemia (CML). The average duration from the establishment of the diagnosis for primary leukemia to the onset of neurological symptoms was 12 months. The most common initial symptom was headache (19 cases). Headache was usually accompanied by nausea and vomiting. Lumbago was experienced as an initial symptom by four patients. Facial nerve palsy was noticed in five patients. Diplopia was also a common symptom. Seizures (Jacksonian type) were seen in one patient. Mental disturbances were seen in two patients, and a loss of consciousness in one. There were five cases of motor weakness in the extremities. Exophthalmos was present in three patients. CSF examination revealed leukemia cells in all cases. The following is a typical case of leptomeningeal involvement by leukemia.

Case 3   3-year-old girl. NCC 154896. Acute myelocytic leukemia.

Swelling of the forehead was noticed by her mother in November 1971. By bone marrow examination, the diagnosis of AML was established. Treatment with vincristine, 6-MP, prednisolone and radiotherapy was received. In August 1973 (21 months after the diagnosis), headache, vomiting, and nuchal stiffness appeared and leukemia cells were detected in the CSF. The symptoms subsided by repeated intrathecal administration of methotrexate over seven months. She died in March 1974. Autopsy revealed leukemia cell infiltration of the pia and arachnoid with hemorrhage. Subdural hematoma due to bleeding from the infiltrated meningeal vessels was also detected.

NEED FOR DIFFERENTIAL DIAGNOSIS

Differential diagnosis of patients with and without a history of cancer should be considered in different ways. In cases with a history of cancer, cerebrovascular disorders are most important. Of 3,603 autopsied cases of patients who died of malignant tumors collected at the National Cancer Center Hospital from 1962 to 1976, the brain was examined in 1,250 cases (34.7%). It was found that 138 cases had intracranial hemorrhage and 54 cases had infarction (Table III-17). Intracranial hemorrhage was found in 47 out of 325 cases (14.5%) with intracranial metastasis, and in 91 out of 925 cases (9.8%) without evidence of intracranial metastasis. The infarctions were found in 18 in 325 cases (5.5%) with metastasis, and in 36 in 925 cases (3.9%) without metastasis. Hemorrhage was found mostly in the form of subarachoid hemorrhage or subdural hematoma, and occasionally in the form of intracerebral hematoma. The hemorrhage generally occurred in the terminal stage of patients, and it became the direct cause of death. One typical case of subdural hematoma was surgically treated.

Case 1   61-year-old man. NCC 147963. Gastric cancer and subdural hematoma.
The patient underwent total gastrectomy for carcinoma of the stomach. He had been treated by oral administration of tegafur (800 mg a day) to prevent the dissemination of carcinoma postoperatively. Three years after surgery, he complained of headache and a gradual progression of right hemiparesis. Angiography revealed the

Table III-17   Intracranial bleeding and infarction in
autopsied cases of cancer patients.

Primary tumor	No. of total cases	No. of intracranial metastasis		No. of bleeding	No. of infarction
Lung cancer	243			13 (5.3%)	14 (5.8%)
		+	111	7 (6.3)	7 (6.3)
		−	117	3 (2.6)	6 (5.1)
		unknown	15	3 (20)	1 (6.7)
Breast cancer	149			4 (2.7%)	6 (4.0%)
		+	46	1 (2.2)	1 (2.2)
		−	100	3 (3)	4 (4)
		unknown	3	0 (0)	1 (33.3)
Gastric cancer	110			6 (5.5%)	3 (2.7%)
		+	13	1 (7.7)	0 (0)
		−	85	4 (4.7)	2 (2.4)
		unknown	12	1 (8.3)	1 (8.3)
Leukemia	97			48 (49.5%)	2 (2.1%)
		+	19	14 (73.7)	1 (5.3)
		−	65	25 (38.5)	1 (1.5)
		unknown	13	9 (69.2)	0 (0)
Sarcoma	102			10 (9.8%)	2 (2.0%)
		+	21	1 (4.8)	1 (4.8)
		−	77	8 (10.4)	1 (1.3)
		unknown	4	1 (25)	0 (0)

presence of subdural hematoma in the left parieto-temporal region. A burr hole was opened and the hematoma was irrigated. The symptoms and signs disappeared and he returned to his job as a school teacher. He remained in good condition for seven years after surgery without any neurological symptoms.

The etiology of hemorrhage varies case by case. Extensive chemotherapy is one of the important causes of hemorrhage.

Many patients were past middle age and atherosclerotic changes of the arteries were also noted. In cases of infarction, the etiology is divided into two categories: ischemia due to thrombosis, and embolism due to metastasized tumor cells. The tumor cells as the cause of embolism are, however, not commonly detected. The clinical diagnosis of infarction or hemorrhage without tumor metastasis in systemic cancer patients was often established erroneously, since metastatic tumors were later found in some cases. Successive CT examinations have made it possible to diagnose those cerebrovascular complications more reasonably and accurately from the metastasis. In cases of hematoma, the density of the hematoma is initially high and becomes low after one week from the time of bleeding.   In cases of infarction, the low density area in CT is always demonstrable.   Alternatively, the mass of metastatic tumors, even if it is small, could be demonstrated as high-density nodules by enhanced CT. Ischemic attacks, TIA or RIND, must also be differentiated from the metastatic tumors. There was a suggestive case of a syncopal attack observed in a gastric cancer patient.

Case 2 30-year-old woman. NCC 114059. Gastric cancer and syncope.
The patient, who had undergone total gastrectomy for stomach cancer three years earlier she complained of gradual headaches and nausea. A few weeks later, she was suddenly attacked by a generalized convulsive seizure. The history and the symptoms initially suggested the presence of metastatic intracranial tumors. RI scintigram and angiography revealed no tumor masses. CSF examination revealed no tumor cells. The blood examination showed hypochromic anemia. At one time serum iron was not measurable. The supplemental iron treatment promptly improved her condition. No further attacks occurred thereafter. She is well now at twelve years after this episode.

An arteriovenous malformation was found in a patient with a history of breast cancer in our series.

Case 3 48-year-old woman. NCC 63118. Breast cancer and cerebral arterio-
venous malformation.
The patient was suddenly attacked by convulsive seizures with unconsciousness two years after mastectomy for breast cancer. Angiography revealed an arteriovenous malformation in the right parieto-occipital area and it was removed. She lived for two years and four months after the craniotomy without any neurological complications, until systemic carcinoma disseminated in her lung.

Differential diagnosis from other types of primary tumors in patients with a history of cancer is quite difficult before surgery. There were three cases of meningioma.

Case 4 45-year-old woman. NCC 166007. Uterine cancer and meningioma.
The patient was attacked by Jacksonian seizures three years after radical surgery for advanced uterine carcinoma. She was found to have a convexity meningioma (1 cm in

diameter) in the left parietal region attached to the dura mater. The tumor was totally removed together with the dura infiltrated by the tumor. She is in good condition, today, nine years after the craniotomy.

It was difficult to differentiate such small tumors from metastatic tumors before surgery. The recent progress of CT imaging, however, makes it possible to differentiate meningioma from the metastatic tumor. In another patient with breast cancer, the presence of meningioma was diagnosed prior to surgery with the aid of CT.

Case 5 65-year-old woman. TU 79123. Breast cancer and meningioma.
The patient, who was mastectomized for breast cancer, complained of headache, right homonymous hemianopsia and right hemiparesis three years after surgery. CT revealed a well-demarcated large tumor mass attached to left side of the tentorium.
The moderately high density tumor mass was further vividly enhanced by intravenous injection of meglumine iothalamate. The homogeneous density and smooth demarcated surface of the tumor suggested the possibility of meningioma rather than metastatic tumors. Angiography also revealed the blood supply to the tumor from the tentorial artery. Histological examination revealed that the tumor was meningotheliomatous meningioma. She is well now, two years after the craniotomy.

There were two cases of astrocytoma verified after histological examination. These cases were difficult to differentiate from metastatic tumors. Abscess is important for differential diagnosis, especially in cases of direct invasion of upper jaw carcinoma. It is important to differentiate infectious meningitis from the leptomeningeal involvement of tumors. There was a case of cryptococcal meningitis in an advanced cancer patient. CSF examinations for bacterial or fungal meningitis gave definite conclusions for these cases. Metabolic encephalopathy such as diabetes mellitus or hepatic coma is generally excluded by routine laboratory examinations. There were two cases of severe vincristine neuropathy. They were rather difficult to differentiate from cerebellar degeneration (Brain et al., 1951; Brain and Henson, 1958), neuropathy (Denny-Brown, 1948) and spinal cord symptoms due to tumor metastasis. Radiation myelopathy generally seen in cases of mediastinal, esophageal and laryngeal cancers is also difficult to differentiate from the metastasis to spinal cord.

In cases without a history of cancer, the problem of differential diagnosis is solved by the general principle of brain tumor diagnosis. The chest x-ray examination is most important in detecting tumors in the lung. General examination and CT findings will offer the most valuable informations about the possibility of intracranial metastatic tumors.

IV. DIAGNOSTIC MEASURES

COMPUTED TOMOGRAPHY

Computed tomography (CT) has brought about great advances for the diagnosis of metastatic intracranial tumors. CT not only gives more accurate information about the figures and charactertistics of the tumor compared with other traditional radiological examinations, but also makes it possible, by repeating examinations, to analyze dynamic changes of the tumor in growth and regression. It is a safe examination, especially for poor-risk patients with increased intracranial pressure. CT clearly demonstrates the shape, size, number of nodules and other characteristics such as the content of the cyst or the vascularity of the tumor, and also the extension of the surrounding brain edema caused by the tumor. From a therapeutic point of view, the design of treatment can be logically established and adjusted by monitoring the exact volume of the tumor, and the effect of radiation or chemotherapy can be accurately measured with the aid of CT. The field of radiotherapy can be accurately controlled. Chemotherapeutic agents will be changed according to the sensitivity of the tumor. Images by CT are becoming clearer and more vivid every year, and the smallest metastatic nodules identified today are in the order of 3 mm in diameter. Besides the views of the axial transverse section, coronal and sagittal sections can now be easily obtained. They are helpful in obtaining much more accurate information about the tumors.

Paxton and Ambrose (1974) first reported on the usefulness of CT for the diagnosis of metastatic intracranial tumors. They have identified 34 out of 35 histologically proven metastatic tumors. The only lesion missed was situated in the high convexity being examined by an axial transverse section. Such a lesion would not be missed today if a coronal or sagittal section is made. Deck and co-workers (1976), as well as Bardfield and others (1977), have reported that CT identified 86 to 100 per cent of all intracranial metastases. In a monograph on CT presented by New and Scott (1975), all of the 24 cases of metastases were identified by CT. The characteristics of several types of metastatic tumors were also presented in the same monograph. The smallest metastatic nodules identified were in the order of 6 mm in diameter. They demonstrated the usefulness of contrast enhancement for the diagnosis of metastatic tumors. Metastatic adenocarcinoma generally appeared on CT scans as dense nodules with absorption ranges from 12 to 30 EMI number. The nodules are generally surrounded by very large volumes of brain edema with diminished absorption (4–14 EMI number). Metastatic malignant melanoma tends to have high absorption values initially ranging in the high 30's, a feature suggestive of hemorrhage in the tumor. Metastatic squamous cell carcinoma generally presents a low density relative to the brain (4-14), with rather smoothly rounded contours with little or no evidence of the surrounding edema. The larger nodules of metastatic adenocarcinoma and malignant melanoma may contain an irregularly low dense central area representative of tissue necrosis. Weisberg (1979) accumulated 190 cases of intracranial metastases, in which 70 cases had single and 120 cases had multiple metastases. In 52 patients, a plain scan showed a single metastasis, but multiple lesions were found after contrast enhancement. In nine patients, the tumor was found only on post-contrast enhancement. There were no characteristic CT patterns specific to each systemic cancer, but squamous cell carcinoma frequently appeared as a low density lesion with a thin peripheral enhancing rim, and adenocarcinoma appeared more often as dense, homogeneous and round-enhancing nodules.

Pattern of CT Findings

Cancer cells generally metastasize from the primary site to the brain by the blood stream, then lodge and make colonies in the capillaries of the brain. The smallest tumor nodule detectable by CT is approximately 3 mm in diameter. It may contain approximately 10^6 to 10^7 tumor cells. Cell kinetic studies suggest that a tumor cell will divide and grow to such a tiny detectable nodule within two months if it is a rapidly growing tumor with a doubling time of two to three days, and there are no host defense mechanisms. The small and tiny tumor nodule appears as a high density spot with or without contrast enhancement (Fig. IV-1A). The tumor nodule grows further in a spheroid or irregular nodulous shape, and appears on CT scans as a small, round or irregular homogeneous mass (Fig. IV-1B). The tumor nodule does not generally contain necrotic tissue inside when its size is less than 1 cm in diameter. A degenerative change starts in the center of the tumor tissue as the tumor grows and the blood supply becomes insufficient at the center of the nodule. The necrotic portion appears on CT scans as a low-density area surrounded by a thin or thick high density rim. It often looks like a ring or a doughnut (Figs. IV-1C and 1D). The ring formation is one of the common appearances of metastatic parenchymal brain tumors on CT scans. The homogeneous or heterogeneous irregular features of the interior portion of the nodule are dependent on the liquified process of the necrotic tissue. It contains solid necrotic tissue in some cases and viscous pus-like or xanthochromic clear fluid in other cases. When hemorrhage occurs in the tumor, it contains hematoma or bloody fluid. It is, however, not easy to differentiate the nature of the low density area. The cyst-like appearance of the sharply marginated and homogenous low density area inside the high density ring does not necessarily reflect the true cystic space, but it often contains a solid necrotic tissue. The tumor grows further and assumes various shapes (Figs. IV-1D and 1E and Figs. IV-2A or 2E). The shape, wall thickness, and the inner structure of the tumor are dependent on the histological type, vascularity or growing speed of each tumor. The tumor forms a multilobulated mass in some cases (Fig. IV-2E). The tumor further enlarges and compresses the surrounding brain tissue causing shifts and deformities of ventricles and the midline. The tumor, on the other hand, stimulates parenchyma and produces extensive brain edema even when the size of the tumor is small. It appears on the CT scan as a low

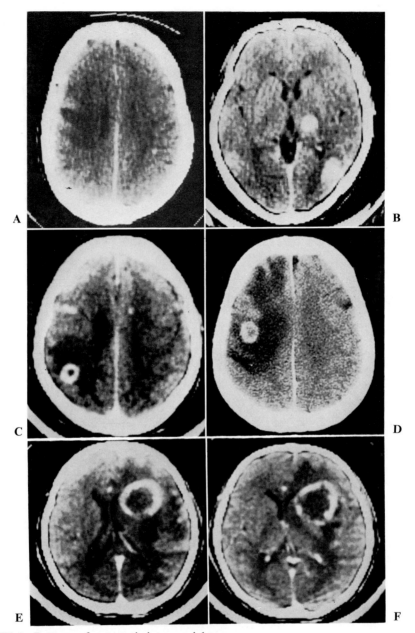

Fig. IV-1 Patterns of metastatic intracranial tumors.

A. A tiny nodule of tumor in the right parietal lobe. Brain edema is present in both hemispheres. The diameter of the nodule is about 3 mm. Lung cancer, adenocarcinoma.

B. Multiple metastases from lung cancer (adenocarcinoma). A round homogeneous nodule (1.5 cm in diameter) in the right thalamus, an irregularly shaped homogeneous nodule attached to the dura mater in the right occipito-temporal region and a partially non-demarcated nodule in the left occipito-temporal region are visualized. Moderate edema is present in both sides.

C. A round, ring-shaped metastatic nodule in the left parietal lobe with extensive edema and a tiny nodule in the right parietal lobe near the falx are seen. Lung cancer, large cell carcinoma (1.5 cm in diameter).

D. A round, ring-shaped metastatic nodule (1.5 cm in diameter) with extensive edema in the left parietal lobe is present. Lung cancer, squamous cell carcinoma.

→

Fig. IV-2 Patterns of metastatic intracranial tumors.

A. A large, irregularly shaped homogeneous tumor nodule attaching to the falx. Breast carcinoma.

B. An irregularly shaped semi-homogeneous tumor nodule in the right parietal lobe. Renal clear cell carcinoma.

C. A large, irregularly shaped tumor mass containing irregular necrotic tissue inside. Lung cancer, adenocarcinoma.

D. An irregularly shaped tumor with a thin enhanced wall. Lung cancer, adenocarcinoma.

E. A large, irregularly shaped multi-lobulated tumor with cysts. The marked shift is demonstrated. Renal clear cell carcinoma.

F. The leptomeningeal involvement of carcinoma. Ventricles are enlarged. Periventricular and arachnoidal tissues are enhanced. The patient also has parenchymal metastases. Brain edema due to the tumor is present in the left hemisphere.

G. The leptomeningeal involvement of retinoblastoma. The infiltration of tumor cells into the subarachnoidal space is demonstrated (Tumor tree formation-Takakura).

H. The leptomeningeal involvement of retinoblastoma. The same patient as shown in G. Infiltration of tumor cells in the wall of both lateral ventricles (periventricular rim) is demonstrated. Hydrocephalus is present.

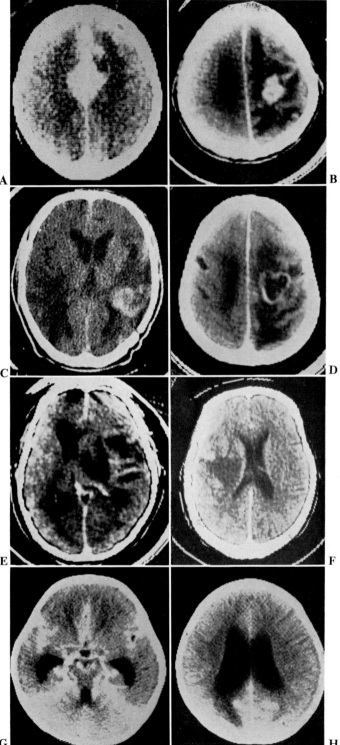

E, F. A large, round, ring-shaped metastatic nodule with extensive edema in the right parietal lobe is seen. The shift of the central axis is present. The tumor contains a necrotic mass (4 cm in diameter). Lung cancer, adenocarcinoma.

density area surrounding the tumor nodule.   Extensive brain edema is another feature of metastatic intracranial tumors.

In cases of leptomeningeal involvement of the tumor, the dilated ventricle with its enhanced rim and the arachnoid appearing in high density are demonstrated (Fig. IV-2F).   In advanced cases, the tumor spreads all over the leptomeninges.   When the tumor grows in subarachnoid space the *tumor tree* is demonstrated by CT.   An example of leptomeningeal involvement from retinoblastoma is shown in Figure IV-2G.   The tumor disseminates all over the ventricular surface and spinal subarachnoid space (Figs. IV-2G and 2H).

Density and Contrast Enhancement of the Tumor

Ambrose and associates (1975a, b) examined 70 cases of intracranial metastatic tumors, in which 64 cases (91 %) had positive CT findings.   Fifty out of 64 cases (78 %) demonstrating abnormal CT showed low density.   Weisberg (1979) reported that the plain CT scan showed a low density lesion in 100 out of 181 patients (55 %) with intracranial metastases diagnosed by CT, and 87 of those cases (87 %) were enhanced after the infusion of a contrast media.   Eighty-one cases showed a high density lesion on the plain CT, and they were always surrounded by low density components. The attenuation coefficient of the high density component was 22 to 34 EMI numbers. The density of the metastatic tumor, however, varies in each examined site.   In the case of a large tumor, the inner portion always has a necrotic mass or fluid which appears as a low density area on CT scans, and the rim generally demonstrates isodensity or slightly higher density compared with the surrounding parenchyma.   In about half of the cases of intracranial metastases, the inner portion of the tumor shows a low density finding as the necrotic process exists.   A careful examination of the CT scan may show a somewhat high density area in some part of the tumor in many cases, especially when the recently developed high-resolution CT is used.   Heterogeneity of density is important.   Only 12 per cent of metastatic nodules showed lower density than the surrounding parenchyma in the entire portion of the tumor.   In other cases, iso- or high density portions in some part of the tumor were demonstrated even though they showed low density in the inner portion of the tumor.   Since it is difficult to detect the entire shape of the tumor when it is isodense, contrast enhancement is always necessary to complete the examination when using plain CT.

Contrast enhancement can be achieved by intravenous rapid infusion of 30 per cent methylglucamine diatrizoate (220 ml for adults and 4 ml/kg of body weight for children).   Deck (1980) reported that contrast enhancement was achieved with an intravenous bolus injection of 100 ml methylglucamine diatrizoate (Conray), with 60 per cent given over two to three minutes.   The patterns of enhancement are demonstrated in Figure IV-3.   Contrast enhancement of metastatic intracranial tumors occurred in almost all cases.   Small isodense tumor nodules are rarely identified using plain CT (Fig. IV-3A-1), and the tumor nodule can be clearly visualized after enhancement (Fig. IV-3A-2).   It is almost impossible to diagnose the presence of the tumor properly in such a case from plain CT alone.   The slightly highly dense mass is demonstrated by plain CT in some cases (Fig. IV-3B-1). Those tumors appear as higher density masses because of the relative contrast with the surrounding low density brain edema. The figure of the tumor nodule can be roughly estimated in such a case, but the actual tumor shape can be vividly visualized only after enhancement, as shown in Figure IV-3B-2. Although more than half of all metastatic tumors appear as isodensity masses on plain CT scans, some tumors appear as high density masses. As an example, an irregularly shaped high density mass was demonstrated by plain CT as shown in Figure IV-3C-1. After enhancement, the ring shaped enhancement was demonstrated (Fig. IV-3C-2). In this case, macroscopic findings at the time of surgery revealed that the irregularly shaped high density mass appearing on the plain CT scan was a solid tumor tissue, and the enhanced ring was a wall structure of the tumor. The low density area surrounded by the ring was a cyst containing xanthochromic fluid. Some other tumors appearing as a high density mass even on plain CT scans are shown in Figure IV-3D-1. The effect of enhancement was not clearly identified in such cases (Fig. IV-3D-2). It was detected only by comparing attenuation coefficients. The figures of the tumor were almost identical on both plain and enhanced CT scans. Irregularly mixed high and low density masses were observed in several cases (Fig. IV-3E-1). Such tumors contain various portions of tumor tissue, necrotic mass or fluid and hemorrhage. In some cases, a clearly marginated high density mass with a small, irregular low density core was demonstrated after enhancement (Fig. IV-3E-2). Tumors demonstrating an iso-, slightly high or low density mass on plain CT scans and marked contrast enhancement, as seen in Figure IV-3A, 3B and 3E, are those that are rich in tumor vascularity. Angiography of the tumor (Figs. IV-3B-1 and 2) demonstrated a marked tumor vascular stain (Fig. IV-4A). On the contrary, tumors not demonstrating clear contrast enhancement (Figs. IV-3D-1 and 2) did not show any clear tumor stain (Fig. IV-4B). This finding is similar to the angiographic pattern of meningioma. The newly formed hematoma in or outside the tumor appears as a high density mass on plain CT scans (Fig. IV-3F-1). The ring formation surrounding the hematoma was demonstrated after contrast enhancement (Fig. IV-3F-2). In this case, the enhanced ring and the small nodule were solid tumor tissues verified at the time of surgery. The whole figure of this tumor looked like the cut surface of an orange. Brain edema is almost always present and appears on CT scans as an irregularly shaped low density area surrounding the tumor. The size of the edematous area is variable and sometimes extends to the entire hemisphere. The peripheral portion of the edematous area extends into gyri-like crab fingers.

Multiple Metastases

Angiography cannot demonstrate the actual figure of a tumor when it is poor in vascularity. The presence of the tumor can be estimated by the indirect findings of the shift or displacement of cerebral vessels. It is difficult to properly diagnose by angiography alone the real locations and figures of multiple metastatic tumors without vascular stains when they are bilaterally or relatively closely situated.

RI scintigraphy was generally considered to be a superior method of examination for the detection of multiple metastases. It was, however, difficult to fully clarify

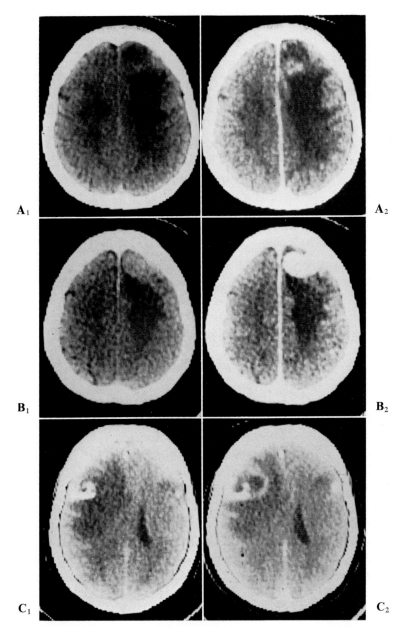

Fig. IV-3   Patterns of metastatic intracranial tumors before and after contrast enhancement.   1) Plain CT, 2) Enhanced CT.
A.   Metastasis from lung adenocarcinoma.
     The isodense tumor mass is hardly visible in the right frontal region on the plain CT scan. The tumor can be clearly visualized in the edematous parenchyme after the enhancement.
B.   Metastasis from lung adenocarcinoma.
     A slightly highly dense area is noticeable in the right frontal cortex.   The oval shaped and clearly marginated homogeneous tumor can be visualized after the enhancement. (See Fig. IV-4A.   The angiogram of this tumor is presented.)
C.   Metastasis from lung adenocarcinoma.
     The irregularly shaped high density mass is seen in the left fronto-parietal region on the plain CT scan.   The newly formed ring adjacent to the irregular mass is visualized after the enhancement.   Macroscopical findings at surgery revealed that the irregularly shaped mass on the plain CT scan was a solid tumor and the ring was a wall structure of the tumor.   The

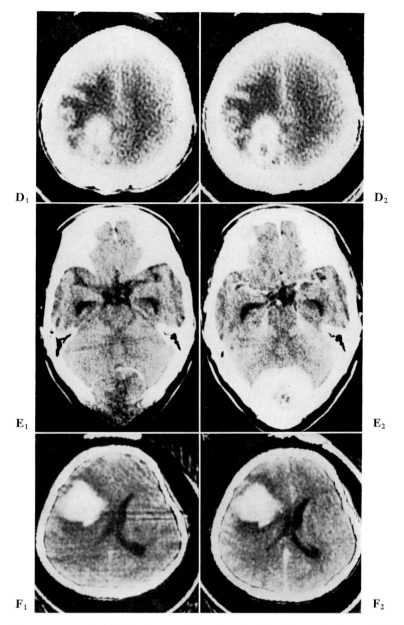

D_1 D_2

E_1 E_2

F_1 F_2

low density area surrounded by the ring was the cyst containing the xanthochromic fluid.   The cyst was not identified by plain CT.

D.   Metastasis from colon adenocarcinoma.

The high density tumor mass is seen on the plain CT scan.   The mass is slightly enhanced, but the enhancement can be hardly detected by the naked eye. (See Fig. IV-4B. The angiogram of this tumor is presented.)

E.   Metastasis from renal clear cell carcinoma.

The irregular, mixed density tumor mass is seen in the occipital region.   It destructs the skull.   The highly enhanced mass with an irregular, low density core is visualized after the enhancement.

F.   Metastasis from osteosarcoma.

The high density mass of a hematoma is seen in the left fronto-parietal region of the plain CT.   No contrast enhancement is noticeable.   The metastatic tumor was located in the hematoma.

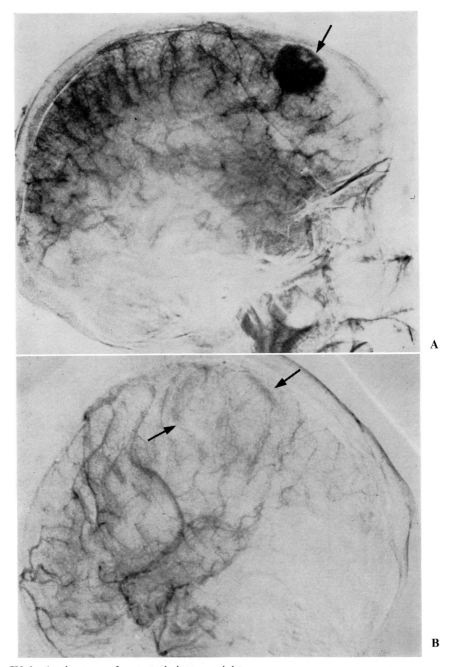

Fig. IV-4 Angiograms of metastatic intracranial tumors.
A. The same patient as shown in Figure IV-3B-1 and 2. The sharply marginated tumor vascular stain is noted in the right frontal region. Lung adenocarcinoma.
B. The same patient as shown in Figure IV-3D-1 and 2. The tumor vascular stain is vaguely seen in the left parietal region. Colon adenocarcinoma.

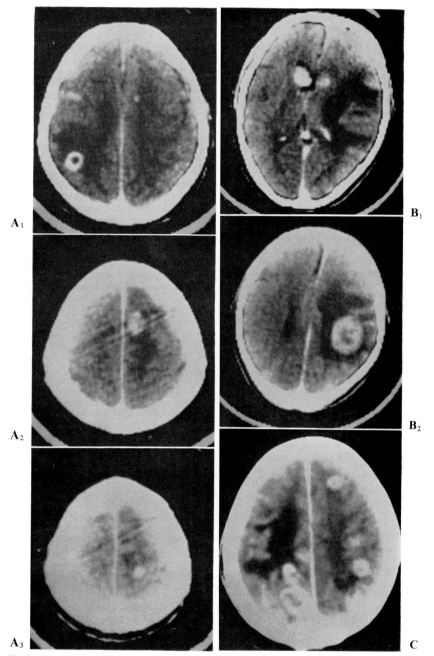

Fig. IV-5 Multiple Metastases.

A(1—3). Seven metastatic tumor nodules can be detected in the three slices. Metastases from lung adenocarcinoma.

B(1—2). Three metastatic tumor nodules can be detected in the two slices. Metastases from lung adenocarcinoma.

C. Multiple metastatic tumor nodules are demonstrated in a single section.

the margin of the tumor from the adjacent edematous brain tissue, and therefore to visualize the actual shape of the tumor. Most problems involved in angiography and RI scintigraphy have been solved by CT. Today CT can visualize all metastatic tumor nodules with diameters of more than 3 mm if the slices cover every field of the brain. Since the coronal CT scan can now clearly demonstrate an image of any tumor situated even in high convexity, there remains no part of the brain where existing tumors cannot be visualized by CT.

Weisberg (1979) reported that 63 per cent of metastatic intracranial tumor patients defined by CT had multiple metastases. In our series during the past two years, 28 out of 51 cases (55%) were multiple metastases. The ratio of single to multiple metastases is dependent on the selection of patients before being referred to various clinics, and therefore it is different from autopsy data.

CT findings of intracranial multiple metastatic tumors are shown in Figure IV-5. In the case illustrated in Figures IV-5A-1, 2 and 3, seven metastatic tumor nodules are detected in three slices of CT. Two round and oval-shaped nodules in the right hemisphere are homogeneous in density. A round nodule in the left hemisphere has a low density core. Three tiny nodules in the right hemisphere with diameters of approximately 3 mm each and an irregularly shaped nodule in the left cortical area are detected. The midline shift is not present since the brain edema is evenly present bilaterally. In the case illustrated in Figures IV-5B-1 and 2, three round- or oval-shaped tumor nodules are detected in two slices of CT. The right to left midline shift is noticeable since the tumor is large and brain edema is extensive in the right hemisphere. The presence of multiple metastases in a single slice of CT is demonstrated in Figure IV-5C.

Biplane CT

Three dimensional views of the CT image provide more accurate information about the anatomical structures of the tumor. Glenn and associates (1975a, b) reported on the capability of CT display concerning the directions of sections other than conventional axial tomography. The coronal and sagittal plane images have also been introduced.

By coronal and sagittal section scans, the location, figure and the relation to the surrounding tissue of the tumors can be more accurately and easily demonstrated. Supra- and infratentorial tumors both in the axial and coronal sections are compared in Figures IV-6A and B as examples. It is noted that the tumor nodule in Figure IV-6B is closely attached to the inferior surface of the tentorium. Surgical approach to the tumor can, thus, be rationally and easily selected by the CT findings. The coronal section scan precisely demonstrates not only the shape of the tumor but also the vertical extension of the tumor. The three-dimensional structure of the accompanying brain edema and the shift of ventricles can also be easily detected. Figure IV-6C gives an example of a metastatic tumor in the right frontal lobe from tonsillar squamous cell carcinoma. The location, irregular shape of the tumor, and shift of the lateral and third ventricles are clearly demonstrated. The coronal and sagittal sections are especially useful in inspecting the skull base structure. The site and shape of the skull base destruction by the invasion of carcinoma are more clearly visualized in the coronal and sagittal sections than in the conventional axial view. Figure IV-6D gives an example of the direct intracranial invasion of carcinoma of the ethmoidal sinuses to the parasellar region. The tumor, containing multiple cysts, is expanding to the supraseller region (Fig. IV-6D-1). It is obvious from the coronal section that the tumor extends to the floor of the third ventricle and pushes it upwards (Fig. IV-6D-2). It is also clearly demonstrated by the axial plane that the right ethmoidal sinuses are filled by the primary tumor which destructs the skull base and extends to the paraseller region (Fig. IV-6D-3). The reconstructed sagittal plane reveals an intracranially extended balloon-shaped mass through the destructed hole of the sellar floor (Fig. IV-6D-4). As seen in the above case, the multiplane images of CT can reveal an almost complete anatomical structure of nasopharyngeal cancers invading the skull base and extending to the intracranial space.

Bone Destruction

Osteolytic lesions by infiltration of a metastatic tumor can be detected by plain craniograms. The whole figure of the tumor in the affected area of the skull is, however, more precisely visualized by CT. Cancer of the breast, thyroid and kidney, as well as various kinds of sarcomas, often metastasize to the skull (Albright, 1944). Nasopharyngeal cancer often directly invades the base of the skull. Full information on the tumor and bone destruction can be obtained by careful examination of CT scans. An example of metastasis to the skull by thyroid cancer is demonstrated in Figure IV-7A. Even though osteolytic lesions are detected in a plain craniogram, CT scan demonstrates not only the metastatic tumor but also the shape of the bone destroyed. Another example of skull metastasis from renal clear cell carcinoma is given in Figure IV-7B. In a case of an uncertain osteolytic lesion in plain craniogram, CT scan will give a definite finding of bone destruction by changing the window levels of CT (Fig. IV-7C). The direct invasion of nasopharyngeal cancer to the base of the skull is clearly shown by coronal or sagittal plane scans, as described above (Fig. IV-6D).

Types of Tumors

Although there are no definite pathognomonic CT patterns in each different histological type of primary tumor, there is a tendency to conduct specific observations related to certain tumors. Hemorrhage often accompanies tumors which are rich in vascularity, such as melanoma, choriocarcinoma or renal clear cell carcinoma. Hemorrhage is easily detected by plain CT as a homogeneous high density mass. Enhancement by contrast media does not occur in the region of hematoma (Fig. IV-8A). Symptoms and signs of hemorrhage appear abruptly like a cerebrovascular accident. Differential diagnosis is easily established by carefully taking the history, as well as by general and specific examinations. For instance, choriocarcinoma is definitely differentiated when a high HCG level in urine or serum is

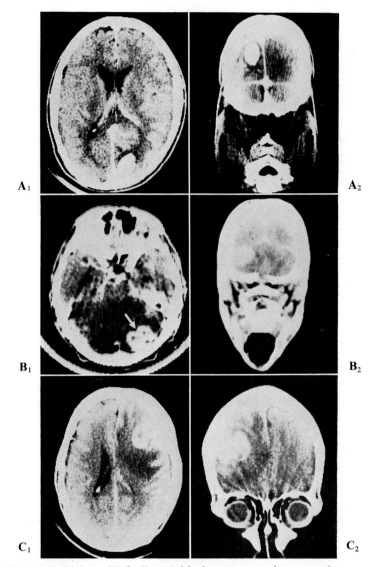

Fig. IV-6   Biplane CT findings (with the contrast enhancement).
A.   A metastatic tumor in the right occipital lobe from renal clear cell
carcinoma.   A-1: axial section; A-2: coronal section.
B.   A metastatic tumor in the right cerebeller hemisphere from lung small
cell carcinoma.   The tumor is closely attached to the inferior surface of
the tentorium.   An arrow indicates the tumor.   B-1: axial section; B-2:
coronal section.
C.   A metastatic tumor in the right frontal lobe from a tonsillar squamous
cell carcinoma.   The location and irregular shape of the tumor and shifted
structure of the ventricles by brain edema are clearly demonstrated.   C-1, 3:
axial section; C-2, 4: coronal section.

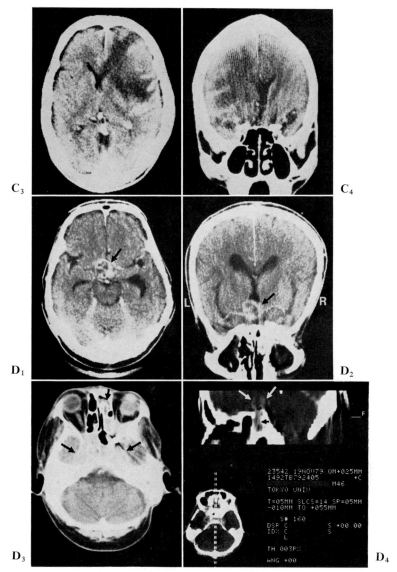

D. A direct invasion of the tumor in the parasellar region from adenoid cystic carcinoma (cylindroma) of the right ethmoidal sinuses.

1) The tumor containing multiple cysts is located in the suprasellar region.

2) The coronal section clearly reveals the tumor extension to the floor of the third ventricle.

3) The right ethmoidal sinus is filled by the tumor. The right eye is an artificial eye ball replaced during the previous operation. The tumor is extended bilaterally from the sellar region.

4) A sagittal section reveals the balloon-shaped intracranial extension of the tumor and the destruction of the sellar floor.

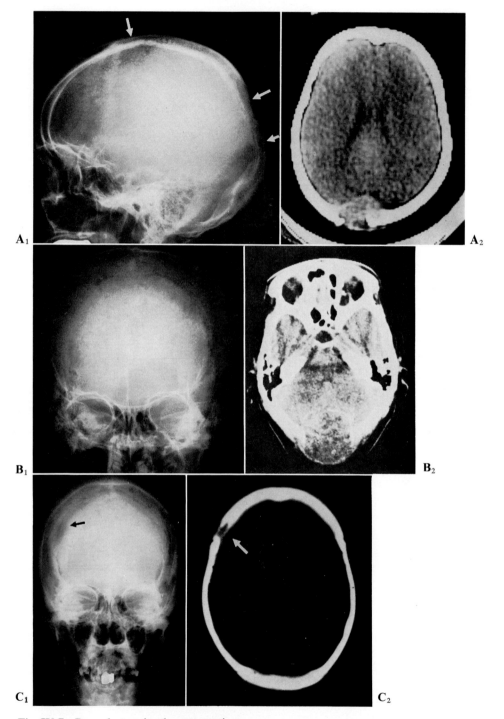

Fig. IV-7 Bone destruction by metastatic tumors.
A. A skull metastasis from thyroid cancer.
1) Osteolytic lesions are shown by the arrows.
2) The CT scan demonstrates the shape of the metastatic tumor and the structure of the bone destruction. A part of the tumor infiltrates the subscutaneous tissue, outside the skull. The internal lamina of the skull is pushed into the intracranial space by the tumor.

detected.   In cases of renal clear cell carcinoma, abdominal CT scan reveals the presence of a renal tumor, as shown in Figure IV-8B$_2$.   Whole body scan is especially useful in detecting retroperitoneal tumors.   Skull involvement is often accompanied by tumors such as breast, thyroid or renal clear cell carcinoma, and various sarcomas, as described in the previous section.

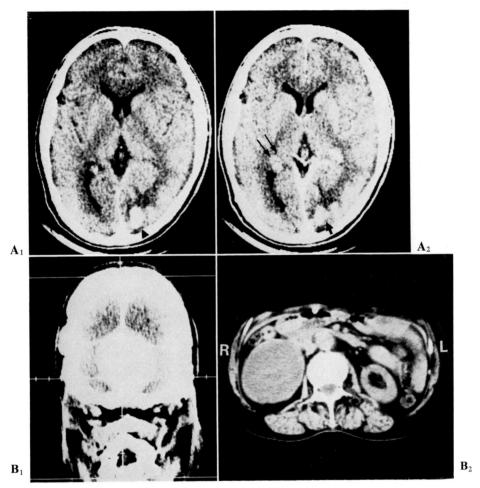

Fig. IV-8   Types of tumors.
A.   Hemorrhagic tumor (Renal clear cell carcinoma).
1)   Plain CT scan reveals hemorrhage(arrow)in the metastatic site in the right occipital region.
2)   Enhanced CT scan.   No effect of the contrast enhancement in the region of the hemorrhage (arrow) is noted.   The small tumor in the left lateral ventricle is enhanced (double arrow).
B.   The search for the primary tumor by whole body CT (Renal clear cell carcinoma).
1)   The enhanced coronal CT scan reveals the round infratentorial metastatic tumor.
2)   The same patient of B1.   The abdominal CT scan reveals the large renal tumor on the right side.

B.   A skull metastasis from renal clear cell carcinoma.
1)   The A-P view of the plain craniogram shows the osteolytic lesion of the skull.
2)   The CT scan without contrast enhancement demonstrates the complete destruction of the bone by a large metastatic tumor having irregular density areas.
C.   Skull metastasis from lung cancer.
1)   An obscure osteolytic lesion (arrow) in the left frontal bone is noted.
2)   An osteolytic lesion (arrow) is clearly demonstrated in CT by changing the window level.

It was reported by Weisberg (1979) that adenocarcinomas appeared as small, round, densely enhanced nodules that were homogeneous or had a small, central low density core. The tumor was surrounded by a low density edema in 72 per cent of 109 cases. The squamous cell carcinomas had a large, low density area with a thin, enhanced peripheral rim in 77 per cent of 40 cases. New and Scott (1975) noted that squamous cell carcinoma generally presented a lower density compared with the brain and rather smoothly rounded contours, with little or no evidence of any surrounding edema. The undifferentiated carcinoma tended to resemble squamous cell carcinoma. From our experience, however, these histological types of adeno-, squamous cell or undifferentiated carcinomas were difficult to differentiate on the basis of the characteristics of CT findings only. Various types of CT findings of adenocarcinomas are shown in Figure IV-9. Peritumoral brain edema is generally observed in every kind of tumor, even in cases of squamous cell carcinoma. CT

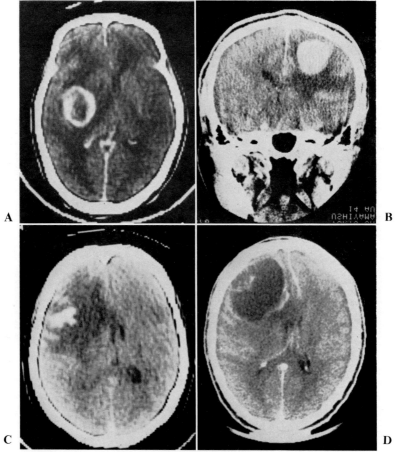

Fig. IV-9   Various types of CT findings of adenocarcinoma (Enhanced CT).
A.   The smooth-bordered, round tumor with a thick enhanced rim and a central low density area representing necrotic tissue with marked surrounding brain edema (lung cancer).
B.   A round, homogeneously enhanced tumor with marked surrounding brain edema (lung cancer).
C.   An irregularly shaped tumor with an irregularly enhanced area (lung cancer).
D.   An irregularly shaped enhanced tumor mass in a large low density area representing a cyst formation with the thin enhanced rim (breast cancer).

findings always vary with the growth of the tumor and with the necrotic processes occurring in most tumors, when the size of the tumor becomes larger than approximately 1 cm in diameter. Tumors of different histological types appear on CT in various shapes. It is therefore extremely difficult to estimate histological types of tumors from CT findings.

Dynamic Aspects of Metastatic Tumors —Development, Growth and Regression—

It is one of the major advantages of CT that the development, growth and regression of the tumor can be easily and accurately followed by repeating examinations.

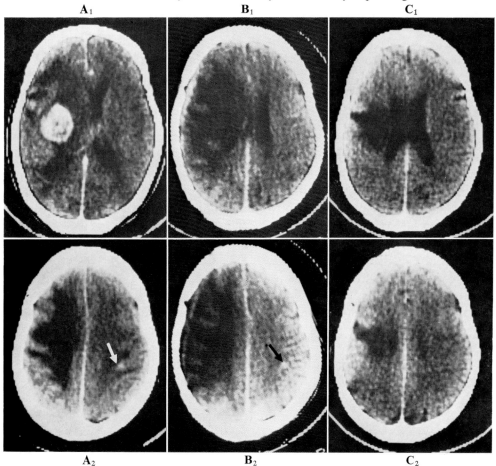

A₁   B₁   C₁

A₂   B₂   C₂

Fig. IV-10 Effects of surgery and chemotherapy. Metastases from lung adenocarcinoma.
A. 1) A large round tumor nodule with a central, irregular, low density area in the left parietal region and a tiny nodule on the right border of the falx were observed before surgery. 2) A small nodule in the right parietal region (arrow) was also noted (April 24, 1979).
B. 1) The large tumor was surgically removed on April 28, 1979. There was still extensive brain edema in the left parietal region at nine days after the surgery.
2) A small nodule in the right parietal lobe was present (May 7, 1979).
C. 1)–2) The remaining tiny tumor nodules have disappeared completely from the CT scan, after the continuous oral administration of tegafur (800 mg/day) for two months (July 5, 1979). The patient has maintained tumor-free for two years now by intermittent administrations of tegafur.

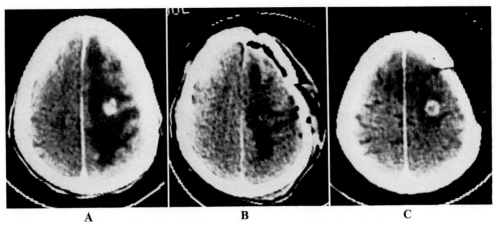

A   B   C

Fig. IV-11   The effect of surgery and the recurrence of metastases from lung adenocarcinoma.
A.   An irregularly shaped tumor nodule with extensive peritumoral brain edema was noticed in the right parietal region (July 5th, 1979).
B.   The tumor was totally removed by surgery on July 10, 1979. The CT scan was taken on the day after surgery.
C.   A new metastatic tumor has developed three months after surgery in the region adjacent to the former nodule (Oct. 3, 1979).

Since not only the tumor itself but also the adjacent brain edema are well detected, a therapeutic schedule for the patient can be logically established.   Because the results of surgery can be precisely visualized, the proper postoperative care can be provided. The administration of glucocorticoid hormone for controlling brain edema is adjusted to the proper dose.   The effects of radiotherapy and chemotherapy had long been evaluated by RI scintigraphy, but it was impossible to accurately distinguish the tumor from the adjacent brain edema.   CT has solved all these problems.

Newly developed tiny metastatic foci are easily detected in the early stages of their appearance (Figs. IV-10 and 11).   Chemotherapy in recent years often proved effective in suppressing such small metastatic tumors.   In the case presented in Figures IV-10 to 12, tiny metastatic tumor nodules remained after surgical removal of the main large tumor.   These disseminated small tumors have been suppressed by combined chemotherapy using tegafur and glucocorticoid (Figs. IV-10 and 12). The sensitivity of tumors to certain chemotherapeutic agents or radiotherapy can be clearly demonstrated clinically with the aid of CT.   On the other hand, tumors which are resistant to radiotherapy or chemotherapy continue to grow rapidly.   In the case presented in Figure IV-11, the recurrence of the tumor is demonstrated. The intracranial metastatic tumor in the left parietal region from lung adenocarcinoma was totally removed by surgery.   The patient received postoperative radiotherapy and chemotherapy using tegafur (800 mg/day p.o.).   The development of a new tumor in the region adjacent to the initial site of metastasis was, however, detected by CT scan three months after the craniotomy.   It is understood that this tumor was resistant to both radiotherapy and chemotherapy using tegafur.

CT can give more precise information on the pathophysiological aspects of the tumor.   The case presented in Figure IV-12 is an example.   A 55-year-old woman underwent a radical mastectomy for cancer in her left breast.   One year and five months later, neurological symptoms of mental retardation and right motor weakness

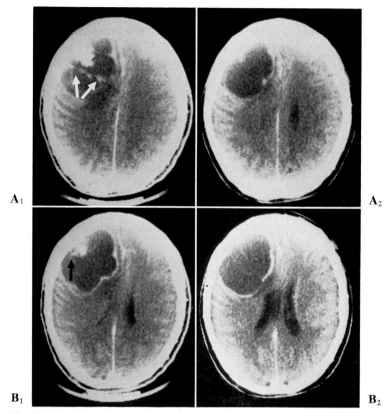

Fig. IV-12 The effect of chemotherapy without surgery or radiotherapy. Metastases from breast carcinoma.

A. 1)–2) A large cystic mass containing irregularly shaped, enhanced high density tumor tissue inside (arrow) was seen in the left frontal lobe (Sep. 27, 1979). The patient was in a semicomatous state with complete right hemiplegia.

B. 1)–2) The size of the cystic area has not changed, but the enhanced mass inside has almost disappeared after the continuous oral administration of tegafur (600 mg/day) and Endoxan (100 mg/day) for four months. Her neurological signs have improved during this period. She has been able to talk and walk since the above chemotherapy (Jan. 26, 1980).

began to develop. When admitted to our clinic, she was in an almost semicomatous state. Complete right hemiplegia was noted. CT scan revealed a large cystic mass containing enhanced high density tumor nodules. Since she had metastases to the lung and various sites of her skeletal system, surgical treatment was not indicated. Chemotherapy with tegafur (600 mg/day, orally), cyclophosphamide (100 mg/day, orally) and prednisolone (80 to 20 mg/day) was initiated. Neurological signs gradually disappeared. The hemiplegia subsided week by week. After four months of continuous chemotherapy, she was able to speak, stand and walk. CT taken at four months after the initial examination revealed that the whole cystic mass had not significantly diminished in size but that the brain edema had significantly subsided. The slightly enlarged ventricles indicated the presence of a minor atrophic change in the brain. The shift of the central axis of the brain had been much improved. The most striking finding was that the enhanced tumor mass located inside the cystic mass had almost disappeared during the four months of continuous chemo-therapy. Since the patient neither underwent surgery nor received radiotherapy, the regression of the tumor as well as the marked improvement of neurological symptoms and signs were due solely to chemotherapy. The sensitivity of the tumor to tegafur, cyclophosphamide and/or prednisolone has definitely been proved. The size of the tumor in the lung also became smaller during the same period. Since the effects of chemotherapeutic agents can be properly evaluated by CT examination, the most appropriate therapeutic schedule can be formulated for each patient. Other examples of therapeutic results on CT findings will be presented in the chapter on treatment.

Differential Diagnosis

The differential diagnosis of metastatic intracranial tumors can generally be established with the aid of the patient's history, clinical symptoms and signs. Com-mon features of CT findings characteristic of metastatic intracranial tumors are as follows:
1) Multiplicity of tumors.
2) Extensive brain edema surrounding the tumor. Even a small metastatic tumor often accompanies a large low density edematous area.
3) Tumors can be generally enhanced by contrast media.
4) A clearly demarcated border and a central low density area representing necrotic changes.

Multiple tumors are rarely found in cases of primary tumors. Multiple menin-giomas in neurofibromatosis can be diagnosed from the slow progression of neurolog-ical signs and symptoms. They rarely demonstrate extensive brain edema. Dermato-logical signs of *café au lait* spots or von Recklinghausen's cutaneous neurofibroma-tosis, if present, will help the diagnosis. A large, homogeneously dense mass without significant surrounding brain edema in CT findings suggests a benign brain tumor such as meningioma. It is also noteworthy that brain edema is often not so extensive in cases of metastatic tumors in the cerebellum. The presence of a diffuse border of the mass, even if it is observed in some part of the tumor, is suggestive of malignant glioma rather than a metastatic tumor (Fig. IV-13A). It is, however, important to note that there are no definite characteristics of metastatic tumors in CT findings. For instance, even a round tumor which is enhanced by contrast media with a demarcated border, a central low density area and extensive surrounding brain edema does not necessarily indicate a metastatic tumor. Glioma, abscess and hematoma often show such CT findings, as shown in Figures IV-13B to D.

The differential diagnosis of a primary brain tumor from a metastatic tumor is especially difficult in patients who have a previous history of cancer. Meningioma is the second most frequent tumor found in cancer patients. A homogeneous and well demarcated mass with no remarkable surrounding brain edema in CT findings is only suggestive for the possibility of meningioma (Fig. IV-13E). The attachment of the tumor to the dura, the skull or the falx is a characteristic feature of meningioma. Angiography will sometimes help to properly diagnose meningioma.

Case 1 48-year-old woman. TU 78192. Uterine carcinoma (carcinoma colli, Ib) and meningioma.

The patient noticed dysmenorrhea and genital bleeding. She was diagnosed as a case of uterine carcinoma and underwent abdominal extensive hysterectomy with bilateral lymphadenectomy on January 19, 1978. Four months later, she was attacked by a fainting sensation similar to a transcient ischemic attack. She also noticed recent memory disturbance which increased gradually, sensory disturbance and motor weakness in the right side. She complained of occasional headache. When the patient was admitted to the clinic, right hemiparesis was evident. Disturbance of recent memory and calculation was noted. Optic fundi revealed a blurred margin of discs. Her visual acuity was almost normal, but right homonymous hemianopsia was present. CT revealed a large, well-demarcated and homogeneously enhanced high density mass in her left occipital region (Fig. IV-13E). It was noted by angiography that the tumor was fed by the left posterior cerebral, posterior meningeal and the meningeal branch of the right occipital artery. Diagnosis of meningioma as a double tumor was established prior to surgery. Occipital craniotomy with the total removal of the tumor was performed on October 11, 1978. All neurological signs showed improvement. Histological diagnosis was meningotheliomatous meningioma.

It is almost impossible to differentiate gliomas in patients having a history of cancer from a metastatic tumor by CT findings alone, without histological verification at the time of surgery. Hematoma due to cryptic angioma or other cerebrovascular accidents can be diagnosed by a clinical course and by repeating CT examinations. Sudden onset of clinical signs and symptoms and their gradual subsidence suggest a cerebrovascular accident. CT demonstrates a high density homogeneous mass in the first few days. A central low density area appears in a week (Fig. IV-13C). The volume of the clot and the surrounding brain edema gradually shrinks. Even though CT findings are similar to those of a metastatic tumor in a certain period, the changing pattern of CT is characteristic of hematoma. It should, however, be borne in mind that metastatic tumors rich in vascularity very often produce hemorrhage and also cause hematoma. It is also important to note that many cancer patients, especially those in the advanced stage, are often attacked by bleeding due to thrombocytopenia or other disturbances of the blood coagulation mechanism produced by chemotherapy.

Cerebral infarction sometimes occurs in cancer patients as a result of tumor emboli, preexisting cerebrovascular disease or abnormal coagulation states (Deck, 1980). The changing pattern of CT findings is identical to the cerebral infarction. The cerebral infarction appears as a low density area not enhanced by contrast media immediately after the accident, but the area will show contrast enhancement 10 days to 3 weeks from the ictus. The time course of symptoms and CT findings will give proper differential diagnosis.

The frequent association of acute or chronic brain abcesses with malignant disease in the lung may be confused with metastatic brain tumors. The CT findings of fungal or tuberculous granuloma also resemble the metastatic tumor of the brain. Multiple abscesses, too, cannot be differentiated from metastatic tumors by CT findings alone. A clinial course, as well as signs and laboratory findings characteristic of infections, will be helpful in diagnosing.

Direct skull base and intracranial invasion of the upper jaw carcinoma is best demonstrated by coronal and sagittal section images. Carcinoma infiltrates and

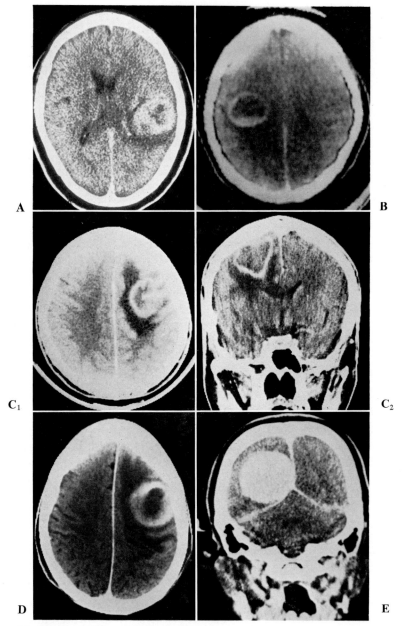

Fig. IV-13 Differential diagnosis.

A. Glioblastoma. The anterior border of the tumor is diffusely infiltrating to the surrounding tissue. The relatively small area of the brain edema is a characteristic of this CT scan.

B. Glioblastoma. It is impossible to differentiate metastatic tumors by the CT findings alone.

C. Hematoma. The CT scan was examined on the ninth day of bleeding due to a cryptic angioma. The findings are similar to a metastatic tumor. C–1: axial section; C–2: cornal section.

D. Abscess. The finding is similar to a metastatic tumor.

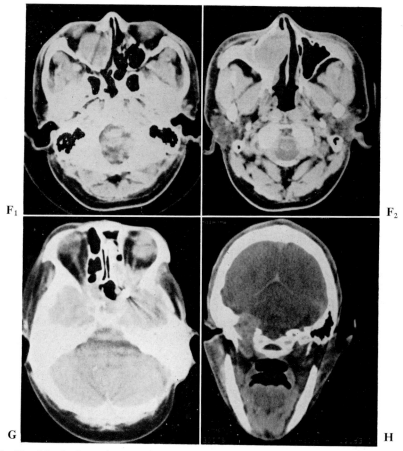

F₁   F₂

G   H

E. Meningioma in a patient who had a history of uterine carcinoma. Hysterectomy was performed four months before the onset of a fainting attack. The CT finding is identical for meningioma. The large homogeneous and well-demarcated tumor is surrounded by brain edema.

F. 1)–2) Maxillary sinus mucocele. The left maxillary sinus is filled by a homogeneous mass. The border of the mass is expanding and shows a round contour. A part of the mass is extends into the orbital cavity causing exophthalmos. The bone surrounding the mass is thinner, but no invasive destruction is noted.

G. Ethmoidal sinus carcinoma. The tumor infiltrates the surrounding tissue, destructs the retro-orbital skull base and extends into the intracranial space.

H. Schwannoma of the fifth nerve. The tumor destructs the pyramis and extends down to the maxillary sinus. The border of the destructed skull base is sharply demarcated. The destructed bone fragment is directed downwards.

destructs the adjacent bone structure, as shown in Figure IV-13G. On the other hand, the non-neoplastic process does not easily destruct the bone. Mucocele, for example, fills the maxillary sinus without significant destruction of the bone (Fig. IV-13F). It grows inside the sinus cavity and expands the surrounding bony structure. The convex form of bone deformity outlining the homogeneous mass without invasive destruction differentiates mucocele from sinus carcinoma. The direction of tumor progression and bony destruction are often visualized by CT. A case of schwannoma of the fifth nerve destructing pyramis and skull base is shown in Figure IV-13H. The downward progression of the tumor can be demonstrated by the direction of the sharpened fragment of the destructed bony structure.

A differential diagnosis of metastatic intracranial tumors and direct invasion of the upper jaw carcinoma will be established by the history, clinical course, symptoms and signs and CT findings. Laboratory data and angiographical findings sometimes give final and conclusive information.

Tuberous sclerosis often demonstrates multiple calcified nodules on CT scans, but it is not difficult to differentiate from metastatic brain tumors by history and symptoms. Seizures without signs of increased intracranial pressure but with mental retardation and possibly cutaneous manifestations of phacomatosis will make a definite diagnosis of tuberous sclelosis.

The CT findings of multiple sclerosis often resemble those of metastatic brain tumors (Cala and Mastaglia, 1976; Aita et al., 1978; Sears et al., 1978; Deck, 1980). The mass enhanced by contrast media is demonstrated during the active phase of multiple sclerosis. The mass will, however, disappear spontaneously in six to eight weeks (Deck, 1980).

Radiation necrosis of the brain often shows CT findings similar to those of a metastatic brain tumor (Rottenberg et al., 1977; Mikhael, 1978; van Dellen and Danziger, 1978). The mass demonstrates iso- or low density enhanced by contrast media and is accompanied by edema, but the CT scan will be normalized with time. Deck (1980) demonstrated a case of eosinophilic granuloma given 10 Gy. of irradiation. It showed a low density area with some surrounding contrast enhancement similar to the finding of the metastatic tumor, but the CT appearance had returned to normal, apart from slight ventricular enlargement three months later.

Radiation or drug-induced leukoencephalopathy also demonstrates a local or generalized low density of white matter accompanied by cerebral atrophy without any contrast enhancement (Peylan-Ramu et al., 1977, 1978; Allen et al., 1978 a, b; Deck, 1980).

ANGIOGRAPHY

The diagnostic value of angiography has greatly changed since the development of CT. Tumor localization as well as the determination of tumor size and shape can be more easily and safely detected by CT scan. Angiography, however, provides information on feeding arteries, draining veins and vascularization of tumors. Surgical treatment of tumors requires such information for safe and proper manipulation by surgeons. The nature of tumor vascularity will help to make possible a more precise diagnosis of histological types of tumors. Angiography also clearly reveals the presence of vascular lesions such as arterio-venous malformation or aneurysm which may complicate intracranial metastasis. Such vascular lesions should be clarified before treatment begins. A case of arteriovenous malformation in a breast cancer patient was in fact found in our clinic, as was reported in the previous chapter.

Technical Note

Since patients having intracranial metastatic tumors are generally a poor risk, the indication of angiography should be cautiously established in consideration of the method of treatment. If there is no surgical indication or need for differential diagnosis for treatment, no angiographic examination should be performed. Gluco-corticoid administration is necessary prior to angiographic examination. Anticon-vulsants should be given as soon as possible when the diagnosis of an intracranial metastatic tumor is established by CT. Convulsive seizures are often induced at the time of angiography without careful medication to control brain edema prior to the examination. Whether to select whole vessel study or one side carotid angiography is dependent on individual cases. The selective angiography of internal and external carotid arteries is sometimes necessary to elucidate the feeding arteries, especially in the cases of skull involvement by the tumor. Serial angiography is always needed since the tumor stain is often invisible in the arterial phase. Angiography is aimed mainly at demonstrating feeding arteries, draining veins and tumor vascularization. A longer injection time using a slightly larger volume of contrast media (15–20 ml in the case of carotid angiography) will demonstrate tumor stains with arterial struc-tures, and it more clearly reveals the relationship between arteries and tumor vessels. The subtraction technique of angiography is always recommended so that tumor vascularization can be more clearly shown.

Angiographic Findings

Tumor Stain (Contrast Accumulation)

Tumor vascularization varies according to the histological type of the tumor. The rich vascular stain in the angiogram of the metastatic tumor is generally seen in cases of renal clear cell carcinoma, melanoma, choriocarcinoma and several types of sarcomas. These tumors have a tendency to cause hemorrhage in the tumor, making it a large hematoma. In those cases, the tumor stain is generally clearly seen even in the arterial phase. More than half of all metastatic tumors show increased vascu-larity (Wickbom, 1953). It is, however, generally difficult to detect tumor stains in the arterial phase in most cases of adenocarcinoma or squamous cell carcinoma. A typical example of serial angiograms of metastatic tumors from lung adenocarcinoma is presented in Figure IV-1. The tumor stain is most clearly visualized in the capillary phase. Tumor stains in most cases are generally not homogeneous nor highly dense like meningioma. They appear faint in the capillary and venous phases, as shown in Figures IV-14 and 15. The tumor stain disappears more rapidly than in meningioma and is visible only for a second. When contrast media injection is pro-longed for more than two seconds, the tumor stain in the capillary phase overlapped with the arterial phase is demonstrated (Fig. IV-16). A relatively well-circumscribed figure of the tumor stain is a differential point from malignant glioma.

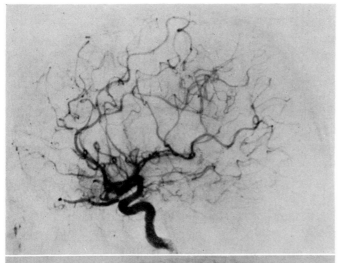

14A

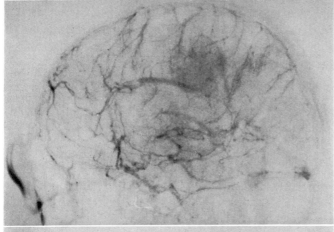

14B

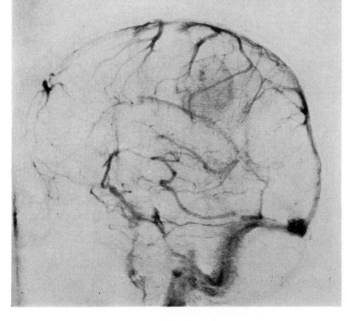

14C

Fig. IV-14 Serial angiogram. Left parietal metastatic tumor from lung adenocarcinoma.
A. Arterial phase.
B. Capillary phase.
C. Venous phase.
D. CT scan.

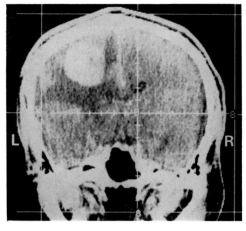

14D

Four patterns of abnormal vascularity have been described (Wickbom, 1953; Lindgren, 1954; Zachrisson, 1963; Newton and Potts, 1974; Taveras and Wood, 1976). (1) Homogeneous tumor stain is similar to that often seen in meningioma. The homogeneity, however, is not as complete as meningioma (Fig. IV-14). (2) There are many irregular vessels with early venous filling such as glioblastoma (Figs. IV-16-18). (3) There is a network of thin, somewhat tortuous vessels, often in a fairly regular arrangement (Fig. IV-19). (4) A relatively avascular central portion of the tumor is shown with a vascular periphery (Fig. IV-15). The last pattern is typical of a metastatic tumor since the central portion of the tumor is filled with a necrotic mass or a cystic fluid. Diagnosis of the multiplicity of tumors, which is not the aim of angiography, should essentially be established by CT. Early venous filling is another characteristic finding of the metastatic tumor, and it is one of the differential points from meningioma. There is no definite correlation between the density or the enhancement of tumors in CT scan and the density of tumor stains in the angiogram.

In most cases, parenchymal metastatic tumors have a round or oval shape and a fairly demarcated margin (Fig. IV-14). Peripheral vessels surrounding the tumor are not as clearly visualized as meningioma. Surgical removal of the tumor therefore is much easier and without bleeding, compared with meningioma. The area surrounding the tumor is encircled by a low density, ring-shaped zone which represents the avascular area of the brain edema or the rim of the encephalomalacia (Figs. IV-14 and 15). When a tumor develops hematoma, the avascular area with compression of vessels is a predominant finding (Fig. IV-20).

Feeding Artery and Draining Vein

Since a metastatic tumor develops from a small embolic site of an artery or a capillary, the feeding artery is single in the early stage of tumor growth. The tumor angiogenesis factor probably stimulates the development of tumor vascularization and connects vessels to other feeding arteries and draining veins. Few feeding arteries are generally demonstrated in a tumor (Figs. IV-16 and 19). The proximal trunks of feeding arteries are usually of normal size or slightly dilated (Figs. IV-16 and 19). In contrast, those that feed arteriovenous malformations are extensively dilated in most cases. The twigs of the arteries around a metastatic tumor are

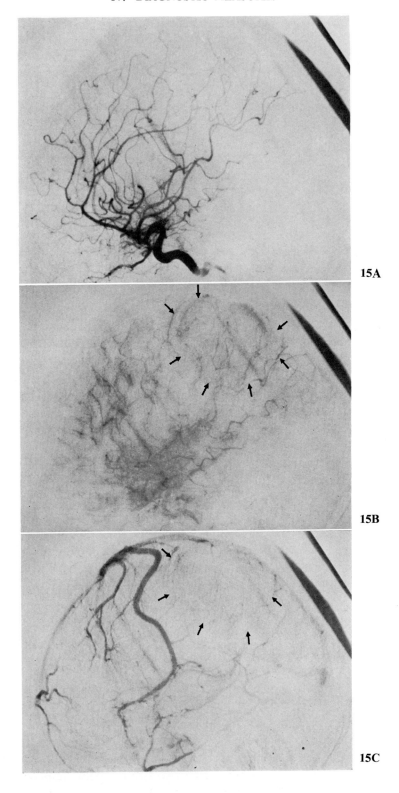

15A

15B

15C

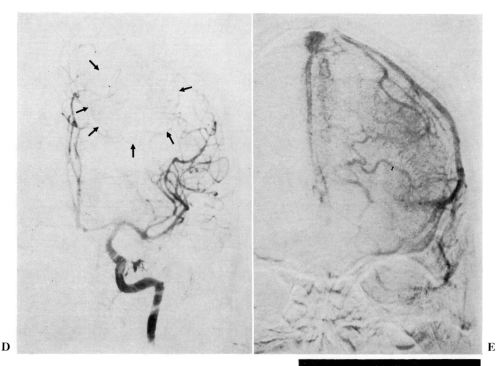

D   E

Fig. IV-15 Serial angiogram. Left parietal metastatic tumor (arrow) from colon carcinoma.
A. Arterial phase.
B. Capillary phase.
C. Venous phase.
D. Arterial phase (A-P view).
E. Venous phase (A-P view).
F. CT scan.

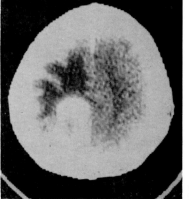

F

stretched or straight, and encircle the tumor. Those that feed on arterio-venous mal-formations are slightly tortuous and can usually be traced directly to the lesion (Newton and Potts, 1974). In some tumors with rich vascularization, such as renal clear cell carcinoma (Fig. IV-17), and some angiomatous sarcomas such as hemangio-pericytoma, feeding arteries are extensively dilated, as in cases of arteriovenous malformation. The ligation or embolization with gelfoam of those feeding arteries prior to surgical removal will help in safe surgical manipulating of the tumor. Such dilated feeding arteries are rarely seen in metastatic tumors of adeno- or squamous cell carcinoma from lung or breast cancer. The tumor, like meningioma, is sometimes fed by branches of the external carotid artery, which are clearly demonstrated by selective angiography (Fig. IV-21).

When the tumor grows in the area surrounding the major arteries or invades the wall of the arteries, the angiographic findings mimic arteritis or arteriosclerotic

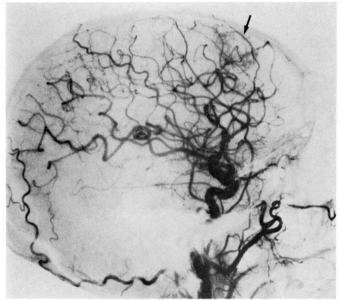

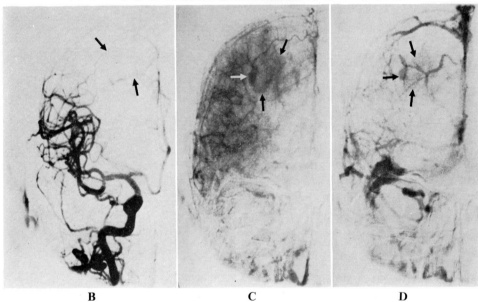

Fig. IV-16 Serial angiography. Right frontal metastatic tumor (arrow) from lung ade-
nocarcinoma.
- **A.** Arterial phase (prolonged injection).
- **B.** Arterial phase.
- **C.** Capillary phase.
- **D.** Venous phase.

Fig. IV-17 Skull metastasis from renal clear cell carcinoma.   →
- **A.** Angiogram, arterial phase (Left).
- **B.** Angiogram, arterial phase (Right).
- **C.** Capillary phase.
- **D.** Venous phase.
- **E.** CT scan.
- **F.** Plain craniogram.

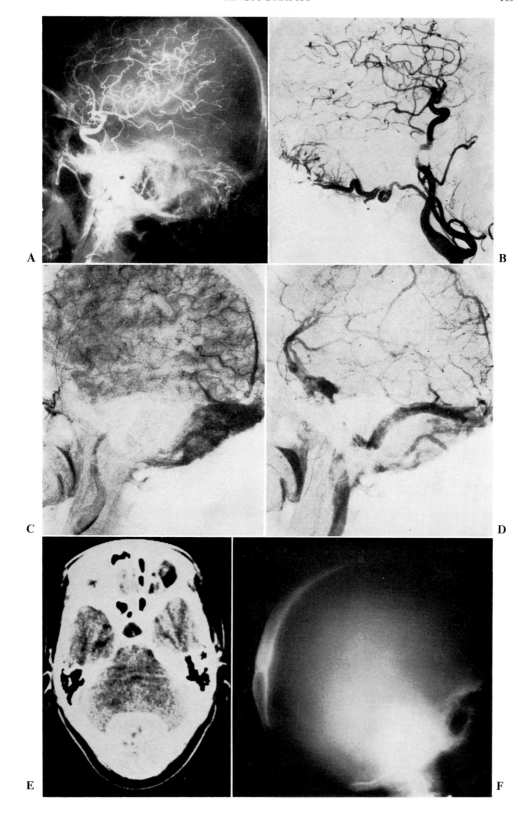

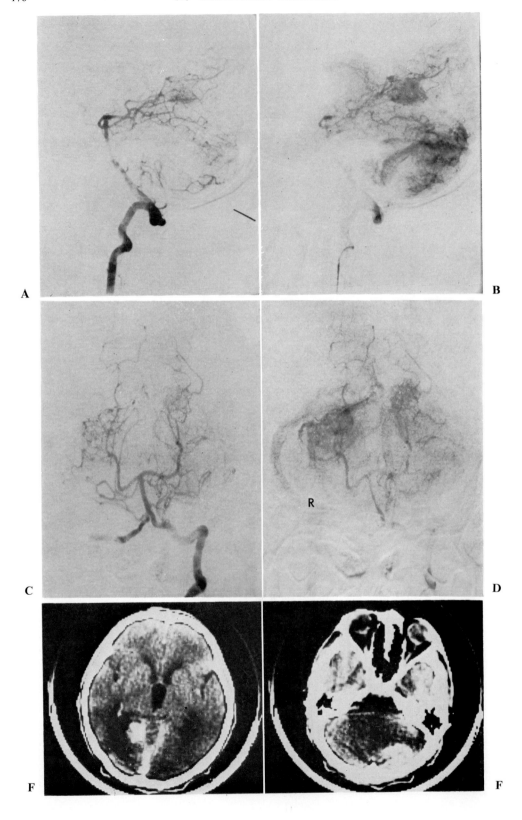

changes (Fig. IV-22).   Invasion by the metastatic tumor into the wall of arteries has been reported by Cowen et al. (1970), Leeds and Rosenblatt (1972), and Newton and Potts (1974).

Stereoscopic angiography clearly demonstrates the three dimensional structure of these feeding arteries and draining veins of the tumor (Sano, 1976).

RI SCANNING

Radioactive isotope (RI) brain scanning was considered the fundamental diagnostic examination for screening of intracranial metastatic tumors before the development of CT.   Since more than half of metastatic brain tumor patients have multiple tumor nodules, the RI scintigram gives more useful information about the locations of those tumors than angiography (Murphy et al., 1969; Constans et al., 1973a).   However, the recent technical progress of CT has overcome all the disadvantages of RI scintigraphy, providing accurate information about tumor location, size, shape, inner structure, characteristics of cysts, the figure and extension of the surrounding brain edema, etc.   CT can detect smaller metastatic tumor nodules than RI scintigraphy.   RI scanning, therefore, is no longer a diagnostic tool in evaluating the presence of intracranial metastatic tumors.

Moore (1948) at the Mayo Clinic first adopted ^{131}I-labeled dio-iodo-fluorescein which was traced by a Geiger-Müller tube, for the detection of brain lesions.   Radioactive substances used in the early days were di-iodo-fluorescein ^{131}I (Ashkenazy et al., 1949; Ter-Pogossian et al., 1952; Davis and Craigmile, 1954; Seman et al., 1954) and radiomercury-labeled chlormerodrin (Neohydrin) ^{197}Hg and ^{203}Hg (Blau and Bender, 1959; Rhoton, Jr. et al., 1964; Goodrich and Tutor, 1965; Ponari et al., 1965; Gold and Loken, 1969).   In 95 per cent of 340 patients suspected of having central nervous system tumors, accurate diagnosis of tumor localization was made possible by scanning using the radioactive di-iodo-fluorescein test and verified by surgery or pneumography (Ashkenazy et al., 1951).   The correct localization was diagnosed in 84 per cent of the tumors by scanning using chlormerodrin (Rhoton, Jr. et al., 1964). Castelli et al. (1968) reported that 217 patients were examined by brain scanning using Neohydrin ^{203}Hg, and 83.4 per cent of these tumors were properly diagnosed regarding their locations.   The localizations of meningioma, glioblastoma and supratentorial metastatic tumors in particular were accurately diagnosed in more than 93 per cent of the cases.   Even basal supratentorial midline cerebral tumors and posterior fossa tumors could be diagnosed in over 90 per cent of the cases by applying Neohydrin (Ostertag et al., 1974).   The short half-life (6 hours) of Technetium^{99m} was introduced for brain scanning by Harper et al. (1964, 1966).   Witcofski and his colleagues

← **Fig. IV-18**   Occipital and infratentorial multiple metastases from lung large-cell carcinoma.
- **A.**   Vertebral angiogram, arterial phase.
- **B.**   Vertebral angiogram, capillary phase.
- **C.**   Vertebral angiogram, arterial phase (A-P view).
- **D.**   Vertebral angiogram, capillary phase (A-P view).
- **E.**   CT scan, supratentorial tumor.
- **F.**   CT scan, infratentorial tumor.

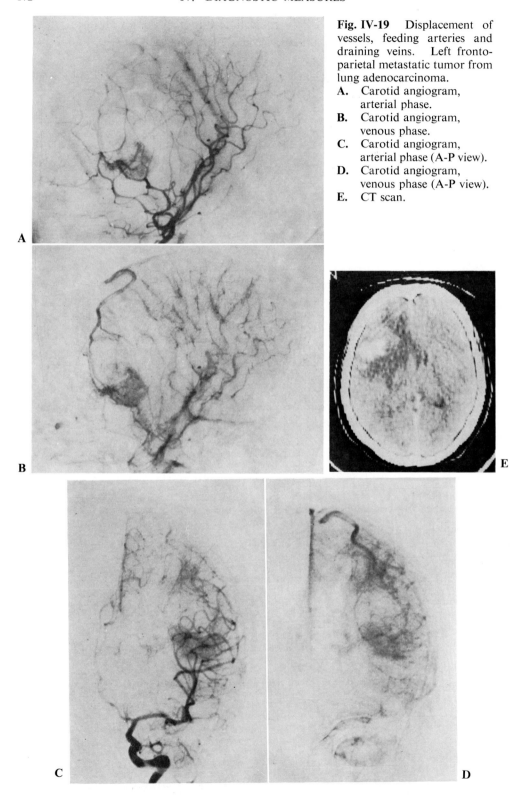

Fig. IV-19   Displacement of vessels, feeding arteries and draining veins.   Left fronto-parietal metastatic tumor from lung adenocarcinoma.
A.   Carotid angiogram, arterial phase.
B.   Carotid angiogram, venous phase.
C.   Carotid angiogram, arterial phase (A-P view).
D.   Carotid angiogram, venous phase (A-P view).
E.   CT scan.

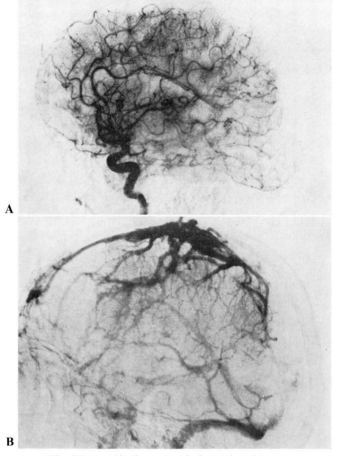

Fig. IV-20 Skull metastasis from thyroid cancer.
A. Angiogram, arterial phase.
B. Angiogram, venous phase.

(1967) reported that 72 out of 95 patients (81.5 %) with proven intracranial neoplasms had positive scans with Technetium[99m]. Because Technetium[99m] in the pertechnetate form is slowly cleared from the blood, the normal intracranial vascular structures, not seen with chlormerodrin [197]Hg or [203]Hg, are depicted on the scan. In a survey involving 625 patients, 54 of 65 patients with proved intracranial neoplasms had positive results by brain scanning using [99m]Tc (Quinn III. et al., 1965). Filson and Rodriguez-Antunez (1968) reported that the overall diagnostic accuracy was 90 per cent by brain scanning after the administration of Technetium[99m] in 95 patients. A consecutive series of 50 patients was studied by simultaneous or close sequential administration of routine diagnostic doses of [203]Hg chlormerodrin and ^{99m}Tc pertechnetate. It was found that the diagnostic accuracy of the two materials were closely parallel, although the general overall accuracy of the pertechnetate was slightly better than that of the mercurials (Croll et al., 1968). Moody et al. (1972) reported that posterior fossa tumors could be diagnosed with accuracy close to that reported for supratentorial tumors by ^{99m}Tc, if the parotid gland was well blocked with perchlorate. One can expect to detect nearly 100 per cent of all meningiomas, over 85 per

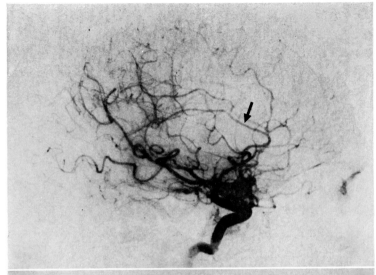

21A

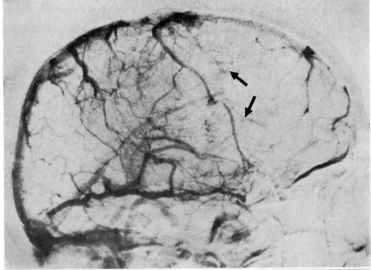

21B

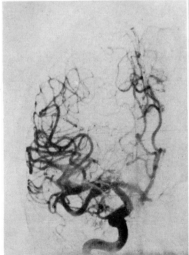

21C

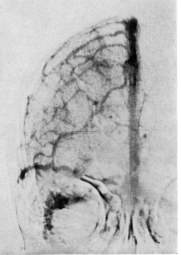

21D

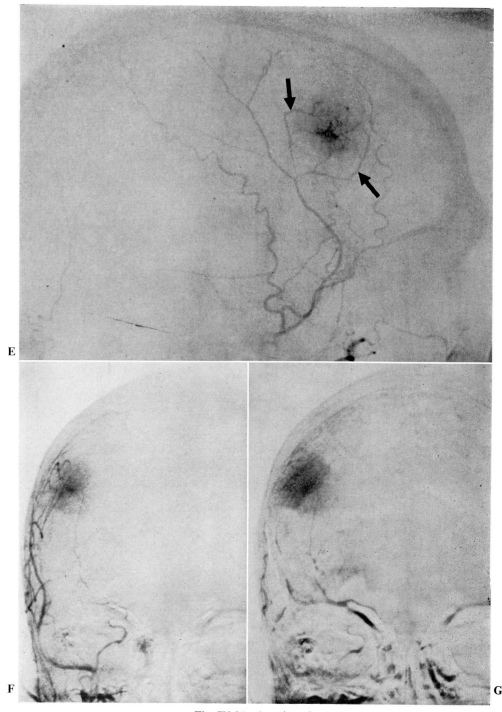

Fig. IV-21 (continued)

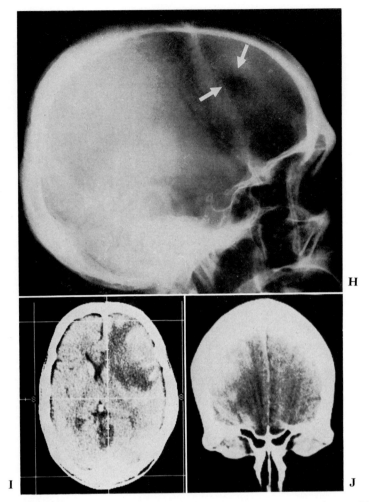

Fig. IV-21 Selective angiogram of the internal and external carotid arteries. Right frontal metastatic tumor with skull invasion from tonsillar squamous cell carcinoma.

A. Internal carotid angiogram, arterial phase.
B. Internal carotid angiogram, venous phase.
C. Internal carotid angiogram, arterial phase (A-P view).
D. Internal carotid angiogram, venous phase (A-P view).
E. External carotid angiogram, arterial phase.
F. External carotid angiogram, arterial phase (A-P view).
G. External carotid angiogram, venous phase (A-P view).
H. Plain craniogram.
I. CT scan.
J. CT scan (Coronal section).

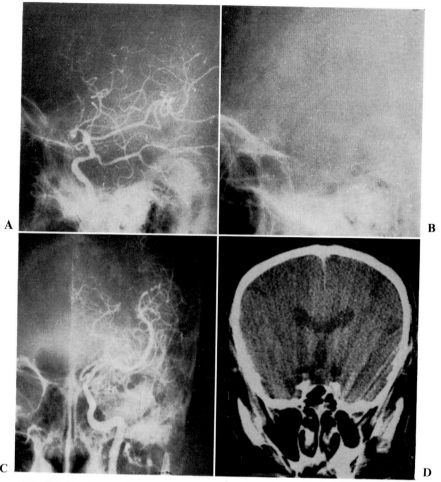

Fig. IV-22 Parasseller metastatic tumor from lung anaplastic carcinoma.
A. Angiogram, arterial phase.
B. Plain craniogram, destruction of sella turcica.
C. Angiogram, arterial phase (A-P view).
D. CT scan.

cent of ependymomas, metastatic tumors and juvenile astrocytomas, and over 80 per cent of acoustic neurinomas. The RI scannings by ^{99m}Tc of the metastatic brain tumors are compared to the CT findings (Fig. IV-23).

The value of repeated scanning for improving the detectability of brain tumors was reported by Gates et al. (1971). Brain scanning was performed on patients during the first hour following the injection of sodium pertechnetate ^{99m}Tc, and the patients were rescanned one to 24 hours later. The detectability of brain tumors was improved from 80 per cent with routine early scanning to 93 per cent with rescanning. The optimal time for repeated scanning was three to four hours following tracer injection. In 40 metastatic brain tumors scanned, 31 patients showed abnormal findings during the initial studies and the remaining nine patients demonstrated abnormal findings at the time of rescanning. Another contribution of RI scanning was that it proved extremely valuable in forecasting the recurrence of the tumor, before it was clinically revealed or detected by other methods (Constans et al., 1973a).

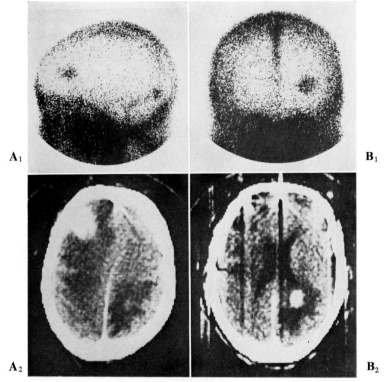

Fig. IV-23   RI scan of multiple metastatic brain tumors from lung adenocarcinoma, and the CT scan of the same patient (^{99m}Tc pertechnetate).
A.   1)   Lateral view of RI scanning.   2)   The axial section of CT reveals
the same tumors in the left frontal and the right parieto-occipital regions.
B.   1)   The antero-posterior view of RI scanning.   2) The axial CT reveals
the same tumor in the right parieto-occipital region.

Cinegammagraphy (cine-scintigraphy) was developed by Ancri (1971, 1972).
He reported that the preliminary results based on 2,000 examinations showed that
this method had the following advantages: 1) low percentage of negative or doubtful
results (2%), 2) high accuracy in the diagnosis of arterio-venous malformations
and meningiomas, and 3) possible improvement in the diagnosis of malignant tumors,
abscesses and intracranial hematomas.   Out of 42 intracranial metastatic tumors,
positive findings were gained for 41 patients, 33 cases of which were exactly diagnosed
according to their histological natures.   Rapid serial scintiphotographs (radioisotope arteriography), as an adjunct to routine brain scanning employing ^{99m}Tc per-
tecnetate, were obtained in over 1,000 patients.   It provided complementary information on the histological nature of the tumor rapidly.   It demonstrated lesions not
visualized by routine scans (Maynard et al., 1969).

Today RI scanning is still a useful tool for screening bone metastases from various malignant tumors (Figs. IV-24 and 25).   Radioactive Gallium^{69} is commonly
employed for this purpose.   The whole body scan is useful in detecting bone
metastases.   Since breast cancer, for instance, often metastasizes to the vertebrae, it
is important to know whether vertebral metastasis is present before the manifestation
of clinical signs and symptoms.   Examples of RI scans of bone metastases are given in
Figure IV-24.

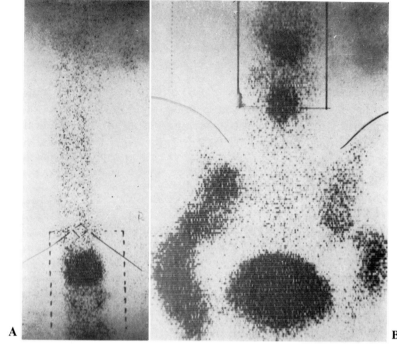

Fig. IV-24 RI scan of bone (^{69}Ga). Multiple metastases are detected in the lumbar vertebrae (L_{1-4}) (A) and iliac bones on both sides (B). Adenocarcinoma from lung cancer.

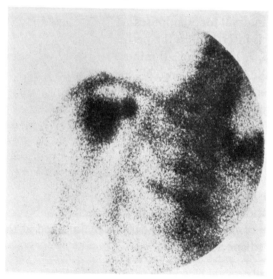

Fig. IV-25 RI scan of bone (^{69}Ga). Multiple metastases are detected in the right scapula and cervical and thoracic vertebrae.
Adenocarcinoma from lung cancer.

Result

The increase of the Hounsfield number was 10 to 15 in normal gray matter and 20 to 25 in the white matter. The CBF was 84 ml/100 g/min in normal gray matter and 21 ml/100 g/min in the white matter. This data is similar to the results obtained by other methods. The normal values of CBF are written in the legend of Figure IV-26. The pattern of those CBF in a patient with a multiple metastatic tumor is demonstrated in Figure IV-26E.

> **Case 1** 65-year-old man. TU 80139.   Multiple metastatic cerebral tumors from gastric cancer.
> The patient was operated on for gastric cancer two years earlier. He then complained of headaches, nausea, poor appetite, weakness of the right upper and lower extremities, and speech disturbance. At the time of admission, he was emaciated and had marked bilateral choked discs with retinal bleeding. Motor and sensory weakness of his right extremities were evident. Large tumor masses in the left parietal and right occipital regions and few small tumor nodules scattered in several parenchymal regions were found by CT. The rCBF was 35 to 64 ml/100g/min in the center of the metastatic tumor and 0 to 14 ml/100g/min in the adjacent edematous brain.

The rCBF is a good indicator determining the therapeutic effects on brain edema and the tumor. The measurement of rCBF by this Xe-CT method is superior to the ordinary ^{133}Xe inhalation method, since the CBF in the gray and white matters are clearly differentiated by this method, and the rCBF in a certain small area of the brain is measured as the absolute value of blood flow. The rCBF clarifies the extent of brain damage due to the metastatic tumors and also gives important information about the reversibility of ischemic brain lesions.

The interest in positron-emission tomography (PET) has been increasing recently. Since the quantitative three-dimensional measurement of radioisotope distribution in tissue can be made, the accurate quantitative measurement of rCBF will be obtained by PET. It offers the opportunity to study hemodynamics as well as tissue metabolism and chemical composition with noninvasive methods. An introductory review of PET is presented by Raichle (1980).

ELECTROENCEPHALOGRAPHY (EEG)

Since Walter (1936) demonstrated for the first time that EEG could be used for the localization of brain tumors, it has become a common diagnostic tool (Ellingson and Lundy, 1962). Some patients with known primary tumors such as lung or breast cancer have demonstrated abnormal EEG changes before any clinical manifestations of metastatic brain tumors (Gastaut et al., 1954 a, b; Rowan et al, 1974). In the case of intracerebral lesions, a high degree of correlation was found between EEG and neurological signs. Even neurologically silent brain metastases were detected by EEG, and very few of those with positive neurological signs were missed by EEG examinations. A tumor size of 2 cm in diameter was thought to be the threshold of detection by neurologic or EEG examination. In 44.5 per cent of 52 cases with intracranial metastases, a correct EEG localization was obtained. Of all lesions measuring more than 2 cm, 81 per cent were correctly detected by EEG, but out of the numerous lesions smaller than 2 cm, only one was detected (Strang and Ajmone-Marsan, 1961).

The diagnostic value of EEG for intracranial metastatic tumors has changed. Today it is no longer an examination aimed at detecting the presence of a tumor but is used as a tool for evaluating the physiological function of the brain regarding seizures due to metastatic tumors, since a quarter of the patients demonstrate convulsive seizures as an early symptom.

The pattern of EEG of metastatic brain tumors is essentially the same as other primary brain tumors. Regarding the change of the basic rhythm of EEG, Bureau-Paillas and Poncet (1974) noted that 24.4 per cent of the cases suffering from intracranial metastatic tumors showed the normal symmetrical basic α rhythm. The asymmetry of basic activity between both hemispheres existed in 51.2 per cent, and diffuse abnormality was noted in 24.4 per cent of the cases.

The focal changes of EEG are composed of slow waves (δ or θ) or paroxismal discharges (spikes or sharp waves). Klass and Daly (1960) described the two categories of slow waves. The arrhythmic (polymorphous) discharge has no fixed rate of waves. It is composed of δ rhythms (slower than 3 Hz). The wave form is irregular and varied. Such discharges usually indicate a relatively severe and acute disturbance of cortical functions and are reliable indicators of the site of the tumor. Figure IV-27 illustrates an example of such arrhythmic discharge at the site of an intracranial metastatic tumor from lung adenocarcinoma. In the other kind of slow

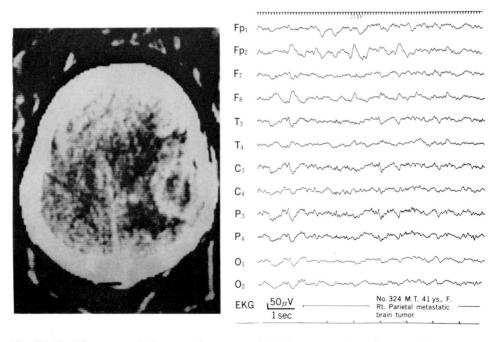

Fig. IV-27 Electroencephalogram of a metastatic brain tumor patient (41-year-old woman. Lung adenocarcinoma). Multiple metastatic tumors are located in the right frontoparietal region. The irregular δ rhythm (arrhythmic) is dominant in the FP_2 lead.

waves, rhythmic discharges (dysrhythmias) are composed of θ or δ rhythms (slow dysrhythmias or monorhythmic deltas). They frequently occur bilaterally and synchronously. These rhythmic discharges are homologous and seen in a remote region from the deeply situated tumor. It is, therefore, referred to as a projected rhythm and is less reliable than the arrhythmic discharge as a tumor site indicator.

Focal changes in EEG were found in 83 per cent of intracranial metastatic tumors (Bureau-Paillas and Poncet, 1974).

They are, however, dependent on the time of examination. In cases of primary malignant brain tumors, the abnormality of EEG may appear throughout the entire hemisphere involved. The frequency of arrhythmic discharges may be higher, and the discharges tend to occur intermittently in histologically more differentiated tumors. It is, however, evident that the histological types of tumors cannot be reliably diagnosed by EEG. The focal arrhythmias which appear in the waking record and persist during sleep are usually associated with superficial cortical lesions; if abnormally slow focal rhythms disappear during sleep, the lesions tend to be situated subcortically (Silverman and Groff, 1957). In cases of deeply situated tumors, the electrical abnormalities are usually dysrhythmic in nature. The discharges are bilaterally synchronous and intermittent. They are increased by hyperventilation and become much more conspicuous if there is some impairment in the patient's alertness.

Seizures are common initial symptoms in intracranial metastatic tumor patients. Paroxismal discharges are seen with seizures. Klass and Bickford (1958) found that in more than 25 per cent of their series of 32 intracranial metastatic brain tumor patients, spike or sharp wave discharges appeared. Bureau-Paillas and Poncet (1974) reported that 27 per cent of their 152 cases demonstrated paroxismal discharges, 12 per cent of them accompanying δ rhythms. They also noted that EEG examinations could detect the susceptibility of seizures before actual clinical attacks. The rate of finding such spikes or sharp waves is less frequent in our clinic today. This is because treatment with anticonvulsant and steroid hormones for the prevention of successive seizures starts immediately after the occurrance of seizures or metastatic tumors are detected, and the dose of the anticonvulsants is controlled by measuring the serum level of each agent. CT for cancer patients showing some minor neurological signs often reveals the presence of intracranial metastatic tumor nodules. Seizures can then be prevented by cautious administration of an anticonvulsant.

Bilateral diffuse abnormalities of EEG were noted in 11 per cent of all cases (Bureau-Paillas and Poncet, 1974). They were composed of θ or δ rhythms and found in cases of leptomeningeal diffuse metastases, infratentorial metastases with hydrocephalus, and multiple metastases. As for supratentorial tumors, correct localization of the tumor was diagnosed in about 80 per cent of the cases. In cases of infratentorial tumors, 86 per cent demonstrated abnormal findings of EEG, 74 per cent of which showed diffuse abnormalities without any laterality.

Since EEG is an easy and harmless examination, it is advisable that EEG and CT be performed as routine examinations, especially for lung and breast cancer patients who are most susceptible to intracranial metastases.

STATIONARY POTENTIAL ENCEPHALOGRAPHY

The existence of the stationary potential of the brain has been demonstrated by experimental and clinical studies (Manaka and Sano, 1979; Sano et al., 1979). The magnitude of the human stationary potential was estimated to be about 20 mV. Brain tumor cells do not possess any stationary potential, and the neuron is considered to be an essential component in generating this potential. The stationary potential is very stable in physiological conditions, but it changes in various intracranial organic lesions and extensive metabolic disorders such as anoxia and generalized convulsive seizures. The stationary potential can be detected through the scalp, and that on the cortex is measured by a high impedance chopper stabilized DC (direct current) amplifier and calomel half-cell electrodes.

The stationary potential encephalogram in normal subjects shows a symmetrical voltage distribution over the hemisphere with the highest potential in the vertex. If the lesion involves the cortex, the stationary potential over the area is negative compared with the normal area in the order of 5 to 20 mV. If the lesion is located in the subcortex, the cortex over the lesion is positive in the order of 5 to 10 mV. When the lesion is an expanding type tumor such as meningioma, the stationary potential shows a "crateriform potential change"; that is negative in the center of the tumor and positive in the surrounding tissue. In cases of intracranial metastatic tumors, they often have multiple stationary potential foci, both positive and negative over the cortex, resulting in irregular patterns on the stationary potential encephalogram (Fig. IV-28).

CYTOLOGICAL EXAMINATION OF CEREBROSPINAL FLUID

Cytological examinations of cerebrospinal fluid (CSF) for detecting malignant tumor cells have been carried out since the begining of this century (Du Four, 1904). It provides information about the presence of atypical cells but rarely demonstrates the histological type of the tumor involved. Since the intracranial pressure of patients suffering from metastatic brain tumors increases markedly, the spinal tap itself is generally contraindicated. Examination of the CSF, however, is required when leptomeningeal involvement by the tumor or infectious meningitis need to be differentiated. Although the definite presence of malignant tumor cells in the CSF indicates the existence of a malignant tumor in the central nervous system, it is evident that a negative cytological examination cannot deny the presence of a tumor in the central nervous system. Glass and his co-workers (1979) reported that immature or reactive lymphocytes in the CSF might mimic lymphoma cells and lead to errors in diagnosis in rare instances of patients with systemic lymphoma and central nervous infection. They also noted that malignant cells appear in the CSF most commonly when leptomeninges are widely seeded by tumor cells, less often when they are focally seeded by

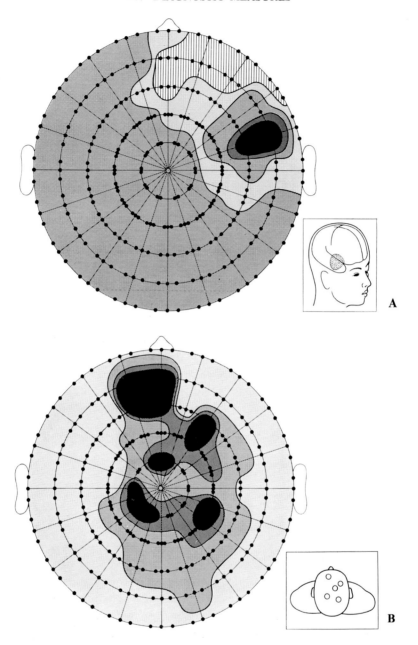

Fig. IV-28 Stationary potential encephalogram.
A. Meningioma. A typical crateriform potential change is seen. The potential of the center of the tumor is negative.
B. Metastatic tumor. The multiple centers of abnormalities are seen.

tumor cells, and almost never when the tumor is located only in the parenchyme. Negative findings cannot exclude diagnosis of leptomeningeal seeding when it is clinically suspected. However, acute lymphoblastic leukemia almost always yields tumor cells in the CSF if meninges are involved. Of the 117 examined patients with a central nervous system tumor with leptomeningeal involvement, 31 (26%) were positive, while only one out of 66 patients with a central nervous system tumor without leptomeningeal involvement had a positive cytological examination. Of 51 patients with leptomeningeal tumors at autopsy, cytology was positive in 30 cases (59%).

To increase the efficacy of the diagnostic value, we have used a cell culture method besides simple cytological examinations of the CSF. The CSF (2–5 ml) is filtered through a millipore filter (0.3 μm pore size), or simply centrifuged when the cells are abundant in order to collect tumor cells. The filter is cut into five to ten pieces and put in Petri dishes containing 3 ml of NCTC 109 culture medium which contains 20 per cent fetal calf serum. The cells are cultured in five per cent CO_2 mixed culture chamber at 37°C. The proliferation of cells is most active about seven days after the start of the culture. The tumor cells are examined with a phase contrast microscope and stained using Giemsa or Papanicolaou's technique. The presence of tumor cells can be identified by this method in more than 40 per cent of the cases, even when the cells are located only in the parenchyma. It is difficult, however, to differentiate the histological type of the tumor except in cases of leukemia. In cases of lymphoblastic leukemia (Fig. IV-29), moderately large cells with scanty cytoplasm and dark-stained nuclei are observed. The size and shape of the cells and nuclei vary and mitotic figures are frequently observed.

In the CSF of malignant lymphoma, an occasional true tissue fragment, rather than mere clustering of cells, helps to distinguish it from leukemia. The moderately large cells in the CSF of malignant lymphoma are nearly all lymphoblasts with

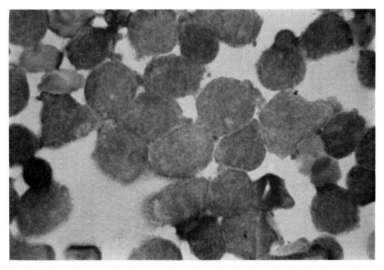

Fig. IV-29 CNS involvement of acute lymphocytic leukemia. Cells from the CSF were collected by centrifugation. Lymphoblasts and prolymphocytes make cellular clusters. The cells are mostly lymphoblasts of various sizes with irregular chromatin clumps and nucleoli, irregular nuclear membranes and scanty cytoplasm (Papanicolaou stain).

multiple, irregular chromatin clumps and nucleoli, clear perichromatin, irregular nuclear membrane and scanty cytoplasm. It is most important that these lympho-blasts are recognized as malignant tumor cells, the nucleoli of which are stained red when examined using Papanicolaou's technique (Rubinstein, 1972). Retinoblastoma often directly invades the intracranial cavity and is disseminated in the leptomeninges and parenchyma of the brain. The tumor cells in the CSF are large, round or oval in shape, with scanty, poorly defined cytoplasm. The nuclei are relatively large and rich in chromatin (Fig. IV-30).

In cases of adenocarcinoma, the cells in the CSF have large chromatin clumps in irregularly shaped nuclei with perichromatin clearing. The culture of the cells in CSF gives more detailed information on the cellular arrangement. At the beginning of the culture, the tumor cells are round or oval and are scattered in the medium. These cells have eccentrically located nuclei with abundant cytoplasm. In a week, the number of cells increases rapidly and they gradually adhere to each other. They finally show a structure similar to an adenomatous arrangement (Fig. IV-31). The pattern of the proliferation of cells in CSF resembles a cell arrangement observed in a surgically removed tissue (Fig. IV-32). The carcinoma cells are initially round and disperse independently into the culture medium from the tissue fragments. As the cells proliferate, they adhere to each other and show a mosaic pattern. When

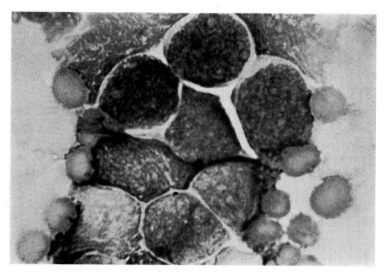

Fig. IV-30 Intracranial invasion of retinoblastoma.
The large cells are round or oval, with scanty or poorly defined cytoplasm. The nuclei are relatively large and rich in chromatin. Mitotic figures are often observed (Papanicolaou stain).

Fig. IV-31 Intracranial metastatic tumor from lung adenocarcinoma.   →
A. Cells from the CSF were cultured in NCTC 109 medium containing 20 per cent fetal calf serum for three days. Relatively large, round or oval cells with eccentrically located nuclei are scattered. Fibroblasts are also present. The perinuclear clear zones are also noted.
B. Cells from the CSF were cultured in the same medium as Figure 31A for seven days. Some cells are closely attached together in a line, similar to the adenomatous structure. The oval nuclei contain multiple nucleoli.
C. Cells from the CSF were cultured for seven days. Round or oval cells of various sizes are scattered with some fibroblasts.

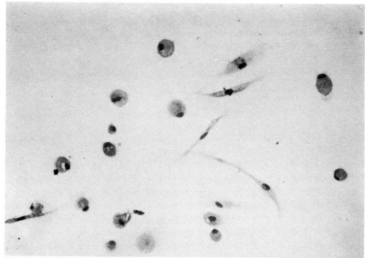

31A

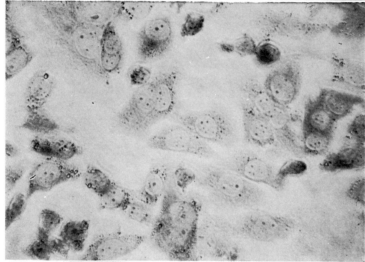

31B

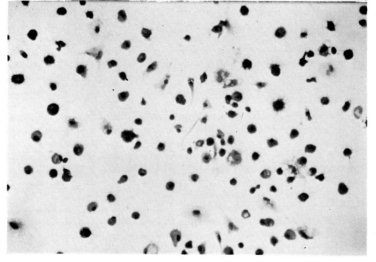

31C

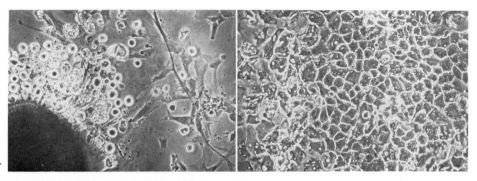

Fig. IV-32 Cultured cells of thyroid cancer.
A. The metastatic brain tumor tissue removed at the surgery was minced, chopped and filtered through platinum mesh and cultured in NCTC-109 medium containing 20 per cent fetal calf serum for seven days. The round tumor cells that dispersed from the tissue fragment are seen in the lower left corner (Phase-contrast microscopic figure).
B. Same cells as shown in Figure A. The cells were cultured for a month. The tumor cells are closely attached together and show a mosaic pattern. On the left side of the picture, secreted colloidal substance is demonstrated.

the cells have a secretory function like thyroid cancer, the colloidal substance produced can be observed around the sheet of cultured cells attached to the surface of the Petridish. The morphological appearance, as well as the functional analysis of the cultured cells, gives more precise information about the nature of the tumor involved when a cytological examination of the CSF is conducted.

TUMOR MARKER

The recent progress in radioimmunoassay and enzyme immunoassay has made it possible to measure a trace amount of tumor marker substances. Substances clinically important as tumor markers today are fetal proteins, some enzymes and hormones. Although they are not specific to the tumors, the measurement of those tumor markers in the serum or other body fluids gives us definite information about the diagnosis, the progression or recurrence of the tumor, and aids evaluation of the therapeutic effect. An example of a typical tumor marker is human chorionic gonadotropin (HCG) in cases of choriocarcinoma. The amount of HCG in the serum or urine of the patient accurately indicates the size of the tumor. When the tumor is excised or effectively treated by chemotherapy or radiotherapy, the level of HCG decreases. A case of choriocarcinoma is presented in the chapter on treatment (p. 276).

Tumor markers routinely assayed today are summarized in Table IV-1. Alpha-fetoprotein (AFP) is fetal serum protein which is synthesized in the fetal liver and yolk sack. It is contained in large amounts in the fetal serum or the amniotic fluid. Hepatoma and teratocarcinoma produce AFP. From a neurosurgical point of view, both germinoma and teratocarcinoma are generally developed in the pineal or chiasmal region. The symptomatology is the same for both tumors. The dissemination of the tumor to the spinal cord, lower vertebral body, and sometimes to the intra-or

Table IV-1   Tumor markers.

Substance	Related tumor
AFP α-fetoprotein	Hepatoma, Teratocarcinoma
CEA carcino embryonic antigen	Embryonic carcinoma
BFP Basic fetoprotein	G.I. tract cancer, Hepatoma
	Breast cancer, Leukemia
	Malignant lymphoma
Malignin	Glioma, Carcinoma
ALP alkaline phosphatase isoenzyme	
R.I. (Regan isoenzyme)	Genito-urinary cancer
N.I. (Nagao isoenzyme)	Ovarial cancer
K.I. (Kasahara isoenzyme)	Hepatoma
Fetal intestinal type	Hepatoma, G.I. tract cancer
Early placental type	Cancer of lung, pancreas and kidney
γ-GTP isoenzyme	Hepatoma
Amylase	Lung and ovarial cancer
HCG human chorionic gonadotropin	Choriocarcinoma
HTC human carcitonin	Thyroid cancer (mucocellular type)
	Lung small cell carcinoma
	Carcinoid, Pheochromocytoma
	(Apudoma)
ACTH	
ADH	Hormone producing tumor
Erythropoietin	Lung and ovarial cancer
PTH	

retroperitoneal cavity occurs mostly in case of teratocarcinoma which produces AFP. Typical germinoma (two cell pattern pinealoma) rarely metastasizes to other organs. Therefore, the measurement of AFP is important when dissemination or recurrence of the tumor is suspected and is useful for differentiating benign germinoma and malignant teratocarcinoma.

Carcinoembryonic antigen (CEA) was first reported by Gold and Freedman (1965). The serum CEA is detected in patients having endodermal carcinoma. False positive CEA in the serum is, however, often found in patients with chronic inflammatory diseases or heavy smokers. The measurement of CEA is useful for evaluating the efficacy of treatment when it is detected. The carcinofetal glial antigen was reported by Trouilass (1972). Basic fetoprotein is a protein found in human fetal serum and the intestine by Ishii (1978). This protein increases in the serum of patients having stomach cancer, colorectal cancer, advanced lung cancer, breast cancer and malignant lymphoma.

Various enzymes are increasing in the serum of cancer patients and the isoenzyme is characteristic of each type of tumor. Alkaline phosphatase has been widely studied and several types are reported to be significant for each type of cancer.

Fishman found the placental alkaline phosphatase in patients with bronchogenic carcinoma and named it Regan isoenzyme (R.I.) after one of the patients. R.I. increases in the serum, especially in cases of genitourinary cancer. Recently, Nagao isoenzyme (N.I.), Kasahara isoenzyme (K.I.), the fetal intestinal-type and early-placental-type of alkaline phosphatase have been reported. N.I. is detected in the serum of ovarial cancer and K.I. is elevated in cases of hepatoma. The fetal intestinal type of alkaline phosphatase is found in the tissue of hepatoma, stomach and colon cancer, but it is not detected in the serum of those patients. Early placental-type alkaline phosphatase has two types, A and B. Type A is not reactive to any anti-alkaline phosphatase. Type B is reactive to anti-liver alkaline phosphatase and is found in cases of lung, pancreatic and renal cancers. γ-GTP has the characteristics of fetal protein. Hepatoma has specific isoenzymes of I' and II' of γ-GTP and can be differentiated from metastatic liver cancer. Hyper-amylasemia without disorders of the pancreas or parotid gland is found in 1) lung or ovarial cancer, 2) post-surgical patients as a transient increase, and 3) immunoglobulin bound amylasemia. Ectopic enzyme production in the lung or ovarial cancer cells is postulated. In very rare cases, excess enzymes are produced in the cells of carcinoma. The next case is an example of excessive LDH-producing lung adenocarcinoma (Takakura et al., 1971).

Case 1 41-year-old man. NCC 126507. Lung adenocarcinoma. Metastasis to brain.

The patient complained of pain in his right chest wall and shoulder at the age of 40. Six months later, he was attacked by an unconscious adversive seizure. Plain chest x-ray examination revealed a tumor in the right pulmonary upper lobe and an osteolytic lesion in his right second rib. Headache, nausa, vomiting and motor weakness of the right extremities soon appeared. The coin-sized tumor in his left pre-motor area was found in a radioisotope scintigram. Laboratory data revealed an extremely high concentration of serum LDH without any abnormal elevation of other enzymes: LDH, 2,100–3,000 U/ml (normal range, 120–200 U/ml); GOT, 3.3–8.2 U/ml (normal range, 5–15 U/ml); GPT, 2.2 (normal range, < 10 U/ml); alkaline phosphatase, 1.6–3.2 U/ml (normal range, 0.8–2.9 U/ml).

Thirty milligrams of prednisolone was administered daily and radiotherapy (megavoltage x-ray) was given to lung (70 Gy.) and brain (49.5 Gy.) Craniotomy was performed. The serum LDH level decreased from 2,900 U/ml before treatment to 2,000 U/ml after radiotherapy and chemotherapy with Mitomycin C, administered intravenously, and it dropped down to a normal level of 160 U/ml immediately after the removal of the metastatic brain tumor.

The serum LDH concentration changed with the progression and temporal regression of the tumor by chemotherapy. But, in his terminal stage, the serum LDH value increased to 5,000 U/ml without an increase of other serum enzymes. He died four months after the craniotomy. The LDH activity of the tumor removed at surgery was 44,000 U/g tissue and at autopsy it was 76,000 U/g tissue (Table IV-2). The LDH

Table IV-2 LDH activity and isoenzyme pattern of a lung adenocarcinoma patient. (NCC 126507, 41-year-old man)

Specimen	Activity of LDH U/ml or g tissue	LDH isoenzyme				
		L_1	L_2	L_3	L_4	L_5
Primary cancer						
Lung tumor	76,000	43.5%	41.9%	12.6%	2.1%	—
Lung (non tumor tissue)	6,800	3.6	19.6	35.7	28.6	12.5%
Metastatic tumor						
Brain tumor (Surgery)	44,000	32.1	38.7	19.6	8.3	1.2
Brain tumor (Autopsy)	37,000	41.2	39.4	15.6	3.7	—
Brain (non tumor tissue)	9,200	41.3	36.0	19.8	2.9	—
Serum						
Early stage	1,800	42.5	51.2	6.3	—	—
Middle stage	5,300	38.7	47.4	11.8	1.2	0.9
Terminal stage	5,200	47.9	45.2	5.3	1.6	—
Normal adult	126–202	21–33	36–46	23–32	1–6	0–5
CSF						
Collected at the time of surgery	3,200	45.4	38.5	10.9	1.7	3.4
Normal CSF	< 15	42–56	30–36	10–19	1–8	0–2

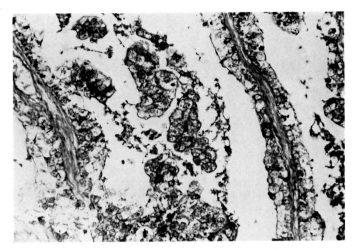

Fig. IV-33 Histological findings of adenocarcinoma (Case 1). Abundant glycogen was found in cytoplasm but disappeared after diastase digestion (Periodic acid Schiff stain).

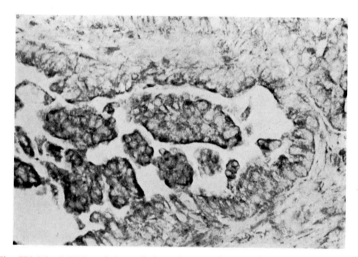

Fig. IV-34 LDH staining of the adenocarcinoma (Case 1). Strong and moderate LDH activities were found in the cytoplasm.

activities of the lung and brain not invaded by tumor were 6,800 U/ml tissue and 9,200 U/g tissue respectively. The LDH isoenzymes of the tumor, serum and cerebrospinal fluid demonstrated the same pattern (dominant L_1 and L_2 types). It was quite different from normal lung or brain LDH isoenzyme patterns. The tumor was histologically diagnosed as papillary adenocarcinoma containing a large amount of glycogen in the cytoplasma (Fig. IV-33). Histochemical staining of the tumor revealed the strong activity of LDH in the tumor cytoplasm (Fig. IV-34). Electron microscopic findings demonstrated the rich mitochondria and glycogen concentration (Fig. IV-35). The autopsy revealed multiple metastases to the brain and disseminated tumors to the pancreas, kidneys, adrenals, thyroid and vertebrae, but not in the liver or heart. There was no special findings in the heart, liver or muscles suggesting abnormal elevation of LDH activity. The excessive production of LDH in the carcinoma cells in this patient was suspected and the activity of LDH in the serum accurately reflected the size of the tumor during the entire course of the disease.

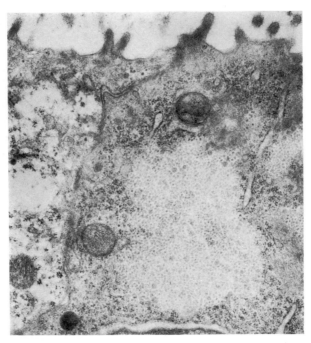

Fig. IV-35   Electron-microscopic findings of the adenocarcinoma (Case 1).   The glycogen has low electron density and does not show a rosette formation.   It is distributed in a large area of the cytoplasm.

Hormones, if present and detected in the serum of patients are good tumor markers.   Human chorionic gonadotropin (HCG) is important in cases of chorio-carcinoma as described previously.   Lung or ovarial carcinomas sometimes have functions producing ectopic hormones.   An ACTH producing tumor causes hypo-potassemia, alkalosis and Cushing's syndrome.   The antidiuretic hormone (ADH) producing tumor is responsible for hypernatremia.   The parathyroid hormone (PTH) producing tumor causes hypercalcemia.   Other hormones produced by tumors include erythropoietin, a colony-stimulating factor that increases white blood cells; prostaglandins, osteoblast-activating factors that stimulate hypercalcemia, gastrin, glucagon, vasoactive intestinal polypeptide (VIP), corticotropin releasing factor (CRF).   These hormones are all polypeptides.   The study of hormone producing tumors will clarify the significance and mechanism of these hormone synthesis in tumor cells and can suggest proper therapeutic plans for the tumors.

V. TREATMENT

PRINCIPLE OF TREATMENT

Metastatic brain tumors are evidently a disease of the central nervous system, but they are also a pathophysiological manifestation of systemic cancer. Therefore, treatment, on one hand, requires neurosurgical techniques to reduce the tumor mass and intracranial pressure and to control brain edema. Selection of chemotherapy, radiotherapy and immunotherapy specific to the central nervous system is essential. On the other hand, treatment also requires a broad knowledge of the oncological characteristics of each primary tumor. Past cases have taught us clearly that simple treatment of the central nervous system alone by surgery or radiotherapy can rarely return the patient to a meaningful life. A multidisciplinary approach to treatment is important for the control of this disease. Cooperative treatment with neurosurgeons and other physicians concerned is of vital importance for each patient.

Once clinical signs of metastasis to the central nervous system appear, the progression of the fatal symptoms is extremely rapid. Without treatment, the patient cannot expect to survive more than few months. Therefore, quick action to establish an appropriate method of treatment for each patient is urgent, not only with regard to oncological characteristics but also the background of the patient's life.

In the first step, the control of brain edema is essential. Surgical treatment should be indicated with extreme care. Thoughtless surgery will give the patient nothing more than a burden. The effects of radiotherapy and chemotherapy should not be overlooked. In the second step, maintenance therapy is indispensable. Chemotherapy and possibly immunotherapy should significantly benefit the patient.

The purpose of treating metastatic brain tumors is to enable the patient to live a useful life as long as possible, and not to induce further suffering by conducting inappropriate treatment. We believe that, in the past, pessimism caused many precious lives to be lost. On the other hand, it is true that optimism has placed unnecessary responsibilities on the patient. The physician must have his own philosophy on how to best treat metastatic brain tumors.

Table V-1 Surgical mortality for metastatic brain tumors.

Author	Mortality (30 days after craniotomy)
Grant (Cushing's series) (1926)	36%
Cushing (1932)	25
Störtebecker (1954)	25 (20 days)
Petit-Dutaillis et al. (1956)	30
Arseni et al. (1956)	30
Leitholf & Kuhlendahl (1957)	33
Bakay (1958)	45
Garde et al. (1958)	48
Simionescu (1960)	38
Brihaye & Martin (1961)	29
Richards & McKissock (1963)	32
Mansuy et al. (1964)	39
Lang & Slater (1964)	22
Støier (1965)	40
Vieth & Odom (1965a)	15 (2 weeks)
D'Andréa & de Divities (1966)	35
Raskind et al. (1971)	12 (2 weeks)
McGee (1971)	26
Haar & Patterson, Jr. (1972)	25 (1932–49)
	10 (1950–54)
	9 (1955–59)
	3 (1960–64)
	11 (1965–69)
Palma (1972)	12
Constans et al. (1973b)	8 (3 weeks)
Paillas et al. (1974a)	29 (before 1956)
	19 (1956–66)
	18 (1966–74)
Maspes (Cited by Paillas et al.) (1974b)	16 (1930–56)
	8 (1956–66)
Salerno et al. (1978)	22
Ransohoff (1980)	10
Gamache et al. (1980)	9
Takakura (Current study) (1981)	14 (1960–75)
	0 (1976–80)

year, and seven patients (4.4%) lived more than five years after surgery.

Radiotherapy has gradually been introduced for treatment of metastatic brain tumors. Combined treatment with surgery and radiation brought better prognosis than surgical treatment alone. Deeley and Rice-Edwards (1968) insisted that radiation should be given to a brain metastasis from lung cancer. McGee (1971) surgically removed the tumor in 27 patients and gave radiation. Fifty-six per cent of them lived more than one year, the longest survival time being more than 32 months after surgery. Magilligan and his co-workers (1976) stated that whole brain radiotherapy was an important factor in prolonging life after extirpation of a brain metastasis. Thirty-two per cent of their patients lived more than one year. Patients with lung cancer who survived more than five years after surgery have been reported by several neurosurgeons. Bakay (1958), Simionescu (1960), and Modesti and Feldman (1975) each reported a case of metastatic lung cancer that survived more than five years, McGee (1971) six years, Raskind et al. (1969) and Tarnoff et al. (1976) seven years, Hendricks et al. (1972) and Haar and Patterson, Jr. (1972) ten years, and Mosberg, Jr. (1976) twelve years. Daniel (1964) reported a lung cancer patient surviving 16 years after craniotomy.

Vieth and Odom (1965a) surgically removed 155 metastatic brain tumors. In their series, seven patients lived more than five years, and three patients lived more than ten years. Salerno et al. (1978) in Montreal have reported the best results in history. They surgically removed both primary tumors and brain metastases of 23 lung cancer patients. Five patients (23%) lived longer than two years and three of them are leading productive lives ten years or more after surgery and radiation therapy.

Modesti and Feldman (1975) of the Veterans Administrative Hospital at the State University of New York stated: "Despite the generally unfavourable statistics with regard to metastasis of carcinoma of the lung to the brain, aggressive treatment of this disorder may have extremely rewarding results in selected instances. Rapid death has been the universal course if no treatment is offered. Radiotherapy with or without administration of steroids has had palliative effects, but long term survival has not been reported. In cases in which metastatic lesions are solitary, as determined by currently available clinical diagnostic procedures and in which the patients general condition is satisfactory to withstand surgery, surgical extirpation of the lesion should be attempted."

The recent advances of CT scanning have enabled precise diagnosis of the metastasis. The multiplicity of metastatic tumors, even if some of them are quite small in size, can be easily detected. The surgical indication today is, thus, selected in a more rational way.

Mode of Surgery and General Prognosis

Since 1960, 616 patients with metastatic brain tumors were refered to our neurosurgical clinics. Two hundred fifty-nine (42.0%) of these patients received surgical treatment (Table V-2), and 115 patients (44.4%) had metastatic brain tumors from lung, and 32 (12.4%) from breast cancer. Cancer of the gastrointestinal tract (20

Table V-2 Surgical treatment and radio-therapy for metastatic brain tumors.

Primary tumor	Total No. of patients	Total No. of surgery	Type of surgery			Surgery alone	Surgery + Radiation
			Total extirpation	Partial extirpation	Decomp-ression		
Lung	278	115	54	40	21	64	51
Breast	100	32	9	17	6	21	11
Gastrointestinal tract	42	20	6	3	11	12	8
Genitourinary organs	42	22	8	8	6	12	10
Thyroid	12	10	7	2	1	6	4
Thymus	2	2	2	0	0	1	1
Parotis	3	2	2	0	0	1	1
Head and neck	16	12	6	5	1	4	8
Skin	6	5	3	2	0	2	3
Retinoblastoma	15	4	0	0	4	0	4
Leukemia	26	1	0	0	1	0	1
Sarcoma	50	17	3	5	9	3	14
Others & unknown	24	17	7	3	7	15	2
Total	**616**	**259**	**107**	**85**	**67**	**141**	**118**

cases), genitourinary organs (22 cases) and various types of sarcomas were other major origins of brain metastasis. As for the mode of surgery, total extirpation of a single brain metastasis was performed in 107 (41.3%), partial extirpation in 85 (32.8%) and decompression or ventricular drainage in 67 (25.9%) patients. Surgery alone was given as therapeutic procedure to 141 patients (54.4%), and surgery combined with radiotherapy was given to 118 patients (45.6%).

The median survival time of patients treated by surgery is summarized in Table V-3. The median survival time of all 259 patients after the onset of neurological signs was 13.2 months, and the median survival time after surgery for brain metastasis was 9.1 months. In patients receiving surgery alone, the median survival time after the onset of neurological signs was 10.9 months. The median survival time after surgery was 6.1 months. In cases treated by surgery and radiation, the median survival time after the onset of neurological signs was 15.9 months, while the median survival time after surgery was 12.5 months. Therefore, the survival time was extended by using combined radiotherapy about five to six months.

Postsurgical survival times differ greatly according to the type of primary cancer (Weller, 1929; Boucot et al., 1959; Cappelen, Jr. et al., 1961; Carbone et al., 1970). Cancer of the parotid gland, other cancers of the head and neck originating mainly from sinuses or the upper jaw, and skin cancer originating from the scalp showed the best median survival times, 44.5, 21.7 and 20.2 months after surgery, respectively. These tumors, however, invaded the skull directly, and did not represent true metastasis. Retinoblastoma invaded the intracranial cavity through the optic nerve and disseminated via the CSF canal. Cancers of the gastrointestinal tract and leukemia showed the worst prognosis, since leukemia and metastasis from stomach cancer generally result in meningeal carcinomatosis.

Surgical mortality and actual survival rates are shown in Table V-4. Postsurgical death in our series was counted on the basis of the number of patients who died within one month after surgery. The surgical mortality of all 259 patients treated by neurosurgical management was 13.9 per cent. It was highest (30.0%) in metastasis from gastrointestinal cancers, since many stomach cancer patients had meningeal carcinomatosis besides nodulous metastases. The surgical mortality of metastasis from lung cancer revealed the lowest figure of 9.6 per cent. In lung cancer, the patients were best selected for neurosurgical management, since brain metastasis from lung cancer is common and we are familiar with how to manage it properly. Surgical mortality rates of breast cancer, urogenital cancer and various other tumors were 15.6, 22.7 and 12.9 per cent, respectively. The surgical mortality, however, was reduced to zero per cent in our clinic after 1976 when CT was introduced for examination. Since then the surgical indication has been well established by the aid of CT.

The postsurgical survival rate (Table V-4 and Fig. V-1) was defined as the ratio of patients alive versus the total number of patients (Berkson and Gage, 1950; Effler and Barr, 1960). Two hundred twenty-three (86.1%) of all 259 patients were alive one month after surgery. The survival rates 1, 2, 3, 4 and 5 years after neurosurgical management were 26.5, 12.6, 4.5, 4.0 and 2.7 per cent, respectively (Tables V-4 and 5).

The long-term survivors who were alive more than five years after neurosurgical

Table V-3 Median survival time of metastatic brain tumors treated by surgery.

Primary tumor	Total No. of patients	Median survival time after onset of neurological signs	Median survival time after surgery	Surgery alone			Surgery + Radiation		
				No. of patients	Median survival time after onset of neurological signs	Median survival time after surgery	No. of patients	Median survival time after onset of neurological signs	Median survival time after surgery
Lung	115	11.2 mos	7.7 mos	64	9.0 mos	5.1 mos	51	13.9 mos	10.9 mos
Breast	32	11.2	7.4	21	9.1	5.0	11	15.1	11.8
Gastrointestinal tract	20	7.5	3.8	12	6.4	2.8	8	9.1	5.2
Genitourinary organs	22	15.9	13.0	12	10.3	7.0	10	22.6	20.2
Thyroid	10	20.8	13.6	6	19.5	12.4	4	22.8	15.3
Thymus	2	16.5	15.0	1	22.0	21.0	1	11.0	9.0
Parotis	2	47.0	44.5	1	32.0	29.0	1	62.0	60.0
Head & neck	12	31.8	21.7	4	33.5	14.5	8	30.1	25.3
Skin	5	24.4	20.2	2	22.0	20.5	3	26.0	20.0
Retinoblastoma	4	10.0	8.3	0	—	—	4	10.0	8.3
Leukemia	1	2.0	1.0	0	—	—	1	2.0	1.0
Sarcoma	17	10.1	6.4	3	4.3	2.7	14	11.4	7.2
Others and Unknown	17	12.8	5.5	14	13.9	5.7	3	7.7	4.7
Total	**259**	**13.2**	**9.1**	**140**	**10.9**	**6.1**	**119**	**15.9**	**12.5**

Table V-4 The surgical mortality and survival rate of metastatic brain tumors treated by surgey.

Primary tumor	Total No. of patients	No. of surgical death	Surgical mortality	Survival rate after surgery (months)											
				3	6	9	12	18	24	30	36	42	48	54	60
Lung	115	11	9.6%	77.5%	42.2%	30.4%	22.5%	8.8%	6.9%	2.9%	2.9%	2.0%	2.0%	2.0%	1.0%
Breast	32	5	15.6	84.6	38.5	26.9	23.1	11.5	11.5	3.8	3.8	3.8	3.8	3.8	3.8
GI tract	20	6	30.0	64.3	35.7	14.3	14.3	7.1	0.0	0.0	0.0	0.0	0.0	0.0	0.0
Genitourinary organs	22	5	22.7	82.4	58.8	47.1	35.3	23.5	17.6	17.6	11.8	11.8	11.8	11.8	11.8
Others	70	9	12.9	77.0	50.8	47.5	36.1	34.4	24.6	9.8	6.6	6.6	6.6	3.3	3.3
Total	**259**	**36**	**13.9**	**76.3**	**44.2**	**34.4**	**26.5**	**17.0**	**12.6**	**5.8**	**4.5**	**4.0**	**4.0**	**3.1**	**2.7**

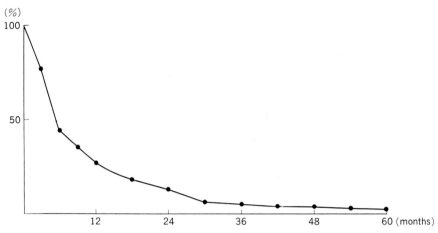

Fig. V-1 Survival rate of patients with metastatic brain tumors treated by surgery
(260 cases).

Table V-5 Long term survival of metastatic brain
tumors treated by surgery (223 cases*).

Year after surgery	No. of patients alive	
1	59	26.5%
2	28	12.6
3	10	4.5
4	9	4.0
5	6	2.7

* Excluding postsurgical death.

Cases that survived more than five years after craniotomy.

1	Uterine ca.	9Y1M*
2	Lung ca.	8Y6M
3	Chorioca.	8Y6M*
4	Maxillary cancer	6Y9M*
5	Breast ca.	5Y2M
6	Parotid ca.	5Y0M

* Still alive in good condition.

management are also listed in Table V-5. The longest survivor is a case of metastatic
uterine cancer (adeno-squamous cell carcinoma) who has lived nine years and one
month after craniotomy, and she is still active today in social life without any
evidence of recurrence. The second longest survivor is a patient with a single metastasis from lung squamous cell carcinoma who lived eight and half years after
craniotomy. Other long-term survivors are cases of choriocarcinoma (brain and lung
metastases, alive and active eight years and six months after craniotomy), maxillary
carcinoma (direct invasion, alive six years and nine months), breast cancer died five
years and two months later) and parotid cancer (a case of direct invasion who died
five years later).

Results of Surgical Treatment of Metastatic Brain Tumors in Each Type of Cancer

Lung Cancer

The mode of surgery and the median survival time of metastatic brain tumors from lung cancer are summarized in Table V-6. Out of the 115 patients treated by neurosurgical management, 54 (47.0%) received total extirpation of the single brain metastasis. Partital extirpation was performed in 40 patients (34.8%) and decompression or ventricular drainage was performed in 21 patients (18.3%).

Surgical mortality is naturally dependent on the mode of surgery. In cases whose brain metastasis was totally removed, the surgical mortality was only 3.7 per cent, while in cases who were treated by partial removal or merely decompression, the operative mortalities were 5.0 and 33.3 per cent, respectively. Median survival time after surgery of the 115 patients was 7.9 months. Median survival time were 11.7 months in totally extirpated cases, 5.3 months in partially extirpated cases, and 3.0 months in the cases merely received decompressive surgery.

Surgery combined with radiotherapy revealed a prolongation of postsurgical life time. Fifty-four patients (47.0%) received postsurgical radiotherapy. Their median survival time was 11.1 months, while 61 patients (53.0%) who received no radiotherapy lived an average of 5.1 months after surgery. The median survival times of patients who received radiotherapy were 18.2 months in totally extirpated patients, 6.0 months in partially extirpated cases and 4.2 months in merely decompressed patients. On the other hand, comparable figures for those patients who did not receive radiotherapy were 6.6 months in totally extirpated cases, 4.5 months in partially extirpated cases and only 2.3 months in decompressed patients.

A major factor in the success of surgery is the number of intracranial metastases. A well-demarcated single metastasis can be removed completely. The prognosis of patients who had single or multiple metastases was compared in cases of lung cancer (Table V-7). The 84 patients having a single brain metastasis demonstrated a median postsurgical survival time of 8.9 months, while the comparable figure for 31 patients with multiple metastases was 4.4 months.

Table V-6 Mode of surgery and Median survival time of metastatic brain tumors from lung cancer.

Mode of surgery	No. of patients	Surgical mortality	Median survival time after surgery	Radiation			
				+		−	
				No. of cases	Median surv.	No. of cases	Median surv.
Total extirpation	54	3.7%	11.7 mos	24	18.2 mos	30	6.6 mos
Partial extirpation	40	5.0	5.3	21	6.0	19	4.5
Decompression	21	33.3	3.1	9	4.2	12	2.3
Total	**115**	**9.6**	**7.9**	**54**	**11.1**	**61**	**5.1**

Table V-7 Median survival time of metastatic brain tumors from lung cancer after surgery (Number of metastases).

Type of metastasis	No. of patients	Median survival time after surgery
Single	84	8.9 mos
Multiple	31	4.4
Total	**115**	**7.7**

Table V-8 Histological type of lung cancer and the median survival time after surgical treatment of metastases to brain.

Histological type	No. of patients	Median survival time after surgery	Radiotherapy + No. of cases	Radiotherapy + Med. surv.	Radiotherapy − No. of cases	Radiotherapy − Med. surv.
Adenocarcinoma	67	7.3 mos	24	10.7 mos	43	5.5 mos
Squamous cell carcinoma	19	14.4	13	17.7	6	7.3
Undifferentiated	21	5.0	11	6.0	10	3.8
Small cell	4	1.5	1	1.0	3	1.7
Large cell	10	6.9	9	7.1	1	5.0
Not specified	7	4.1	1	1.0	6	4.7
Total	**107**	**8.2**	**48**	**11.5**	**59**	**5.4**

* Cases of decompressive surgery without verification of histological types are excluded. All those cases died in short time after surgery.

The histological type of the lung cancer also has an influence on the prognosis of the brain metastasis (Table V-8). The histological type of the brain metastasis was verified in 107 patients. Median survival times after surgery of the various histological types were 7.3 months in adenocarcinoma, 14.4 months in squamous cell carcinoma and 5.0 months in undifferentiated carcinoma. Squamous cell carcinoma demonstrated the best median survival period. The prognosis of undifferentiated carcinoma, especially in small cell carcinoma, was poor. There might be no indication of surgical management of a metastatic brain tumor from small cell carcinomas of lung cancer. The details of the prognosis of each histological type, treated by surgery combined with radiotherapy, are summarized in Table V-8.

Breast Cancer

It is well known that breast cancer is a highly hormone-dependent tumor and that more than half of the patients are hormone sensitive. The details of hormonal treatment for brain tumor metastasis from breast cancer will be discussed later. Table V-9 gives a summary of the mode of surgery, surgical mortality and the median survival time of patients with metastatic brain tumors from breast cancer.

The surgical mortality of all 32 patients was 9.4 per cent. There was no post-surgical death in cases whose metastases were totally extirpated. Surgical mortalities were 11.8 per cent for partially extirpated tumors and 16.7 per cent in cases that were merely decompressed.

Table V-9 Mode of surgery and median survival time of metastatic brain tumors from breast cancer.

Mode of surgery	Total No. of patients	Surgical mortality	Median survival time after surgery	Radiation			
				+		−	
				No. of cases	Med. surv.	No. of cases	Med. surv.
Total extirpation	9	0%	15.8 mos	6	16.6 mos	3	14.3 mos
Partial extirpation	17	11.8	4.2	4	4.8	13	4.0
Decompression	6	16.7	3.6	1	11.0	5	2.1
Total	**32**	**9.4**	**7.4**	**11**	**11.8**	**21**	**5.0**

The median survival time after neurosurgical management was 7.4 months. The same figure for totally extirpated cases was 15.8 months, 4.2 months in partially extirpated cases, and 3.6 months in decompressed cases.

Effects of combined radiotherapy for prolongation of life span are summarized in Table V-9.

Cancers of the Gastrointestinal Tract

Stomach cancer is the most common malignancy in Japan, while colon or rectal cancers are less frequent compared with European countries, the United States or Canada. Out of a total of 20 patients treated with neurosurgical management, ten cases (50%) involved metastases from stomach cancer.

The median survival time from the onset of neurological signs was 2.6 months in cases treated without neurosurgical management, while it was 8.3 months in cases treated with surgery (Table V-10-1).

Intracranial metastases of liver carcinoma or hepatoma are very rare. Even though the median survival time after the onset of neurological signs was 13.0 months and longer than cases of other origin, there is no statistically significant difference in survival times among the cancers in this group. The median survival time after neurosurgical management for cancers of the gastrointestinal tract was 3.7 months.

The median survival time after surgery in cases of stomach cancer was 2.7 months. This poor prognosis might be attributed to its pathological type of dissemination. Half of the patients with stomach cancer demonstrated meningeal infiltration of malignant cells accompanied by solitary metastatic nodules in the parenchyma.

Cancers of Genitourinary Organs

Out of 42 patients with genitourinary cancers, 17 patients showed brain metastasis from uterine carcinoma, and 14 patients had renal clear cell carcinoma (hypernephroma, Grawitz's tumor). Choriocarcinoma is not very common now, since it is well controlled and can often be cured by chemotherapy with Actinomycin D and methotrexate.

The median survival time from the onset of neurological signs of the 42 patients with genitourinary cancers was 11.0 months. In cases treated without

Table V-10-1 Survival time of metastatic brain tumors from cancers of gastrointestinal tract.

Primary tumor	Total No. of patients	Median survival time from the onset of neurological signs	Surgical treatment −		Surgical treatment +			Effect of Radiation
			No. of cases	Median surv. after the onset of neurol. signs	No. of cases	Median surv. after the onset of neurol. signs	Median surv. after surgery	
Esophagus	6	6.7 mos	2	3.5 mos	4	8.3 mos	5.5 mos	Rad + — (0)* Rad − 5.5 mos (4)
Stomach	26	4.0	16	2.6	10	6.2	2.7	Rad + 5.9 (4) Rad − 0.5 (6)
Colon & rectum	7	4.5	3	3.0	4	7.0	3.3	Rad + 2.5 (2) Rad − 4.0 (2)
Liver	2	13.0	0	—	2	13.0	6.5	Rad + 6.5 (2) Rad − (0)
Pancreas	1	1.0	1	1.0	0	—	—	Rad −
Total	**42**	**4.8**	**22**	**2.6**	**20**	**8.3**	**3.7**	**Rad + 5.2 (8)** **Rad − 2.8 (12)**

Table V-10-2 Survival time of metastatic brain tumors from cancer of genitourinary organs.

Primary tumor	Total No. of patients	Median survival time from the onset of neurological signs	Surgical treatment −		Surgical treatment +			Effect of Radiation
			No. of cases	Median surv. after the onset of neurol. signs	No. of cases	Median surv. after the onset of neurol. signs	Median surv. after surgery	
Kidney	14	12.1 mos	6	9.6 mos	8	13.9 mos	10.3 mos	Rad + 1.0 (1)* Rad − 10.9 (7)
Urinary bladder	2	10.5	0	—	2	10.5	8.5	Rad + 8.5 (2) Rad − (0)
Uterus	17	9.9	9	2.7	8	18.0	14.8	Rad + 22.7 (5) Rad − 1.5 (3)
Chorioca.	4	21.0	1	2.0	3	27.3	26.0	Rad + 74.0 (1) Rad − 2.0 (2)
Testis	4	2.5	3	3.0	1	1.0	0.1	Rad + (0) Rad − 1.0 (1)
Prostate	1	11.0	1	11.0	0	—	—	Rad + (0) Rad − (0)
Total	**42**	**11.0**	**20**	**5.2**	**22**	**16.3**	**13.4**	**Rad + 22.8 (9)** **Rad − 6.6 (13)**

* Number in parentheses indicates the number of patients.

neurosurgical management, it was 5.2 months. The median survival time was 16.3 months in cases treated with surgery. The figure after neurosurgical management was 13.4 months. In cases of metastatic brain tumors from choriocarcinoma, the median survival time after surgery was 26.0 months, the longest of all. It is attributed to one case with a good postsurgical course. The patient is alive today at eight years after craniotomy, recurrence being prevented by combined chemo-radio-immuno-therapy. The median survival times after surgery were 10.3 months in cases of renal carcinoma, 8.5 months in cases of carcinoma of the urinary bladder and 14.8 months in cases of uterine carcinoma. Table V-10-2 summarizes the effects of combined radiotherapy on the median survival time.

Miscellaneous Cancers

Thyroid cancer is sensitive to internal radiotherapy using radioactive iodine, ^{131}I, after pretreatment with TSH. The prognosis of patients having brain metastases from thyroid cancer is better than that for lung, breast or gastrointestinal cancers. The median survival time after the onset of neurological signs was 20.8 months and that after surgery 13.5 months. Five out of ten patients treated with neurosurgical management lived more than one year, and three of them more than two years.

Head and neck cancers rarely metastasize to the brain via vascular routes but generally directly invade the intracranial cavity and compress the brain. These cancers can be removed or controlled rather easily by radiotherapy, since the tumor is located on the surface of the brain. The median survival time of head and neck cancer cases was 31.3 months after the onset of neurological signs, and 21.9 months after neurosurgical management.

The prognosis of patients with intracranial metastasis of various sarcomas is generally poor. Only two cases of metastasis from alveolar soft part sarcoma lived more than two years after surgery. The other case of metastasis from liposarcoma lived more than one year. Some sarcomas are, however, sensitive to radiation and chemotherapy, and it is expected that chemo-radiotherapy will better control tumor progression in the future. The median survival times of metastatic brain tumors from miscellaneous origins are summarized in Table V-3. The median survival times of metastatic brain tumors treated with or without neurosurgical management were compared. This comparison has, however, no significance, since the neurosurgical management was always performed when the surgical indication was established. The median survival time after the onset of neurological symptoms was 5.2 months in 357 cases treated without surgery and 13.2 months in 259 cases treated with surgery. Survival times after the onset of neurological symptoms in cases treated without surgery were: 4.0 months in lung cancer, 4.4 months in breast cancer, 2.7 months in gastrointestinal cancer and 5.2 months in genitourinary cancer cases. The figures in cases treated with surgery were 11.2 months in lung cancer, 11.2 months in breast cancer, 7.5 months in gastrointestinal cancer, and 15.9 months in genitourinary cancer patients.

Indication

The indication for surgical management is dependent on the state of intracranial metastasis, the primary tumor and the general condition of the patient.

The State of Intracranial Metastasis

The best indication is a single and solitary metastasis (Meyerson and Reynolds, 1967) located in a region accessible to surgical manipulation. Even if the tumor is located in a subcortical area just on the Sylvian fissure, the tumor can usually be removed from either the anterior or posterior side of the Sylvian fissure without any major damage to the cortex of motor or sensory areas. The patient generally demonstrates amazingly good recovery from the motor or sensory dysfunction. When the tumor is located in the brain stem, there is no surgical indication at all. Even in multiple metastases, if they are accessible for surgery, it might sometimes be possible to remove them (Shimizu et al., 1976). We have a patient with metastases from lung cancer who survived four and half years in good condition after two operations on both supra- and infratentorial tumors.

The following case of metastatic brain tumor from lung adenocarcinoma suggested the possibility of surgical management for multiple metastases.

> **Case 1** 62-year-old woman.   UT 79109.
> Lung adenocarcinoma, multiple metastases to both hemispheres of brain.
> Left pulmonary upper lobectomy was performed for lung cancer in November 1977. In January 1979, she began to notice motor weakness of her right upper and lower extremities and difficulty of speech. She was admitted to our clinic on April 26, 1979. She was alert, but right hemiplegia and complete motor aphasia were evident. Marked bilateral choked discs were noted. CT revealed a large metastatic tumor nodule in her left parietal lobe surrounded by extensive brain edema. A tiny tumor nodule in the right border of the falx and a small nodule surrounded by brain edema in the right parietal lobe were also detected (Fig. IV-10A). The total removal of the major tumor mass in her left hemisphere was performed on April 28, 1979. The tumor nodule in the right parietal lobe was clearly seen on a CT scan taken on May 7, 1979. After the surgery, she was given chemotherapy with tegafur (800 mg administered orally a day) for two months without radiotherapy. The remaining tumors have disappeared completely from the CT scan after the chemotherapy (Fig. IV-10B, C). Her neurological symptoms gradually ameliorated and she began to talk and walk slowly. She was in good mental condition in November 1980 without evidence of recurrence of brain metastasis at one year and seven months after the craniotomy.

In cases of meningeal carcinomatosis, there is usually no surgical indication. Only when a hydrocephalic condition is noted, the ventricular drainage or the insertion of a catheter both for removal of cerebrospinal fluid and application of chemotherapeutic agents is indicated. Surgery is not indicated in diffuse metastases. Decompressive surgery without removal of the tumor or ventricular drainage for patients demonstrating increased intracranial pressure is hazardous and contraindicated. It must be kept in mind that surgery for a metastatic tumor should aim for the total extirpation of the intracranial tumor mass. Biopsy should be avoided when diagnosis could be made in other ways. It should also be remembered that in most cases, steroid hormones could control extensive brain edema and that chemo-radio-therapy can extensively regress the tumor. If the limitations of surgery are well realized by surgeons, the benefit of surgical treatment for metastatic brain tumors will be increased.

Condition of the Primary Tumor

In cases whose primary tumors are cured or suppressed almost completely, there are indications for neurosurgical management of brain metastasis. If the primary tumor is active and progresses rapidly, there is no indication for brain surgery. For lung cancer patients, squamous cell carcinoma or adenocarcinoma can be considered for brain surgery. There is, however, no surgical indication for undifferentiated carcinoma, especially in cases of small cell carcinoma.

In cases of slow-growing carcinoma such as thyroid cancer, a surgical indication for brain metastasis is worthwhile to consider, even when the primary cancer remains. The biological characteristics of each tumor is another main factor employed to establish indications for surgical treatment of brain metastasis. For instance, in cases of choriocarcinoma, even when the primary tumor disseminates to various organs, there might be a chance to cure the disease by chemotherapy. In such a case, a craniotomy should be considered for removing the emergent condition of increased intracranial pressure.

General Condition

In general, the presence of liver metastasis is a limiting factor for neurosurgical management. Cachexia, decreasing renal and liver functions, leukopenia, thrombocytopenia, severe anemia and a bleeding tendency are also limiting factors for further treatment. Diabetes mellitus should fully be examined, since a large amount of glucocorticoid is generally administered to patients with brain metastasis before and after surgical treatment.

The indications and contraindications for surgical treatment of metastatic intracranial tumors are summarized as follows:
1) Indications
    a. State of primary tumor.
       The primary tumor is cured or to be cured. It can at least be properly controlled for a long period.
    b. Good general condition of the patient.
    c. No metastasis to other vital organs.
       No metastasis to the liver nor presence of uncontrollable tumors in the lung.
    d. State of metastatic intracranial tumor.
       Single and solitary metastasis.
       Easily accessible for surgical removal.
       In a case of multiple metastases, surgical treatment is generally not

accepted, but if a major tumor nodule can be removed and other small tumors can be controlled by radiation or chemotherapy, it is worthwhile to perform craniotomy.

2) Contraindications
   a. Diffuse or disseminated intracranial metastases.
   b. Poor general condition.
   c. Presence of metastasis to other vital organs especially to the liver and lung.
   d. Progressive and uncontrollable expansion of the primary tumor.

Surgical Management

Preoperative Care

It is very important to devise ways to manage brain edema associated with a metastatic tumor. The extent of edema can be accurately measured by CT. Most symptoms generally disappear soon after the administration of glucocorticoids, and the dose of steroid hormones depends on the degree of severity. A suggestive initial dosage of steroid hormone administration is as follows:

Rp	Prednisolone	40 to 60 mg/day
Rp	Betamethasone	8 to 16 mg/day
	or Dexamethasone	8 to 16 mg/day

The daily dose is decreased according to the subsidence of symptoms. The regular maintenance dosages are prednisolone 20 mg/day and betamethasone or dexamethasone 4–6 mg/day. When a patient shows severe symptoms such as consciousness disturbances or continuous vomiting or nausea, mannitol or glycerol should be given intravenously. When patients demonstrate dehydration, the infusion of an electrolyte-balanced solution is necessary.

A suggestive regimen for infusion is

Mannitol (20%)   200 ml   intravenously (speedy infusion),
followed by slow infusion of

Electrolyte-balanced solution   500 ml
Hydrocortisone   200 mg
(or prednisolone   40 mg   } for the intial
or dexa- or betamethasone   4 to 8 mg } infusion.
with an antiemetic or a sedative (slow infusion).

It is quite common that patients with metastatic brain tumors show convulsive seizures. Anticonvulsants should be always given orally. The most common prescription is

Rp   { Phenobarbital   100 mg
     { Diphenylhydantoin   300 mg
                                Three times a day, after meals.

In severe cases, oxygen inhalation helps to relieve the increased intracranial pressure.

Surgical Technique

When the skin incision is started, 200 to 500 ml of mannitol is given intravenously. A sufficient amount of steroid hormones should also be given before the surgery. After finishing craniotomy, hyperventilation is started before excision of the dura mater. By these three procedures, hazardous swelling of the brain can be properly controlled. The tumor is usually situated subcortically and the surface of the brain shows an extensive edematous appearance (Plate V-1, p. 212). Tapping is necessary to identify the depth of the tumor and also to evacuate any cystic or necrotic fluid (Plate V-2, p. 212). The nature of cystic fluid varies in each case. It sometimes contains clear xanthochromic or bloody fluid, or viscous pus-like necrotic fluid. The evacuation of cystic fluid will often help further surgical removal of the tumor. Corticotomy is performed in the next step to reach the surface of the tumor. The tumor is usually well demarcated from the normal brain with a layer of necrotic brain tissue. Although some textbooks suggest the use of a finger to enucleate the tumor in case of metastatic neoplasms, it is not advisable. If the tumor is situated under the Sylvian fissure, finger manipulation will cause a permanent neurological deficit. If the tumor is removed in a gentle way like a meningioma, using fine-tipped suction and covering the surrounding brain with a cotton pledget, quick recovery of the patient from neurological symptoms will be expected. Neurosurgeons should perform surgery gently even through it is a metastatic brain tumor. Hemostasis is easy when the tumor is totally removed (Plate V-3, p. 213). It should be noted that some types of metastatic tumors such as renal clear cell carcinoma are highly vascular and need meticulous manipulation such as in cases of meningiomas.

Whenever the surgical indication is established and the design of surgery planned, the surgeon should try to remove the tumor completely. Even if the metastatic tumors are multiple, it is worthwhile to try to remove all of major tumor nodules, if possible (Plate V-4, p. 213). Partial removal of the tumor or biopsy or simple decompression will not benefit the patient. All or none is the basic philosophy for operating on metastatic tumors.

In rare cases, ventricular drainage for removal of excess cerebrospinal fluid and administration of chemotherapeutic agents is applicable to meningeal carcinomatous infiltration accompanied by a hydrocephalic state.

The choice of craniotomy or craniectomy depends on the condition of the edematous brain. The use of an artificial dura mater should be avoided if possible, since it is soft and can sometimes cause brain damage at the edge of the patients' dura mater if extensive postoperative brain swelling occurs. Fascia lata or lyophilized dura mater is advisable for use in those cases.

Postoperative Care

An adequate oxygen supply and glucocorticoid administration are indispensable for subsiding postoperative brain edema. Patients are usually put in oxygen tents for two days postoperatively. Mannitol is sometimes used for a few days, but only when the intracranial pressure is considered to be high. Complications generally do not occur if the tumor is totally extirpated.

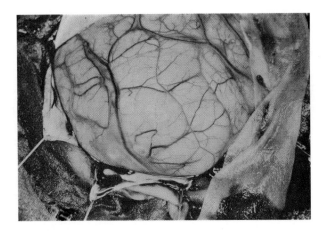

Plate V-1   Edematous brain cortex due to metastatic brain tumor.   The
tumor is subcortically located.

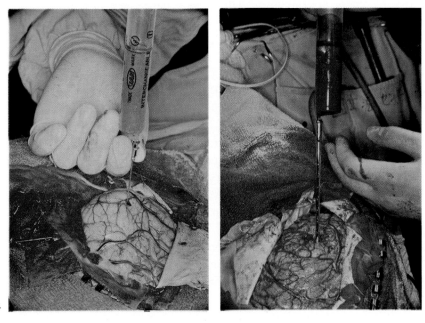

Plate V-2   Tapping of the metastatic tumor.   Xanthochromic (A), bloody
(B) or often necrotic, pus-like fluid is aspirated.

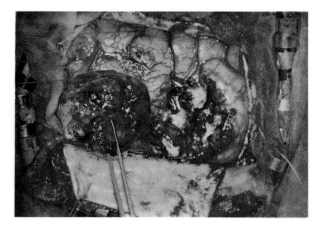

Plate V-3 Removal of a metastatic tumor from lung cancer. A well-demarcated tumor was extirpated.

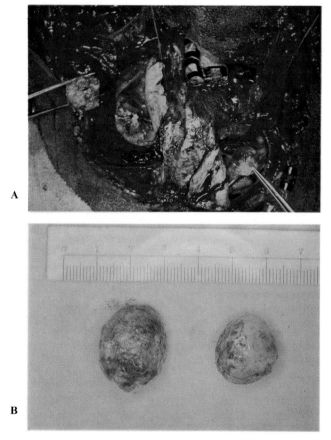

A

B

Plate V-4 Removal of double metastases from breast cancer. The tumors were simultaneously enucleated from both sides of the occipital lobes (A). Extirpated tumors (B).

RADIOTHERAPY

Historical Note

Radiotherapy for metastatic brain tumors started more than half a century ago. In earlier days, both x-ray and local radium application were utilized for radiotherapy. In 1931, Lenz and Freid reported the results of radiotherapy in five patients suffering from metastatic brain tumors from breast cancer. Three of these patients had shown an increased intracranial pressure. In the first case, the headache disappeared after four months of x-ray treatment. Recurrence was then noted, and radiotherapy again brought temporary relief. In the second case, the headache was relieved for six months. In the third case, the headache and Jacksonian convulsive seizures disappeared following the application of a small amount of radium and x-ray treatment to the opposite side of the brain. These three cases survived 11, 18 and 20 months respectively after the onset of neurological symptoms. The remaining two cases showed localized neurological symptoms without increased intracranial pressure. One patient demonstrated improvement of clinical signs following a small radium pack, while the other showed no improvement following x-ray therapy. Dyke and Davidoff (1942) reported three cases treated by radiotherapy. In the first case, the patient's return to social life was accomplished. In the second case, marked relief of symptoms was noted, and in the third case, no improvement whatsoever was demonstrated. Richmond (1949) reported eight cases including three cases of lung cancer. Symptomatic relief was obtained in five cases. Since brain metastases appear frequently in multiple sites and often in the form of disseminated type or meningeal carcinomatosis, irradiation of the entire brain became a regular therapeutic procedure. Burford (1950), Holmes and Schulz (1950) reported that symptomatic palliation was obtained with a tumor dose of 20 to 30 Gy. by whole brain irradiation.

A large series of radiotherapy for metastatic brain tumors were sequentially reported by Chao et al. (1954), Chu and Hilaris (1961) and Nisce et al. (1971) of the Department of Radiotherapy at Memorial Hospital in New York. Chao and his associates first published the results of radiotherapy for 35 metastatic brain tumor patients, collected during the period from 1949 through 1953. Twenty-four out of the 38 treated cases showed worthwhile palliation. Chu and Hilaris gathered 218 cases treated between 1954 and 1958. Radiation consisting of a total dose of 30 Gy. was given in three weeks duration to the whole brain. In 35 cases, radiation was not completed, and 12 cases could not be followed up. Among 158 evaluable cases, 123 (78%) demonstrated improvement with an average remission period of 4.7 months and an average survival time of 6.6 months after the onset of symptoms. The longest survival time recorded was 27 months from the onset of symptoms. Nisce et al. (1971) reported the results of more recent cases treated during the period from 1961 through 1968. The study was aimed at determining the effects of higher dose levels for better response rates and the duration of remission by such radiotherapy. The entire brain was irradiated in 560 cases, including 220 cases (39.3%) of breast cancer and 141 cases (25.2%) of lung cancer. Half of the cases were treated by ortho-voltage irradiation, and the rest were treated either by telecobalt or linear accelerator. In the majority of cases, 30 to 40 Gy. were given over a period of three to four weeks. Steriod hormones were given during radiation to evaluate the adjuvant effects. Among a total of 560 cases, 139 patients died before the completion of treatment, and 45 cases could not be included in follow-up studies. The remaining 376 cases were analyzed for the response to radiation. Three hundred two patients out of the 376 cases (80%) showed improvement of their symptoms. The mean duration of remission was five months (the median duration of remission: three months). Half of the patients demonstrated major improvements. The average duration of remission of breast cancer was six months and that of lung cancer and melanoma was five and three months, respectively. All patients who did not complete radio-therapy died within three months after the onset of the symptoms. Twenty per cent of the patients responded favorably and survived more than one year. Ten per cent of them survived more than two years. Twenty-five per cent of breast cancer, 15 per cent of lung cancer and 10 per cent of melanoma patients survived more than one year. Autopsy of 91 patients revealed that 60 per cent showed multiple brain metastases. The longest survival time recorded was five years after the onset of symp-toms. On the whole, 302 out of 560 cases (53.9%) and 302 out of 376 evaluable cases (80.3%) demonstrated improvement by radiotherapy. Forty-seven cases received a second course of radiation, and 21 (44.7%) again showed symptomatic improvement with a mean duration of four months. Only three patients received a third course of radiotherapy. There was no significant difference in effects between the total doses of 30 Gy. in three weeks and 35 to 40 Gy. in the three- to four-week period. A total dose of under 27.5 Gy. in the three week period, however, showed poor prognostic effects. It was also concluded that corticosteriods produced immediate symptomatic im-provement in a majority of the patients and facilitated the administration of irradia-tion. It did not, however, influence the overall results of radiotherapy. Nisce gathered a total of 816 patients treated at Memorial Hospital. One fourth of the patients could not complete radiotherapy due to their terminal conditions. Seventy-five per cent of the patients terminated the full course of radiotherapy, which proved effective. Order et al. (1968) gathered 108 cases, of which 56 patients received whole brain irradiation consisting of 25 to 30 Gy. Palliation was noted in 60 per cent of the patients.

The effects of surgical treatment and radiotherapy were compared by several investigators Støier (1965) surgically treated 96 patients, 22 of which received craniotomy and radiotherapy. The average survival time of patients receiving surgery alone was 5.5 months. The figure for patients receiving both surgery and radiation was 6.0 months. Thus, it has been concluded that radiotherapy does not result in any extension of the average postoperative survival period. Hazra et al. (1972) collected 35 cases with metastatic brain tumors. Radiation was given to 25 cases and their mean survival time was 27.8 weeks after radiotherapy. Surgical treatment was performed in ten cases with a mean survival time of 16.6 weeks. It was concluded, on the contrary, that surgery could not be considered the treatment of choice owing to the limited number of cases. The role of surgery in the treatment of metastatic brain tumors was discussed in the previous section.

The side effects of radiation have also been studied by many researchers. In animal experiments, Clemente and Holst (1954) noted the destruction of neurons, neuroglia and the blood-brain barrier of the monkey after radiation. Ross et al. (1954) reported his findings on cerebral edema, but Redmond et al. (1967) did not observe cerebral edema after clinical doses of radiation. Both noticed that in animals acute neurologic abnormalities and behavioral changes were caused by brain irradiation. Hakansson (1967) observed no change in ventricular pressure after a dose of 2 to 4 Gy. a day. Young et al. (1974) reported an increase in cerebrospinal fluid pressure caused by radiation in patients suffering from carcinomatous meningitis. Post radiation necrosis of the brain and spinal cord is fully realized. In general, the total dosage over 50 Gy. is hazardous to the nervous system. It is, however, not known whether the necrosis is due to the occlusion of small vessels which induces secondary infarction of the brain, or whether there are direct effects of radiation on the cells of the nervous system (Posner, 1971).

Recently, higher dose treatment has been introduced in several clinics. High-dose, short-term radiotherapy has been advocated for palliation of cerebral metastases, because it shortens the hospitalization of patients with a limited life expectancy. Hindo et al. (1970) of Presbyterian Hospital in St. Louis conducted a single, large-dose increment radiotherapy (10 Gy. of ^{60}Co to the whole brain) on 54 patients. Sixty-five per cent of the patients demonstrated a significant symptomatic improvement, and their average survival time was 5.6 months. Three patients, however, died within 48 hours after radiotherapy. Deutsch et al. (1974) gave 30 Gy. in 10 fractions to the whole brain and added 9 Gy. in three fractions to localized metastatic regions. Eighty-eight patients were treated between 1962 and 1971 in the University of Pittsburgh. Radiotherapy was completed in 65 out of a total of 88 cases, in which nine patients (13.8%) died within one month, and 45 patients (69.2%) within six months. Six out of 31 (19.3%) lung cancer and two out of 21 (9.5%) breast cancer patients survived more than one year. Young et al. (1974) evaluated rapid course radiotherapy. Group A, consisting of 83 patients, received 15 Gy. in two treatments (7.5 Gy. a day) in three days. Group B consisting of 79 patients received the ordinary-scheduled therapy of 30 Gy. in 15 days. Neurological amelioration was produced in 57 per cent of Group A and 62.3 per cent of Group B. The median duration of survival time was 59 days in Group A and 116 days in Group B (p<0.02). Complications consisting of headache, nausea, fever, etc. were observed in 49.4 per cent of Group A and 15.2 per cent of Group B (p<0.01). Cerebral herniation during radiotherapy was observed in six cases from Group A and in three from Group B.

Therefore, it seems that the rapid course radiotherapy is rather hazardous and less effective than ordinary scheduled radiotherapy. The only merit is the reduction of the treatment period. Montana et al. (1972) also reported on the results of short course radiotherapy. He gave 20 Gy. (4 Gy. five times in four elapsed days) or 18 Gy. (6 Gy. three times in two elapsed days). Both of these doses correspond to 1,200 rets*. Fifteen cases also received surgical treatment, but the remaining 47 cases

---

* Rets (Rad equivalent therapy): The concept permits a comparison of various treatment schedules consisting of different total doses, treatment times and number of fractions (Winston et al., 1969).

received only radiotherapy. The survival rates of the patients were 59 per cent at three months, 28 per cent at six months and 12 per cent at one year after treatment. Montana concluded that radiotherapy for metastatic brain tumors was better than surgical treatment with respect to therapeutic cost and operative mortality. From the above reports and from recent studies by Shehata et al. (1974), Hendrickson (1975, 1977), and Harwood and Simpson (1977), it was seen that patients suffering from metastatic brain tumors could tolerate a dose of 10 Gy. in one treatment, 30 Gy. in 10 treatments, and 20 Gy. in five treatments as effective palliative doses. Fitzpatrick and Keen (1980) reported the result of retrospective and randomized prospective study on brain metastases at the Princess Margaret and Ontario Cancer Foundation. Treatment consisted of total brain irradiation with 10, 20 or 30 Gy. in one, five or ten exposures. The prognosis was poor and similar for all treatment groups. The median actual survival time for lung, breast and other cancer patients was 100, 170 and 100 days, although a few patients lived over one year. The only real benefit was in improved neurologic and intellectual levels, which lasted for one-half of the patient's remaining life. They concluded that the optimum treatment for patients with a poor prognosis is 10 Gy. in a single exposure and for others 20 Gy. in five daily fractions. Optimum treatment is defined by them as treatment which provides the maximum benefit to the patient and at the minimum cost.

Constans et al. (1973b) reported the results of their findings regarding 167 cases of metastatic brain tumors. Simple radiation treatment was given to 31 patients: 22 of them received high dose therapy (concentré), and the remaining nine patients received ordinary treatment. Combined surgical and radiotherapy was given to 40 patients. In concentrated radiotherapy, 17 Gy. in two to three days were administered, and three weeks later, the same dose of radiation was applied. In the group treated with simple radiotherapy, the average survival time was six months, with the longest time being 18 months. In the group of patients who underwent combined therapy, the average survival time was ten months, and three out of 41 patients lived more than 30 months after surgery. Some radiologists stressed the advantages of radiotherapy over surgery with regard to lower cost, shorter hospital stay and possibilities of treatment in outpatient clinics (Richards and McKissock, 1963; Lang and Slater, 1964).

Table V-11   Outcome of radiation therapy for metastatic brain tumors.

Series		No. of cases	Med. survival time (months)	One year survival
Lenz & Freid	(1931)	5		40.0%
Chu & Hilaris	(1961)	158	6.6	
Nisce et al.	(1971)	376	6.0	16.0
Young et al.	(1974)	83*	2.0	
		79	4.0	3.0
Posner	(1974)	42	4.0	10.0
Støier	(1965)	96	6.0	
Deutsch	(1974)	65		12.3
Deeley & Rice-Edwards*	(1968)	61	9.0	14.0
Montana et al.**	(1972)	62		12.0
Constans et al.	(1973b)	31 rad. only	6.0	
		rad. + Surg.	10.0	

*   Lung cancer   **   Rapid-course therapy.

Specific types of cancers were also analyzed to confirm the effects of radiotherapy. Deeley and Rice Edwards (1968) treated 88 lung cancer patients. Prognosis was much better in patients whose primary tumors were initially treated before neurological manifestations appeared. Prognosis for squamous cell carcinoma is better than that for anaplastic carcinoma. When primary lung cancer was properly treated, patients could sometimes live for a long period. Daniel (1964), Harr and Patterson, Jr. (1972), Mosberg Jr. (1976), Turnoff et al. (1976), and Salerno et al. (1978) reported on cases of metastatic brain tumors from lung cancer who survived more than ten years by receiving surgery and radiotherapy. Prognosis for metastatic brain tumors from breast cancer is much better than in cases of lung cancer. It seems, however, that it is not dependent on the radiosensitivity of tumor cells but on the biological behavior of breast cancer such as hormonal dependency or the rate of progression. Renal clear cell carcinoma can be most effectively treated by radiotherapy (Vieth and Odom, 1965a; Lang and Slater, 1964). The results of radiotherapy that appeared in the literature are summarized in Table V-11.

Investigations have recently been made into methods to potentiate the effects of radiation. In order to obtain better therapeutic results, the effect of combined chemotherapy and radiotherapy was evaluated by several investigators. Radiotherapy combined with doxorubicin hydrochloride (Adriamycin) and CCNU for metastatic brain tumors from lung cancer (15 squamous cell, 4 adeno-, 3 oat cell and 2 large cell carcinomas) was reported by Chan and his colleagues (1980). Cyclophosphamide was given to patients with oat cell carcinoma. Doxorubicin hydrochloride (40 to 50 mg/m^2) was administered intravenously every three weeks, whereas CCNU (50 to 60 mg/m^2) was simultaneously given orally on day 1 and every six weeks. Cyclophosphamide (300 mg/m^2) was added on day 1 and every three weeks for oat cell carcinoma. Radiotherapy to the whole brain was given concomitantly with the chemotherapy. The radiation dose to the brain was 20 Gy., given in five consecutive days and repeated after three weeks rest. The total 40 Gy. was delivered in five weeks. Among the 22 evaluated patients, the neurologic functional response was complete in 82 per cent and partial in 18 per cent. Three months after completion of treatment, 15 patients shownd normal isotope brain scans and five patients showed 50 per cent improvement. The median survival time was eight months. The regimen of this report was based on the radiosensitizing effect of doxorubicin hydrochloride (Cortes et al., 1974). The halogenated thymidine analogue BUdR (5-bromo-2'-deoxyuridine) has been introduced by Sano and his associates (1968) and used for the treatment of malignant brain tumors including metastatic brain tumors. Nitroimidazole compounds such as metronidazole and misonidazole (Ro-07-0582) have also been introduced as potent hypoxic cell sensitizers. These compounds were studied to check their radiosensitizing effects through animal experiments and clinical evaluations (Committee for Radiation Oncology Studies, 1976; Urtasun et al., 1976a, b; Dische et al., 1977; Sheline et al., 1979). Nitroimidazoles are expected to improve the effects of radiotherapy for metastatic brain tumors, and, randomized Phase III studies for the evaluation of misonidazole combined with radiation in the treatment of patients with brain metastases are being conducted in the United States. Another approach to potentiating the effects of radiotherapy is the regulation of the tumor cell cycle. Synchronization of the tumor cell cycle of chemotherapeutic agents prior to radiotherapy has been studied in our clinic (Shitara et al., 1976, 1978). The rationale for this treatment as well as how it is conducted will be discussed later. Favorable effects of radiotherapy for the management of metastatic brain tumors are fully established today. Further research should be conducted in the next decade for the development of more sophisticated methods of radiotherapy.

Results of Radiotherapy—Our Experience

Methods

A linear accelerator was used in most cases. A total dose of 30 to 40 Gy. was irradiated to the whole brain, and 20 Gy. were often added to local sites of metastatic tumors. A dose of 1.8 to 2 Gy. a day was used and in some cases, the dose started from 0.5 Gy. and gradually increased to 2 Gy. a day, according to the patient's general condition and intracranial pressure. Radiation was given five days a week and terminated in three to four weeks. When local radiotherapy was additionally given, two more weeks were necessary for the entire course of radiotherapy. Glucocorticoids were generally administered before and during radiotherapy (Horton et al., 1971) to control brain edema (prednisolone 20–30 mg/day, dexamethasone or betamethasone 4–8 mg/day). The administration of mannitol was not required in most cases. Simple radiotherapy, however, is not frequently utilized today since combined chemoradiotherapy has proved to bring about better neurologic amelioration and regression of tumors on CT scan.

Results

Recent CT scans clearly revealed the actual suppressive effects of tumor growth. Out of 616 patients, 215 received radiotherapy: 97 of these received radiotherapy alone and 118 cases received radiotherapy combined with surgery. Survival rates of both groups are summarized in Table V-12. Of 215 patients treated with radiotherapy, 31.8 per cent of them survived one year, 12.6 per cent two years and only 6.5 per cent survived three years after the onset of neurological symptoms. The group of patients treated with combined surgery and radiotherapy lived longer than those who were treated with radiotherapy alone. Survival rates one, two and three years after the onset of neurological signs were 14.4, 7.2 and 2.1 per cent in the group treated only by radiotherapy, and 45.6, 16.9 and 10.2 per cent in those treated by radiotherapy with surgical management.

Table V-12 shows the survival rates of metastatic tumors of different primary origins. No patient lived more than one year without surgery and/or radiotherapy. These figures clearly demonstrate the effects of treatment on prolongation of life, but at the same time, they indicate the limitations of radiotherapy.

Histological changes after radiotherapy are shown in Figures V-2 and 3. The figures demonstrate the histological pattern of anaplastic carcinoma, intracranially

Table V-12 Long-term results of radiotherapy for metastatic brains tumors. Survival rate for each type of primary tumor.

Primary tumor	Surgical treatment	No. of patient	Survival rate (%)				
			3 mos	6 mos	1 year	2 years	3 years
Lung	Total	102	83.3	54.9	25.5	7.8	3.9
	Surgery −	51	70.6	35.3	7.8	3.9	2.0
	+	51	96.1	74.5	43.1	11.8	5.9
Breast	Total	21	90.0	80.0	50.0	15.0	5.0
	Surgery −	10	80.0	70.0	50.0	20.0	0.0
	+	11	90.9	81.8	45.5	9.1	9.1
Gastrointestinal tract	Total	12	83.3	41.6	25.0	0.0	0.0
	Surgery −	4	50.0	0.0	0.0	0.0	0.0
	+	8	100.0	62.5	37.5	0.0	0.0
Genitourinary organs	Total	19	94.7	68.4	26.3	15.8	10.5
	Surgery −	9	88.9	44.4	11.1	11.1	0.0
	+	10	100.0	90.0	40.0	20.0	20.0
Others	Total	61	85.2	63.9	39.3	21.3	11.5
	Surgery −	23	82.6	52.2	17.4	8.7	4.3
	+	38	86.8	71.1	52.6	28.9	15.8
Total	Total	215	85.6	60.5	31.8	12.6	6.5
	Surgery −	97	75.3	42.3	14.4	7.2	2.1
	+	118	94.1	75.4	46.6	16.9	10.2

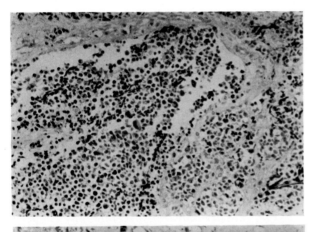

Fig. V-2 Anaplastic carcinoma invaded the left frontal base from the maxillar region. The surgical specimen.

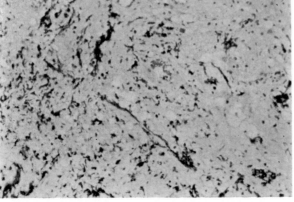

Fig. V-3 The effects of radiotherapy. Autopsied material from the above case (Fig. V-2). The necrotic tissue with scattered degenerated tumor cells was demonstrated six months after radiotherapy.

invaded from the left maxillar region. After partial removal of the tumor, the patient received radiotherapy of 50 Gy. Six months after the completion of radiotherapy, the patient died and an autopsy was performed. The main tumor mass showed necrosis associated with scattered degenerated cancer cells.

Synchronized Chemo-radiotherapy

Rationale

It has been noted that the radiosensitivity of tumor cells is dependent on cell cycle phases, in which G_2-M phases are most sensitive (Terashima and Tolmach, 1963; Tolmach et al., 1965; Dewey and Humphery, 1972; Sinclair, 1972; Terashima, 1974). From cell kinetic studies of tumors, the cell population in each cell cycle has been roughly calculated (Hoshino et al., 1972, 1975). A large proportion of tumor cells, e.g. 60 to 70 per cent, is occupied by G_0 or a dormant cell population; it is sensitive to neither radiation nor chemotherapy. Within cycling cells, a cell population of G_2 or M phases is rather small (10 per cent or less). Since, the cell population in G_2 or M phases, which is thought to be the best target for radiotherapy, is approximately three to four per cent of all tumor cells, simple radiation is considered quite inefficient. The cell cycle dependency of various chemotherapeutic agents has also been studied by Sinclair and Morton (1963), and has been categorized in three groups: S-phase specific, S-phase specific with self limitation, and cell cycle non-specific agents. The effectiveness of both radiation and chemotherapy might be potentiated if the cell population in every part of a cell cycle phase could be synchronized to the target cell cycle phase by suitable pretreatment. On the other hand, it is noteworthy that certain kinds of alkaloids, such as colchicine or colcemid, can stop cell progression at the mitotic phase of a cell cycle. Therefore, it was postulated that these substances might accumulate and increase the cell population in the M phase. The effects of cellular synchronization using colcemid as pretreatment for combined chemo-radiotherapy were studied. It was found that colcemid could accumulate cells in G_2-M phases three times more than non-treated tumor cells (Shitara et al., 1976). Thus, it was expected that the effects of radiation might be potentiated. A clinical trial of synchronized chemo-radiotherapy has been undertaken. Several chemotherapeutic agents were screened to study synchronizing effects and it was found that vincristine, ACNU (Nimustine) and VM-26 (epipodophyllotoxin) are suitable for this purpose.

Experimental Results

Basic experiments were initiated using an *in vitro* model. Cultured rat glioma C_6 cells were incubated *in vitro* in RPMI 1640 medium containing 20 per cent fetal calf serum and vincristine as an M-phase blocking agent. After 24- and 72-hour contact with vincristine, an increased cellular population of G_2 and M phases was clearly demonstrated in the DNA histogram of tumor cells using flow cytometry (Fig. V-4). The synchronized effects of VM-26, vincristine and ACNU on glioma C_6 cells *in vitro* are summarized in Table V-13.

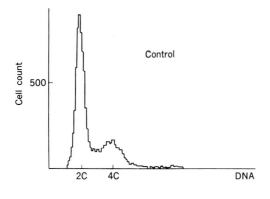

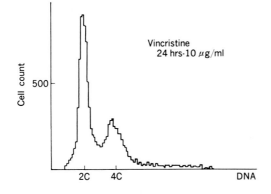

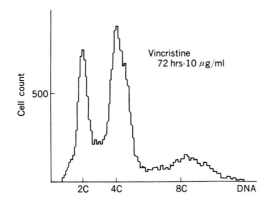

Fig. V-4 DNA histogram of rat glioma C6 cells treated with vincristine *in vitro*. The nuclei of cultured cells stained with ethidium bromide were analysed by flow cytometry. The 2C peak indicates the cells in G_0 and G_1 phases. The 8C peak is composed of fused nuclei or cells in the polyploid cell cycle induced by vincristine. Top: Control cells before treatment. Middle: Cells contacted with vincristine (10μg/ml) for 24 hours. Bottom: Cells contacted with vincristine (10μg/ml) for 72 hours.

Experiments using animal tumor models were undertaken to clarify the synchronized effects *in vivo*. Fisher rats inoculated with glioma C_6 cells to the brain were treated with vincristine and ACNU. Doses of these chemotherapeutic agents were adjusted to the dose applicable to human patients (Byfield, 1972). Synchronizing effects of tumor cells *in vivo* were also demonstrated (Fig. V-5). Similar experiments *in vivo* using adenocarcinoma of the lung (Sato lung cancer) inoculated to the brain of Donryu rats also revealed accumulating effects of cycling cells into G_2 and M phases. The results of these experiments suggest that concomitant chemotherapy with vincristine, ACNU or VM-26 can potentiate the effects of radiation in the suppression of brain tumors.

Table V-13 Synchronized effect of VM-26, vincristine and ACNU on glioma C_6 cells determined by computer-aided flow-cytometric analysis.

	Concentration	Time (h)	Rate of cell numbers in each cell cycle phase		
			$G_0 + G_1\%$	$S\%$	$G_2 + M\%$
VM-26	1 µg/ml	24	23.9	5.0	71.1
		72	23.4	33.2	43.4
	10	24	46.5	11.9	41.7
Vincristine	10	24	61.4	18.7	19.9
		72	26.0	26.4	47.6
	1	24	59.6	18.8	21.6
		72	52.2	21.0	26.8
ACNU	100	24	66.8	16.5	16.5
		72	41.1	18.4	40.5
	10	24	53.3	16.6	30.1
		72	23.3	29.9	47.2

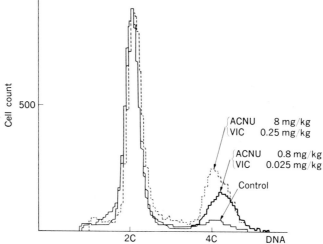

Fig. V-5 DNA histogram of intracerebrally inoculated rat glioma C_6 cells, treated by intravenous administration of ACNU and vincristine. The tumor was removed at 72 hours after injection. A marked increase of cells in G_2 and M phases is noted by the administration of the chemotherapeutic agents.

Clinical Methods

Vincristine (0.02 mg/kg body weight) is intravenously injected on days 1 and 2 of treatment, and ACNU (1 mg/kg body weight) is given intravenously on days 2 and 3. Radiation starts on the same day on which therapy begins. On days 4 and 5 of treatment, the dosage of radition is increased to 3 Gy. a day and then reduced to a daily dose of 1.5 Gy. from the second week. In the fourth week the same course of chemotherapy is repeated. After two to four weeks rest the similar boost course is repeated. Therefore, two to three courses of chemotherapy are given to a patient during the entire period of radiotherapy. The total dose of radiation is around 50 to 60 Gy. White blood cell and thrombocyte counts and liver function should be examined every week, and if some side effects of chemotherapy are noticed, then the second or third course of chemotherapy is skipped or the dosage reduced.

In some cases, VM-26 is used instead of vincristine and ACNU for the same purpose. VM-26 (1 mg/kg body weight) is intravenously administered for three consecutive days with the same schedule as that for radiotherapy.

Result of Clinical Application

The tumor suppressing effects of synchronized chemo-radiotherapy were evaluated by CT, neurological signs and symptoms.

> **Case 1** 67-year-old man. NCC 208475. Multiple metastatic brain tumors from lung adenocarcinoma.
>
> The patient received 40 Gy. by simple radiation. The size of the tumor enlarged during this radiotherapy. Then, synchronized chemo-radiotherapy with vincristine and ACNU (20 Gy.) was additionally given. The tumor regressed markedly with neurological amelioration (Fig. V-6). This case demonstrated clearly the effect of radiosensitization of the chemotherapy.

> **Case 2** 51-year-old man. NCC 190620. Metastatic brain tumor from renal clear cell carcinoma.
>
> The patient had received a nephrectomy for renal clear cell carcinoma. He had progressively developed left hemiparesis. Carotid angiography (CAG) revealed a coin-sized vascular tumor stain in the right postparietal region. After synchronized chemo-radiotherapy with vincristine and ACNU, the tumor stain disappeared in six weeks and the hemiparesis subsided (Fig. V-7).

Metastatic Tumor (Lung Ca.)
(Adeno Ca.)

    A   B   C

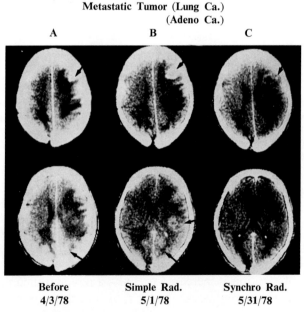

   Before   **Simple Rad.**   **Synchro Rad.**
   4/3/78   **5/1/78**   **5/31/78**

Fig. V-6 The effect of synchronized chemo-radiotherapy. Case 1. 67-year-old man. Metastatic brain tumors from lung adenocarcinoma.
A. Before radiotherapy.
B. After simple radiation, 40 Gy.
C. After adding synchronized chemo-radiotherapy (20 Gy.) with vincristine and ACNU.

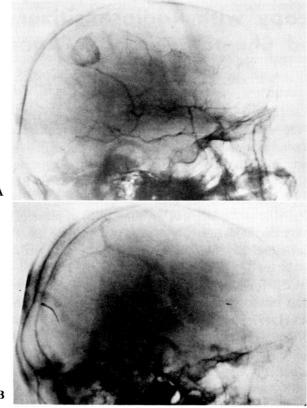

Fig. V-7 The effects of synchronized chemo-radiotherapy. Case 2.
45-year-old man. Metastatic brain tumor from renal clear cell carcinoma.
A. Before radiotherapy.
B. After synchronized chemo-radiotherapy (40 Gy.).

One hundred two cases of malignant brain tumors including 19 cases of metastatic brain tumors were treated by synchronized chemo-radiotherapy. The results of this treatment in the induction stage are summarized in Table V-14. Satisfactory regression of the tumor as seen on the CT scan and neurological amelioration have been achieved in about 35.2 per cent of the cases. The response to radiotherapy was noted in 74 out of 102 cases (72.5 %).

Table V-14 Effects of synchronized chemo-radiotherapy.

Type of tumor	No. of patient	Excellent	Good	No response
Metastatic tumor	19	7	8	4
Glioblastoma	45	18	11	16
Other glioma	38	11	19	8
Total	**102**	**36** (35.2 %)	**38** (37.3 %)	**28** (27.5 %)

Excellent: Marked regression of tumor size on CT scan (> 50 %) and neurological amelioration.

Good: Marked regression of tumor size on CT scan or neurological amelioration.

No response: No regression of tumor size on CT scan (< 50 %) and no neurological amelioration.

Table V-15-1 Effect of radiotherapy with intrathecal administration of BUdR and chemotherapeutic agent.

Age	Sex	Chart no.	Primary tumor	Type of tumor	Operation	Chemotherapeutic Agent	Radiation dose (Gy.)	Survival time***	Grade of temporary recovery
4	M	NCC 123871	Retioblastoma	Multiple	Drainage	Mtx* 30 mg / BUdR 3,000 mg	30	11 mos	Home life useful
32	M	NCC 135269	Thymoma	Multiple supra-infra.	Partial	Mtx 17 mg / BUdR 3,000 mg	30	16	Home life useful
50	M	NCC 43903	Lung Adeno.	Multiple	Partial	MMC** 11 mg / BUdR 1,300 mg	50.5	14	Home life useful
46	F	NCC 124829	Lung Adeno.	Diffuse	Partial	MMC 10 mg / BUdR 2,500 mg	50	14	Home life useful
40	M	NCC 86996	Lung Adeno.	Single	Partial	MMC 18 mg / BUdR 3,800 mg	50	10	Social work
51	F	NCC 118941	Breast	Meningeal ca.	Decomp.	MMC 8 mg / BUdR 1,200 mg	40.5	15	Home life useful
58	F	NCC 58949	Breast	Meningeal ca.	Decomp.	MMC 16 mg / BUdR 2,400 mg	50	9	Poor
37	F	NCC 118785	Breast	Diffuse & Pituitary	Partial	MMC 15 mg / BUdR 5,000 mg	50	12	Home life useful

Table V-15-2 Effect of radiotherapy with intraarterial infusion of BUdR and antimetabolite (BAR therapy).

Age	Sex	Chart no.	Primary tumor	Type of tumor	Operation	Chemotherapeutic Agent	Radiation dose (Gy.)	Survival time***	Grade of temporary recovery
51	M	NCC 11038	Lung Undiff.	Single	Partial	5FU 1,500 mg / BUdR 4,000 mg	12	2 mos	Poor
53	F	NCC 104958	Lung Adeno.	Multiple	None	5FU 50 mg / BUdR 3,000 mg	10	9	Poor
58	M	NCC 122422	Lung Small cell	Single	None	5FU 2,250 mg / BUdR 2,100 mg	31	1	Poor
54	M	NCC 114535	Lung Squamous cell	Single	Subtotal	5FU 1,250 mg / BUdR 12 g	40	21	Social work
36	M	NCC 154769	Lung Adeno.	Multiple	Partial	Mtx* 1,500 mg / BUdR 10 g	50	33	Home life useful
44	M	TU 67004	Lung Undiff.	Single	Partial	Mtx 100 mg / BUdR 8,800 mg	20	3	Poor
30	M	TU 690223	Malignant Lymphoma	Multiple	Partial	Mtx 20 mg / BUdR 10 g	50	6	Home life

* Mtx: methotrexate.   ** MMC: Mitomycin C.   *** Survival time after the onset of neurological symptoms.

and Actinomycin D. Wilms' tumor is also sometimes curable. Intracranial involvement of leukemia can be prevented or suppressed for months or years by intrathecal administration of methotrexate. Although achievements in the field of chemotherapy for brain metastases in the past have been depressing, better management of the disease can be expected in the future.

Subsequent to Klopp's report (1950) of fractionated intra-arterial injection of nitrogen mustard for cancer patients, treatment of brain tumors by intracarotid administration has been reported by French et al. (1952), Sullivan et al. (1953), McCarthy (1965) and Hatiboglu and Owens (1961). French reported on two cases of metastatic brain tumors. The marked improvement of right hemiplegia in a patient with metastasis from bronchogenic carcinoma was noted after the first intracarotid injection of nitrogen mustard (20 mg/kg). This improvement, however, lasted only for five weeks and a second injection resulted in a fatality. A second patient with multiple metastases in the brain from bronchogenic carcinoma died of acute cerebral edema 15 hours after the injection, never regaining full consciousness. Microscopic sections of the small metastatic nodule in the left hemisphere of the first case showed considerable necrosis of the metastasis, which was not seen in a similar nodule in the cerebellum. Nevertheless, the area surrounding the affected nodule—in fact, the larger part of the entire left hemisphere—showed extensive demyelinization and gliosis, resulting from the earlier injection of nitrogen mustard seven weeks before, as well as petechial hemorrhages and edema of the whole brain from the second injection. It was concluded that nitrogen mustard was too toxic for the normal brain tissue for giving the effective dose to brain tumors.

Sansone reported in 1954 that the intrathecal administration of aminopterin palliates meningeal leukemia and the subsequent use of methotrexate (amethopterin) for this condition has proven more effective and less toxic. Similar results following the intrathecal administration or intraventricular perfusion of methotrexate for treatment of CNS involvement for leukemia and other brain tumors have been reported by several investigators (Whiteside et al., 1958; Hyman et al., 1962; Rieselbach et al., 1962; Newton, Jr. and Sayers, 1965; Rubin et al., 1965, 1966).

Sullivan et al. (1959, 1961) reported the continuous intracarotid infusion of methotrexate with intermittent intramuscular citrovorum factor administration for the treatment of cancer patients. Methotrexate does not penetrate the blood-brain barrier, and the distribution of methotrexate in the brain tissue after intra-arterial and intrathecal administration has been investigated by Ojima and his co-workers (1966). The concentration of methotrexate in the brain tissue increases twenty-fold after intrathecal administration, compared with intra-arterial infusion. Methotrexate seems to be the first chemotherapeutic agent which has proved truly effective for the suppression of the intracranial invasion of tumors.

As for pyrimidine antagonists, extensive experience with the continuous intra-arterial administration of 5-fluorouracil (5-FU) and 5-fluoro-2'-deoxyuridine (FUdR) was reported by Sullivan (1962). A malignant astrocytoma treated by intra-arterial infusion of 5-FU, however, showed no objective response. Takeuchi et al. (1968) reported on the significant tumor-suppressing effects of intra-arterial 5-FU infusion on some metastatic brain tumors when they were simultaneously treated with radiotherapy.

The parenteral administration of 5-FU to mice with subcutaneously implanted melanomas resulted in inhibition of the growth of the experimental tumors, but there was no effect on the growth of the intracerebral tumors at equivalent levels (Kotsilimbas et al., 1966). This evidence suggested that 5-FU could not penetrate the blood-brain barrier. On the contrary, 5-FU and azauracil produced central nervous depression with ataxia and electroencephalographic abnormalities following systemic administration, strangely suggesting that 5-FU or some metabolic derivatives do cross the blood-brain barrier (Bering, Jr. et al., 1967). Intrathecal administration of 5-FU (2.5 mg/kg) killed rats within 48 hours, indicating penetration of 5-FU to the brain tissue beyond the CSF-brain barrier. Judging from the toxicity in experimental animals, intrathecal administration of 5-FU was not considered advisable (Jinnai et al., 1967). Although 5-FU has been demonstrated to have tumor-suppressing effects on several cancers such as breast, gastrointestinal, uterine and ovarial cancers, there was no report on the significantly proven effectiveness for brain tumors. Wilson and de la Garza (1965) reported three cases of cancers metastasized to the brain which were treated with 5-FU and Endoxan. They found some amelioration in two breast cancer patients, but another case of digestive tract cancer showed no improvement in clinical symptoms.

In 1966, Hiller and his co-workers in the Soviet Union synthesized a new chemotherapeutic agent, 1-(2-tetrahydrofuryl)-5-fluorouracil (tegafur = Ftorafur = Futraful, FT-207) (Blokhina, 1970). This is a masked compound of 5-FU which is less toxic than 5-FU. Tegafur is lipid soluble. Apinis and Purin found in 1973 that it penetrates the blood-brain barrier (Blokhina et al., 1972). It is given either orally or intravenously and is effective for adenocarcinoma such as breast, lung and gastrointestinal cancers. We found that tegafur was quite effective in some cases of metastatic brain tumors (Kohno et al., 1976c).

Alkylating agents such as cyclophosphamide (Endoxan) and triethylene-thiophosphoramide (Thio-TEPA) can penetrate the blood-brain barrier. There was, however, no report describing their definite suppressive effects on gliomas. Nevertheless, cyclophosphamide has proved to be effective for malignant lymphoma, leukemia, Ewing's tumor, rhabdomyosarcoma, ovarian carcinoma, head and neck cancer, breast cancer, etc. (Clarysse et al., 1976; Livingston and Carter, 1970), and is widely used for the treatment of these neoplasms. However, there have been only a few papers reporting on the effects of cyclophosphamide for the treatment of metastatic brain tumors. Holcomb et al. (1964) treated two cases, and Rose et al. (1964) also treated two cases of metastatic brain tumors with cyclophosphamide without any amelioration of neurological symptoms.

The following case reports which represent the effectiveness of cyclophosphamide on brain metastases appeared in the literature (Constans and Cioloca, 1974).

Case 1 51-year-old woman (Wilson and de la Garza, 1965). Breast cancer.
Metastases to the brain with inoperable primary breast cancer. All neurological symptom disappeared after cyclophosphamide administration. Intracranial hypertension appeared a few months after the cessation of cyclophosphamide administration, and the chemotherapeutic agent was changed to 5-FU. Although 5-FU caused the side effects of leukopenia and stomatitis, the patient regained neurological amelioration. The effectiveness of cyclophosphamide lasted for five months, and that of 5-FU lasted six weeks.

Case 2 53-year-old woman (W.L. Wilson and de la Garza, 1965). Breast cancer.

Four years after mastectomy, brain metastases appeared. They regressed using cobalt therapy, and all neurological signs disappeared after cyclophosphamide administration. No mention was made of the duration of the effectiveness or survival time.

Case 3 Woman (Wagenknecht, 1973). Breast cancer.

Four years after surgery for primary breast cancer, multiple brain metastases with bone and lung dissemination appeared. Treatment with cyclophosphamide with methotrexate and prednisolone brought clinical remission with decreased intracranial pressure. Remission lasted for ten months.

Case 4 64-year-old man (W. L. Wilson and de la Garza, 1965). Lung cancer.

Brain metastases caused facial palsy and brachial monoplegia. Treatment with cyclophosphamide brought complete remission that lasted for five months, but the length of survival time was not reported.

Davis and Shumway (1961) treated 97 brain metastases (31 lung and 66 breast cancers) with Thio-TEPA, some of which responded to treatment, but the results were not conclusive.

Nitrosourea compounds cross the blood-brain barrier and are now the most widely used compound for the treatment of malignant gliomas. Since Venditti et al. (1964) reported on the suppressive effects on advanced L1210 leukemia of mice, various experiments for the treatment of brain tumors have been conducted. Clinical trials of 1,3-bis(2-chloroethyl)-1-nitrosourea, (BCNU) proved effective in the treatment of glioma. Phase II evaluations of BCNU by Walker and Hurwits (1970), and Wilson et al. (1970) demonstrated that it provides a response rate of approximately 50 per cent in the late stage of recurrent gliomas. A controlled, prospective and randomized study evaluated the effectiveness of BCNU and/or radiotherapy in the treatment of patients who were operated on and had histological confirmation of anaplastic glioma by Walker et al. (1978). The median survival times of patients in the valid study group (VSP) was, with the best conventional care, 14 weeks (adequately treated group = ATG: 17.0 weeks); 18.5 weeks for BCNU (ATG: 25.0 weeks); 35 weeks for radiotherapy (ATG: 37.5 weeks); and 34 weeks for BCNU and radiotherapy (ATG: 40.5 weeks). These results suggested that radiotherapy significantly prolonged the life span, although BCNU did not show any increase in life span over radiation-treated patients. There was a significantly greater surviving fraction of patients at the end of 18 months among those who received combined therapy.

Few papers reporting on the effects of BCNU on metastatic brain tumors are available (Kohno et al., 1976a, b). Fewer et al. (1972) treated four patients of metastatic brain tumors from melanoma with BCNU alone (3 cases) and BCNU with VM-26 = epipodophyllotoxin (1 case). A case of amelioration of neurological symptoms was noted. The survival time, however, was not described, and the significant effectiveness could not be concluded. Three other metastatic brain tumor cases were treated with BCNU alone without any response. Matsutani et al. (1972) also treated a case of metastatic brain tumor from lung cancer with BCNU, without any benefit. Misset (1973) reported on cases of metastatic brain tumors, including malignant lymphoma treated with BCNU and VM-26. He cited four cases of amelioration. Besides BCNU, CCNU [1-(2-chloroethyl)-3-cyclohexyl-1-nitrosourea] was introduced for the treatment of malignant brain tumors (Hausen et al., 1971; Hausen, 1972). Rosenblum et al. (1973) reported on three cases of metastatic brain tumors treated with CCNU, and observed two cases of amelioration.

Case reports representing the effectiveness of CCNU on brain metastases (Rosenblum et al., 1973) are as follows:

Case 5   61-year-old woman. Lung cancer.
Multiple cerebral metastases were not removed surgically. The patient received radiotherapy and corticosteroid therapy. CCNU (130 mg/m^2) was given in two courses. Neurological symptoms remained unchanged for three and a half months. Gradual progression then occurred and the patient died 12 months after the onset of neurological symptoms.

Case 6   46-year-old man. Lung cancer.
A single brain metastasis was removed and radiotherapy was given. CCNU (150 mg/m^2) was given in four courses. A neurological examination revealed no abnormal signs after six months. The patient died of pulmonary trouble 16 months after the onset of neurological symptoms.

Shapiro (1980) reported the results of chemotherapy using nitrosourea for lung cancer metastasized to the brain. Of seven patients treated with BCNU after radiotherapy, only one patient improved and remained stable for five months before deteriorating, while the other six patients all showed progressive disease without CNS response. Of seven melanoma patients treated with BCNU, two of them responded for four to nine months. He also treated 14 other metastatic brain tumor patients with CCNU. Only one patient who responded showed improvement in normal neurologic examinations for eight months. The overall results indicate an approximately 20 per cent response rate.

Shapiro also reported on 31 cases out of 45 of meningeal metastases treated with intrathecal administration of methotrexate. All five lymphoma patients improved, including two who received chemotherapy without radiotherapy. Of the solid tumors, 85 per cent of the patients improved; breast cancer demonstrated the best results with 13 of 16 patients responding. Even some of the lung cancer patients responded for a short period of time.

Misset (1973) reported on three cases of metastatic brain tumors treated with BCNU and VM-26. VM-26 (60 mg/m^2) was given on days 1 and 2 for synchronization, and BCNU (70 mg/m^2) was given on days 3 and 4 of the three week course. The results were not satisfactory. The first case showed tumor regression of more than 50 per cent with incomplete remission. The second case showed tumor regression of less than 50 per cent with incomplete remission, and in the third case, tumor regression of more than 50 per cent was noted without remission. Constans and Cioloca (1974) used a similar protocol. They administered VM-26 (50 mg, intravenously) on days 1 and 2 and CCNU (100 mg, orally.) on days 3 and 4 of a one-month course repeated for at least six months. VM-26 blocks the cell cycle at mitosis, and it is used for synchronization and possibly recruitment. They treated ten cases of metastatic brain tumors (6 breast, 2 renal, and 1 lung cancer, and 1 melanoma) by this scheduled chemotherapy. Three out of ten patients survived longer than six months (alive, 8, 10 and 12 months).

Several antibiotics were also used. Kofman and Einsenstein (1963) treated 22 metastatic brain tumor patients with Mithramycin, but the results were not conclusive. Mitomycin C proved effective for lung and gastrointestinal cancers and was widely used for metastatic brain tumors in our clinic. Bleomycin was also used in several cases and proved effective in some special cases (Takakura, 1971). Aoyagi et al. (1971) reported on a tumor regression lasting for three years in a case of nasopharyngeal cancer invading the intracranial cavity, which was treated by local administration of Bleomycin, Mitomycin C, and 5-FU. We have seen a case of scalp cancer successfully treated with Bleomycin and radiotherapy. Bleomycin, however, has demonstrated effectiveness in only a few cases.

By reviewing literature concerning the chemotherapy of metastatic brain tumors (Table V-16), it is realized that the significant effectiveness of the therapy is still uncertain. The biological characteristics and drug sensitivity of metastatic tumors are largely different from gliomas. Since brain metastases are a part of disseminated cancer, it is important to note that chemotherapeutic agents should be used from the viewpoint of systemic cancer treatment.

Table V-16 Chemotherapy for metastatic brain tumors.

Chemo-therapeutic agent	Combined chemo-therapeutic agents	Primary cancer	Author	Year	No. of patients	No. of amelio-ration
BCNU	Vcr.	Melanoma	Fewer et al.	1972	4	1
BCNU			Fewer et al.	1972	3	0
BCNU		Lung	Matsutani et al.	1972	1	0
BCNU		Lung, melanoma	Shapiro	1980	14	3
BCNU	VM26	Reticulosa. etc.	Misset	1973	9	4
CCNU		Lung	Rosenblum et al.	1973	3	2
CCNU			Newman & Hansen	1974	19	—
CCNU		Lung, melanoma etc.	Shapiro	1980	14	2
ACNU	Vcr.	Miscellaneous	Shitara et al.	1978	11	9
VM-26		Lung	Sklansky et al.	1974	1	1
VM-26	CCNU	Miscellaneous	Constans & Cioloca	1974	10	—
Procarbazine		Lung etc.	Kumar et al.	1974	2	1
Endoxan		Lung	Holcomb et al.	1964	2	0
Endoxan		Lung	Wilson et al.	1966	1	1
Endoxan	Mtx	Breast	Wagenknecht	1973	1	1
Thio–TEPA		Breast, Lung	Davis & Shumway	1961	97	?
5FU		Digestive	Wilson et al.	1966	1	0
5FU	Endoxan	Breast	Wilson et al.	1966	2	?
5FU		Miscellaneous	Takeuchi et al.	1968	?	?
5FU			Kirsch	1973	20	?
Tegafur		Miscellaneous	Kohno et al.	1976c	25	11
Mtx		Miscellaneous	Matsutani et al.	1976	21	13
Mtx			Garfield & Anthony	1973	1	0
Mtx		Meningeal meta.	Shapiro	1980	31	27
Mtx	BUdR	Miscellaneous	Sano et al.	1968	2	0
Mtx	BUdR	Miscellaneous	Takakura et al.	1972	5	4
5FU	BUdR	Lung	Takakura et al.	1972	4	1
MMC	BUdR	Miscellaneous	Takakura et al.	1972	6	5
Bleomycin	5FU, MMC	Maxiller ca.	Aoyagi et al.	1971	1	1
Bleomycin	Vcr.	Scalp ca.	Takakura et al.	1972	2	1
Mithramycin		Miscellaneous	Kofman & Einsenstein	1963	22	8
Adriamycin	CCNU	Lung	Chan et al.	1980	24	18
Thalidomide			Brihaye	1963	2	0

Chemotherapeutic Agents Sensitive to Various Types of Cancer

The sensitivity of chemotherapeutic agents to each type of cancer is an important and basic factor in the treatment of the metastatic brain tumors (Table V-17).

Lung Cancer

A therapeutic schedule for lung cancer metastases depends on the local characteristics of the tumor, reserve of pulmonary function, host factors such as cardiac, hepatic and renal functions and the histological type of the tumor (Zelen, 1973). A five-year survival rate is the highest in squamous cell carcinoma (Selawry and Hansen, 1973) and the lowest in small cell anaplastic carcinoma (oat cell carcinoma, Mountain et al., 1974). The five-year survival rate of small cell carcinoma was less than 1 per cent. The effects of therapy with surgery and radiation were clarified by the Medical Research Council of Great Britain (Miller et al., 1969), but the effects of chemotherapy on lung cancer are still limited. Cyclophosphamide and CCNU were widely used, proving most effective in small cell carcinoma but for a short duration (Kaung et al., 1974; Durrant et al., 1971; Selawry, 1974; Green et al., 1969; Edmonson and Lagakos, 1974; Hansen et al., 1976). Rates of effectiveness of chemotherapeutic agents are given below (Carter et al., 1977). For adenocarcinoma, squamous cell carcinoma and large cell carcinoma:

> CCNU 41%
> Cyclophosphamide 29%
> Methotrexate 25%
> Adriamycin 24%
> Mitomycin C 30% (Taguchi, 1977)

In Japan, Mitomycin C is commonly used and several combined forms of chemotherapy have been suggested (Ohta et al., 1980). Recently, the chemotherapeutic agents most frequently being used are tegafur and ACNU.

For small cell carcinoma:

> Cyclophosphamide + CCNU 35%
> Cyclophosphamide + CCNU + Methotrexate 56%
> Adriamycin 36%

Breast Cancer

Survival time in cases of breast cancer generally depends on the size of the cancer, its histological type, presence of lymph node metastases, anatomical site of the tumor, etc. (Fisher et al., 1968, 1969). Today, advanced breast cancer is treated with combined hormonal therapy and chemotherapy. Schedules of therapy are dependent on age, the state of menstruation, postoperative remission period, the degree and site of metastasis and the growing speed of the tumor. The selection of hormonal treatment is decided based on the following three periods:

1) Patients who have menstruation.
2) Patients in the menopausal period.
   (six months to five years after the cessation)
3) Patients in the post menopausal period.
   (more than five years after the cessation)

Oophorectomy is a common hormonal treatment for premenopausal patients (Kennedy, 1974). The rate of effectiveness is 20 to 40 per cent. For patients of the second group, chemotherapy is the first choice for treatment, and rate of effectiveness by androgen treatment is about 13 per cent (Cooperative Breast Cancer Group, 1964). For the patients of the third group, treatment by estrogen is the first choice. The rate of effectiveness is about 50 per cent (Kennedy, 1974). For this group, either chemotherapy and anti-estrogen treatment are also effective (Legha and Carter, 1976).

For initiating hormonal therapy, attention should be paid to the hormone dependency of each tumor. The patient should be carefully checked every two to three weeks for the growth of the tumor. The best result of control is obtained by examining the estrogen receptor of the primary tumor.

Breast cancer is responsive to cyclophosphamide, 5-FU, Adriamycin, methotrexate, vincristine, etc. (Carter, 1974, 1976). Greenspan (1963, 1966) developed a combined chemotherapy and later Cooper (1969) made a regimen using cyclophosphamide, methotrexate, 5-FU, vincristine and prednisolone (CMFVP). The most common combined chemotherapy is CMF (cyclophosphamide, methotrexate, 5-FU) therapy. The combined chemotherapy with Adriamycin and vincristine is also reported to be effective (DeLena et al., 1975). The rate of effectiveness is approximately 50 per cent for every combined treatment. The combined treatment with cyclophosphamide and Adriamycin (Salmon and Tones, 1974; Jones et al., 1975) and cyclophosphamide and Adriamycin with large-dose methotrexate (Mattsson et al., 1977) was also reported to be effective. The rate of effectiveness of hormonal therapy is about 30 per cent each for estrogen, antiestrogen and androgen therapy.

Cancers of Gastrointestinal Tract

In Japan, gastric cancer is the most predominant cancer, but the mortality and the incidence of gastric cancer in the United States has been decreasing year by year (Comis and Carter, 1974a; Hawley et al., 1970). The most common chemotherapeutic agents for the treatment of gastric cancer are 5-FU and Mitomycin C (Comis and Carter, 1974b). The response rate of 5-FU is about 20 to 26 per cent (Moertel and Reitemeier, 1967; Brennan and Vaitkevicius, 1960). Although Mitomycin C is the most widely used agent, its effects on hematopoiesis and renal functions is a limiting factor for the use of significant doses (Jones, 1959; Lui et al., 1971). Nitrosourea (BCNU, CCNU, methyl CCNU) and Adriamycin were also reported to be effective for gastric cancer (Moertel, 1973, 1975). Combined treatments with Mitomycin C + 5-FU, or 5-FU + BCNU or methyl CCNU have shown better results than single chemotherapy (Kovach et al., 1974; Baker et al., 1975; Moertel et al., 1976; Okei, 1977). Tegafur, however, is used most often.

Proposed combined chemotherapies for other gastrointestinal tracts such as rectal and esophageal cancers are listed in Table V-17.

Table V-17 Chemotherapeutic agents suitable for each cancer.

	Cancer	Chemotherapeutic agents
Lung	Small cell	CYC + CCNU (35%)*
		CYC + CCNU + MTX (56)
		ADR (29), Hexamethylmelamine (36), TGA
	Adeno. Sq. Large	ADR (24), CYC (29), MTX (25), CCNU (41)
Breast		CYC + MTX + 5FU (53)
		ADR + CYC (70), TGA
		ESTROGEN (30), ANDROGEN (30), Anti-EST (30)
GI	Stomach	5FU + BCNU (41), 5FU + mCCNU (40)
		MMC (30), TGA
	Esophagus	BLEO (20–30)
	Colorectal	5FU + mCCNU + VIC (30)
		5FU + mCCNU (30)
	Hepatoma	5FU (37), ADR (70), 5FU + BCNU (37)
	Pancreas	5FU (28), MMC (27)
GU	Chorioca.	
	(low malig.)	MTX (95), ACTD (95), VBL (95)
	(high malig.)	MTX + ACTD + CHLORAMBUCIL (70–80)
		MTX + 6MP (70–80)
	Cervical ca.	MTX (16), CYC (15), 5FU (21), VBL (23)
	Endometrial ca.	PROGESTERONE (30–40)
	Ovarium	MELPHALAN (47), CYC (44), CHLORAMBUCIL (51)
	Bladder	ADR (35), 5FU (35)
	Prostate	ESTROGEN (8–90), CYC (31), ADR (26)
	Renal clear cell	PROGESTERONE (20), VBL (13), HYDROXYUREA (35), TGA
	Testis	VBL + BLEO (75)
		VBL + BLEO + CPDD (100)
Others		
	Adult soft tissue	ADM + DTIC (42), ACTD (20)
	sarcoma	CYC (20), VBL (20)
	Head & neck ca.	MTX (40), BLEO (31), CYC (36), ADR (23), TGA
	Children	
	Rhabdomyosarcoma	VIC + ACTD + CYC (60), ADR (38)
	Ewing's sarcoma	VIC + ACTD + CYC (100), ADR (50)
	Neuroblastoma	CYC + VIC (40), ADR (40)
	Osteogenic sarcoma	MTX (large dose) + citrovorum factor rescue (40)
	Wilms' tumor	ACTD + VBL (60), ADR (63)
	Melanoma	DTIC (24), BCNU (18), INTERFERON
	Skin ca.	5FU (80), BLEO, INTERFERON

* Number in parentheses indicates the response rate that appeared in Carter, Bakowski and Hellmann, eds. *Chemotherapy of Cancer* 1977.

** This table shows only a guide for chemotherapy.

*** Chemotherapy for leukemia and malignant lymphoma is omitted, since the advancement of the chemotherapy is so rapid and not suitable for listing here.

CYC: cyclophosphamide,   MTX: methotrexate,   TGA: tegafur,
ADR: adriamycin,   MMC: Mitomycin C,   BLEO: Bleomycin,
ACTD: Actinomycin D,   VCR: vincristine,   VBL: vinblastine,
CPDD: Cis-platinum diamine dichloride,   DTIC: dacarbazine imidazole carboxamide.

Cancers of Genitourinary Organs

One of the most distinguished examples of chemotherapy for cancers is the treatment of choriocarcinoma by methotrexate, Actinomycin D and vinblastine (Hertz et al., 1961; Bagshaw, 1963; Hammond et al., 1967, 1973; Lewis, 1976). The effectiveness has been proved in 95 per cent of the patients. In more than 90 per cent of the cases, the patient can be cured or a complete remission of the tumor can be obtained by the use of these chemotherapeutic agents.

Chemotherapeutic schedules for uterine carcinoma are different for cervical and endometrial carcinoma. For cervical carcinoma, methotrexate, cyclophosphamide, 5-FU or vincristine are effective for 15 to 23 per cent of the patients. For endometrial carcinoma, the hormonal treatment using the progesterone group such as hydroxy-progesterone, medroxyprogesterone or megestrol acetate, suppress tumors in about 30 to 40 per cent of the patients.

Renal clear cell carcinoma can be treated either by hormonal treatments with medroxyprogesterone or by chemotherapeutic agents such as hydroxyurea, vinblastine, tegafur etc.

Miscellaneous Cancers

Chemotherapeutic agents suitable for other cancers are listed in Table V-17.

Chemotherapy for Metastatic Brain Tumors in our Series

Effects of Chemotherapies in General

Three hundred twenty-nine out of a total 616 patients received some kind of chemotherapy. Of these, 118 patients received chemotherapy alone. Eighty-two patients were treated with surgery and radiotherapy, 57 patients were treated with surgery alone, and 72 patients with simple radiotherapy (Table V-18). Chemotherapeutic agents used for the treatment of metastatic brain tumors in our clinic are listed in Table V-19. Hormones used for the treatment of breast cancer have been omitted from this table. Mitomycin C was one of the agents most frequently used in Japan for the treatment of lung, breast and gastric cancers. Cyclophosphamide (Endoxan) is the most common chemotherapeutic agent for the treatment of breast cancer. 5-FU and tegafur are also widely used. ACNU has recently been introduced for the chemo-radiotherapy of brain tumors (see previous section on radiotherapy).

The effects of chemotherapy for the treatment of metastatic brain tumors are summarized in Table V-20. It is, however, difficult to conclude whether chemotherapy can prolong the life of patients. Surgery and radiotherapy play major roles in extending the lifespan of the patients. The effects of chemotherapy for metastatic brain tumors from lung cancer is summarized in Table V-21. Chemotherapy could extend the lifespan of the patients by two to three months. The longest survivors were in a group treated with surgery, radiotherapy and chemotherapy.

Table V-18 Chemotherapy for metastatic brain tumors.

Primary tumor	No. receiving chemotherapy	Chemotherapy combined with			Chemotherapy alone
		Surgery	Radiation	Surg. + Rad.	
Lung	120 cases	17	33	31	39
Breast	85	19	9	9	48
Others	124	21	30	42	31
Total	**329**	**57**	**72**	**82**	**118**

Table V-19　Chemotherapeutic agents used at our clinic for treatment of metastatic brain tumors.

Chemotherapeutic agents	Total No. of cases	Lung cancer	Breast cancer	Other cancers
Mitomycin C	97	63	23	11
Bleomycin	17	9	0	8
Adriamycin	15	8	1	6
Daunomycin	1	0	0	1
Actinomycin D	4	0	0	4
Chromomycin A_3	26	16	0	10
Cyclophosphamide	66	27	28	11
Thio-TEPA	2	1	1	0
5-FU	38	23	12	3
Tegafur	39	18	10	11
Methotrexate	26	3	1	22
6MP	2	0	0	2
Vincristine	35	14	3	18
Vinblastine	1	0	0	1
VM-26	2	1	1	0
ACNU	23	17	1	5
BCNU	7	5	0	2
CCNU	4	1	0	3
m-CCNU	2	0	1	1
Others	16	5	1	10

Table V-20　Effect of chemotherapy for metastatic brain tumors*.

Treatment		No. of cases	Survival time after the onset of neurological signs
None		129	2.2 mos
Chemotherapy alone		118	4.1
Radiation	without chemotherapy	38	4.3
	with chemotherapy	72	8.3
Surgery	without chemotherapy	83	10.0
	with chemotherapy	57	11.6
Surgery + Radiation	without chemotherapy	37	16.4
	with chemotherapy	82	15.9

Table V-21　Chemotherapy for metastatic brain tumors from lung cancer.

Treatment		No. of cases	Survival time after the onset of neurological signs
None		78	2.1 mos
Chemotherapy alone		39	5.3
Radiation	without chemotherapy	13	3.4
	with chemotherapy	33	6.7
Surgery	without chemotherapy	47	8.4
	with chemotherapy	17	10.8
Surgery + Radiation	without chemotherapy	20*	17.3
	with chemotherapy	31	11.7

* Including the longest survival case who had lived for eight and half years after the craniotomy.

Table V-22 Chemotherapy including hormonal therapy for metastatic brain tumors from breast cancer.

No. of patients receiving chemotherapy and/or hormonal therapy	Chemotherapy alone	Hormonal therapy alone	Chemotherapy and hormonal therapy
85	11	31	43

Table V-23 Chemotherapy for metastatic brain tumors from breast cancer.

Treatment		No. of cases	Survival time after the onset of neurological signs
None		9	1.7 mos
Chemotherapy alone		48	3.1
Radiation	without chemotherapy	2	6.0
	with chemotherapy	9	13.2
Surgery	without chemotherapy	2	2.0
	with chemotherapy	19	9.8
Surgery + Radiation	without chemotherapy	2	3.8
	with chemotherapy	9	17.6

Table V-24 Chemotherapy for metastatic brain tumors from cancers other than lung and breast cancers.

Treatment		No. of cases	Survival time after the onset of neurological signs
None		42	2.5 mos
Chemotherapy alone		31	4.3
Radiation	without chemotherapy	23	4.6
	with chemotherapy	30	8.6
Surgery	without chemotherapy	34	12.6
	with chemotherapy	21	13.9
Surgery + Radiation	without chemotherapy	15	16.8
	with chemotherapy	42	18.6

In the cases of breast cancer, 85 out of the 100 patients received chemotherapy and/or hormone therapy (Table V-22). The beneficial effects of hormone-chemotherapy are evident in cases of breast cancer (Table V-23).

In other cancer cases, the tumor-suppressing effects of chemotherapy are evident, and the life span of the patients were prolonged by a few months, compared with those treated without chemotherapy (Table V-24).

Cyclophosphamide (Endoxan)

Cyclophosphamide was used in the treatment of 45 metastatic brain tumors in our clinic. The median survival time from the onset of neurological signs is shown in Table V-25. Fifty-five per cent of the 287 patients not treated with chemotherapy received surgery and/or radiotherapy; their median survival time was 6.5 months. On the other hand, 62 per cent of the patients treated with cyclophosphamide received

Table V-25   Effect of cyclophosphamide on metastatic brain tumors.

Primary cancer	No. of cases	Median survival time	Treated with				Without chemotherapy	
			Surg. + rad	Surgery	Radiation	None	No. of cases	Median survival time
Lung	10	7.9 mos	1	5	2	2	158	6.0 mos
Breast	27	6.5	3	8	1	15	15	2.6
Others	8	13.6	3	3	2	0	114	7.8
Total	**45**	**8.1**	**7**	**16**	**5**	**17**	**287**	**6.5**

surgery and/or radiotherapy. Their median survival time was 8.1 months. Therefore, the effects of cyclophosphamide on extending the median survival time is less than 1.5 months. The effects of cyclophosphamide are clearly noticeable only in breast cancer patients. Of 27 breast cancer patients treated with cyclophosphamide, 12 cases (44%) received surgical treatment and/or radiotherapy. Their median survival time was 6.5 months. On the other hand, in the 15 patients treated without chemotherapy, six cases (40%) received a surgery and/or radiotherapy, and their median survival time was only 2.6 months. It can thus be expected that cyclophosphamide be effective in extending the life span for metastatic brain tumors due to breast cancer.

Mitomycin C

Mitomycin C is widely used for the treatment of lung, breast and gastrointestinal tract cancer. It sometimes shows dramatic supressive effects on primary lung cancer on a chest roentgenogram by bronchoarterial infusion. Several combined chemotherapies with Mitomycin C have been proposed. FAMT (5-FU-Endoxan-Mitomycin C-Chromomycin A_3) therapy is an example, but it is difficult to prove the better therapeutic effects of the combined chemotherapy over a single chemotherapy. A comparison was made between the effects of the single Mitomycin C administration and the combined FAMT therapy (Table V-26). Fifty-six patients received the single Mitomycin C therapy, whereas 36 patients received the FAMT therapy. Although the ratio of those having surgery and radiotherapy in the group treated with the single Mitomycin C therapy was slightly higher than those in the FAMT-treated group, the mean survival time was longer in the group treated with Mitomycin C

Table V-26   Effect of Mitomycin C and FAMT* administration for metastatic brain tumors.

Primary cancer	MMC** (Single chemotherapy)				FAMT (Combined chemotherapy)			
	No. of cases	No. of surgery	No. of radiation	Median survival time	No. of cases	No. of surgery	No. of radiation	Median survival time
Lung	39	13	27	7.5 mos	19	5	8	6.9 mos
Breast	11	3	4	6.9	11	3	1	3.7
Others	6	5	4	16.1	6	4	4	15.6
Total	**56**	**21**	**35**	**8.3**	**36**	**12**	**13**	**7.4**

  *   FAMT = 5-FU, Cyclophosphamide, Mitomycin C and Chromomycin A_3.
 **   MMC = Mitomycin C.

alone. There was, thus, no evidence demonstrating that combining chemotherapy is superior to single chemotherapy.

Tegafur

Although the systemic or intracarotid infusions of 5-FU could not produce any significant suppressive effects on the metastatic brain tumors, tegafur was occasionally noticeably effective in tumor regression.

The tegafur-glucocorticoid therapy is one of the most effective chemotherapeutic regimens today for metastatic brain tumors. The effects of tegafur on the survival time for metastatic tumor patients are shown in Table V-27. Forty-four patients were given tegafur orally. Compare this data with those shown in Table V-25 on the effects of cyclophosphamide. The median survival time for the 44 patients was 11.5 months. This is three months longer than the group treated with cyclophosphamide. The ratio for the patients who had surgery and/or radiotherapy is almost equivalent to that for the group treated with cyclophosphamide. Tegafur is less toxic than 5-FU. It can be given orally on a long-term basis with only minor side effects.

The patients' response to tegafur is listed in Table V-28. Tegafur was given orally every day at a dose of 600 to 800 mg/day. The total dose of tegafur ranged from 2.1 to 161 g. In almost all of the cases that were effective, the total dose was more than 30 g. Thirty per cent of the patients showed excellent response to the treatment in which the neurological amelioration lasted more than three months, and another 27 per cent of the patients demonstrated neurological amelioration which lasted for more than one month. The total response rate was 57 per cent.

Case 1   63-year-old man. NCC 131084. Lung squamous cell carcinoma.
The patient was admitted as a result of a progressive increase in intracranial pressure and convulsive seizures. The RI scintigram revealed a metastatic tumor in the left

Table V-27   Effect of tegafur on the survival time of metastatic brain tumors.

Primary cancer	No. of cases	Median survival time	No. of patients treated with			
			Surg. + Rad.	Surg.	Rad.	None
Lung	23	11.3 mos	4	4	10	5
Breast	10	6.5	1	1	2	6
Others	11	16.5	5	2	4	0
Total	**44**	**11.5**	**10**	**7**	**16**	**11**

Table V-28   Effect of tegafur on metastatic brain tumors.

Surgery	Rad.	No. of cases	Excellent	Effective	Not respond.
+	−	7	3	3	1
	+	10	4	4	2
−	−	13	4	1	8
	+	14	2	4	8
Total		**44**	**13** (30%)	**12** (27%)	**19** (43%)

parieto-temporal region. He responded well to tegafur (103 g in 198 days) and betamethasone treatments. Headache, nausea and marked choked discs soon disappeared. He was able to return to work, and four and a half years afterwards, he still had not had a relapse of his old symptoms. He did not have a craniotomy, radiotherapy or any other chemotherapy except for immunotherapy with BCG and levamisole. The metastatic brain tumor could not be verified histologically, but a CSF examination revealed the presence of tumor cells.

Case 2   57-year-old man. NCC 178357. Lung squamous cell carcinoma.

The patient was admitted for left hemiparesis, convulsive seizures and an increase in intracranial pressure. The metastatic tumor in the right parietal lobe was removed. He received tegafur (more than 200 g in one year), betamethasone and BCG immunotherapy. The remission continued for about two years and then a recurrence appeared. He died of a metastatic brain tumor three years after craniectomy.

Case 3   57-year-old man. NCC 170308. Lung adenosquamous cell carcinoma.

The patient was admitted for dizziness and an increase in intracranial pressure. The RI scintigram revealed a metastatic tumor in the cerebellum. He received tegafur (295 g in more than one year) and betamethasone therapy. His symptoms quickly disappeared and the remission was maintained for more than a year and a half. There was a recurrence of the tumor and he died after the radiotherapy. Autopsy revealed the presence of a necrotic tumor mass in the same region where the tumor was detected by the RI scintigram in the initial stage.

Cases of metastatic brain tumors from lung adenocarcinoma (Fig. IV-10) and breast cancer (Fig. IV-12) also demonstrate the tumor suppressing effect of tegafur.

These clinical cases demonstrated the effectiveness of the combined tegafur and glucocorticoid therapy. The patients maintained good health and were able to carry out their work normally for more than a year. No other chemotherapeutic agents have demonstrated such effectiveness.

The side effects of tegafur are summarized in Table V-29, and these are limiting factors for the continuation of this chemotherapy. Mild leukopenia and elevation of the serum GOT, GPT, and LDH levels are most common. Exanthema and stomatitis appeared in about 10 per cent of the patients. These side effects, however, are relatively mild compared with other chemotherapeutic agents, and more than half of the patients could tolerate the long-term administration of tegafur.

Tegafur appears in the serum three hours after oral administration of the maximal dose, and in the CSF one hour later. The concentration in the CSF maintains a higher level than that in serum for three hours, and then decreases gradually to almost the same as the level of the serum. It was noted in animal experiments that the activity of tegafur and the active form of 5-FU remained for 24 to 48 hours in the CSF and brain after the administration of tegafur (Fujita et al., 1976).

Table V-29   Side effects of tegafur.

Exanthema	9.7%
Stomatitis	9.7
Anorexia	6.5
Malaise	3.2
Leukocytopenia (< 4000)	10.0
Thrombocytopenia ($< 10^5$)	10.0
GOT (> 45u.)	30.0
GPT (> 30u.)	25.0
LDH (> 380u.)	60.0

Nitrosourea Compounds

No definite results have been obtained for the suppressive effects of BCNU, CCNU and methyl-CCNU on metastatic brain tumors, since the number of patients treated with these nitrosourea compounds was limited (Table V-19). Seven patients (5 lung, 1 rectal, 1 renal clear cell carcinoma) received BCNU, and three of them responded slightly (2 lung, 1 renal carcinoma). Nevertheless, the period of remission was less than two months. Four patients (lung, rectal, skin, and nasopharyngeal carcinoma) received CCNU orally and only one nasopharyngeal cancer patient responded for a few months. There was no remission observed in the two metastatic brain tumor patients treated with methyl-CCNU.

ACNU was administered to 23 metastatic brain tumor patients (17 lung, 1 breast, 2 gastric, 1 uterine and 2 other carcinomas), 16 of whom were concomitantly treated with vincristine and radiotherapy (synchronized chemoradiotherapy—see previous section on radiotherapy, p. 221). Tumor regression on CT scans and neurological amelioration were observed in seven out of the 19 patients treated with radiotherapy combined with ACNU and vincristine. On the other hand, only one out of seven patients treated without radiotherapy responded. Tumor regression was verified in a lung cancer patient undergoing ACNU treatment (63-year-old man, adenocarcinoma, NCC No. 188906). This patient had brain and liver metastases. The complete regression of the tumor on CT scan and the rapid decrease of the serum GOT, GPT and LDH levels after the administration of ACNU and vincristine (vincristine 3 mg and ACNU 100 mg/3 days course) were observed (Figs. V-8 and 9).

The above results suggest that single chemotherapy with a nitrosurea compound rarely suppresses the growth of metastatic brain tumors. Nevertheless, the combined chemotherapy with vincristine and the further concomitant use of radiotherapy might be quite effective for controlling metastatic brain tumors.

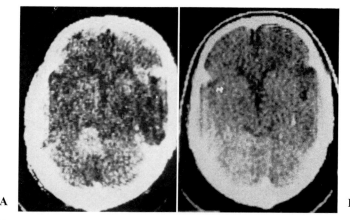

A   B

Fig. V-8 The effect of combined chemotherapy with ACNU and vincristine on metastatic brain tumor from lung cancer. (Adenocarcinoma, 63-year-old man, NCC 188906)
A. CT scan taken before treatment.
B. CT scan taken two months after chemotherapy. No radiotherapy was given.

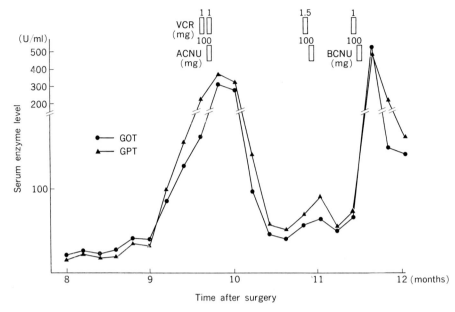

NCC 188906. S.S. 63 M Lung Ca., brain meta., liver meta.

Fig. V-9 The effect of combined chemotherapy with ACNU and vincristine and BCNU on the liver metastasis (same case as Fig. V-8). The rapid decrease of the serum enzyme level (GOT and GPT) was observed after chemotherapy.

Glucocorticoid Therapy

Treatment of Brain Edema

Since Galicich and his associates reported on the preventive effects of dexamethasone for brain edema caused by brain tumors and neurosurgical operations, glucocorticoid has been widely used for the treatment of brain edema in the field of neurosurgery (Galicich and French, 1961; Galicich et al., 1961; Rasmussen and Gulati, 1962; Jelsma and Bucy, 1967; Reulen et al., 1973). Brain edema in the surrounding tissue of the tumor is generally more extensive in metastatic brain tumors in comparison with glioma. Perhaps, it is partly due to impaired respiratory functions and lower oxygen content in the blood caused by primary or secondary lung tumors. Kofman et al. (1957) reported that the use of prednisolone resulted in the amelioration of the clinical symptoms caused by metastatic brain tumors due to breast cancer.

It is widely known that corticosteroid hormones dramatically interrupt the early clinical manifestations of brain metastasis. Today, almost all patients receive some kind of glucocorticoid therapy. Prednisolone, hydrocortisone, dexamethasone or betamethasone is used for the treatment. As an example, improvement in clinical manifestations due to the use of dexamethasone is shown in Table V-30. Almost all 26 cases responded well to the treatment in some symptoms and signs. If a patient does not respond to a high dose of glucocorticoid, then it is suggested that the patient

Table V-30 Effect of dexamethasone on clinical manifestations of metastatic brain tumors (26 cases).

Clinical manifestation	No. of cases	No. with improvement
Headache	22	18
Conscious disturbance	17	13
Choked disc	15	10
Hemiparesis	12	7
Nausea, Vomiting	9	9
Memory disturbance	5	3
Disorientation	4	4
Speech disturbance	4	3
Agraphia	3	3
Delusion	3	3
Convulsive seizure	3	3
Acalculia	2	2
Dizziness	1	1
Visual disturbance	1	1

is in the terminal stage. Glucocorticoids reduce the cerebral edema adjacent to the tumor and increase the cerebral blood flow. The common method for the administration of glucocorticoid is to start with a high dosage of glucocorticoid (such as dexamethasone or betamethasone 16 mg/d or prednisolone 60 to 120 mg/d) and then reduce to the maintenance dosage gradually. The following administrative method was suggested by Lokich (1975) for the glucocorticoid therapy. A few days after commencing steroid therapy (dexamethasone, 16 mg daily in divided doses), local therapy (surgery or radiotherapy) is initiated. Subsequently, the glucocorticoid reduction is carried out at seven-day intervals (25% each) for 28 days, at which time an every other-day steroid regimen is given with near physiologic maintenance doses; by the 35th day, all steroid therapy is discontinued. If symptoms return due to withdrawal, the therapy should be restarted with an increase in the dosage. Many neurosurgeons often realize that neurological manifestations recur when the administration of glucocorticoid is discontinued. From these experiences, the continuous administration of glucocorticoid was considered. The aim of this type of continuous treatment is to ease the burden of the patients for as long as possible, and to assist in other forms of therapy. Few patients in our clinic received large amounts of glucocorticoid continuously for months. Four patients with metastatic brain tumors received more than 1,000 mg of dexamethasone (Table V-31). When continuous glucocorticoid administration is started, the prevention of infections and gastrointestinal ulcers should be considered. Examinations of hematology, serum glucose, electrolytes and blood pressure are necessary. All of the patients were feeling much better without anxiety,

Table V-31 Cases treated with continuous and large doses of dexamethasone.

Age	Sex	Primary cancer	Daily dose (mg)	Duration (days)	Total dose (mg)	Survival time (months)	Effect
41	M	Lung (adeno.)	20–10	120	1,695	10	+
51	M	Lung (adeno.)	10–4	135	1,054	14	+
48	F	Lung (adeno.)	10–3	330	2,298	14	+
23	M	Alv. soft part sarcoma	30–10	180	2,430	12	+

and were free from prior headaches and nausea. They also showed better appetite, the lack of which was one of the side effects of glucocorticoid. It is especially noteworthy that almost no supressive effects on the hematopoietic functions occurred (Table V-32). The white blood cell and lymphocyte counts did not significantly decrease. Glucocorticoid is generally thought to reduce the immunological functions, and therefore, it is better not to use glucocorticoid for long time. It is, however, important to note that a larger amount of glucocorticoid is required for suppressing the immunological functions and that the regular doses of glucocorticoid rarely influence lymphocytic functions even though it is given continuously. It might not be necessary to discontinue the glucocorticoid therapy even after the immunological treatment has commenced, and the benefits of administering glucocorticoid should be considered more seriously. In our series of metastatic brain tumors, more than 500 patients received some kind of glucocorticoid therapy, but there was no case showing serious immunological dysfunction due to glucocorticoid administrations.

The side effects of glucocorticoid therapy are summarized as follows:

Electrolyte balance: The decrease of potassium rarely occurred. Serum electrolytes, however, should be checked, especially in the early stage of the glucocorticoid therapy when a large dose of glucocorticoid is administered.

Diabetes mellitus: Preexisting diabetes mellitus often worsened. In such a case, concomitant use of insulin was required. Patients with a normal level of serum glucose rarely demonstrated an abnormally high glucose level after the administration of glucocorticoid.

Table V-32   Blood examination after long-term administration of dexamethasone.

a.   23-year-old man.   Alveolar soft part sarcoma.   Multiple brain metastases.

	Before treatment	Days after treatment				
		10	16	33	47	60
Total cumulative dose (mg)	0	150	210	380	520	650
WBC ($\times 10^3$)	7.4	10.6	7.5	9.8	12.8	10.9
Lymphocyte count (per cu mm)	2,035	2,226	900	1,568	1,920	2,562
RBC ($\times 10^4$)	475	409	525	483	524	484
Hb (g/dl)	14.7	14.9	15.9	15.5	15.1	14.9
Thrombocyte ($\times 10^4$)	36.5	35.5	17.9	20.3	23.1	25.2

b.   48-year-old woman.   Lung cancer, Adenocarcinoma. Multiple brain metastases.

	Before treatment	Days after treatment				
		15	50	110	160	240
Total cumulative dose (mg)	0	130	330	390	670	1,450
WBC ($\times 10^3$)	5.9	5.2	9.0	3.6	8.6	5.3
Lymphocyte count (per cu mm)	944	1,794	1,890	1,224	645	1,431
RBC ($\times 10^4$)	267	310	360	321	330	356
Hb (g/dl)	8.6	9.4	12.1	10.7	13.4	12.5
Thrombocyte ($\times 10^4$)	18.4	—	18.7	—	14.5	24.5

Serum cholesterol: It often increased moderately. Patients with high levels of cholesterol should be checked frequently.

Blood: No effects on the red blood cell count or hemoglobin were observed. Lymphocyte counts decreased temporarily, when a large amount of glucocorticoid was administered. Long-term administration of glucocorticoid (a moderate daily dose) did not influence the lymphocyte count. Blood coagulation, prothrombin, fifth factor, fibrinogen, plasmin and thrombocytes were not influenced.

Gastrointestinal ulcer: Few patients demonstrated melena in the terminal stage. No patients showed hematemesis.

Constipation: It frequently occurred, and medicine to relieve the constipation was required.

Infection: When patients had preexisting infectious foci, it required the concomitant administration of antibiotics.

Blood pressure: No patients showed a dangerous increase in blood pressure.

Psychosis: No patients showed paranoia or psychotic symptoms. On the contrary, preexisting delusions and overexcitement, which are rather common for patients with metastatic brain tumors, disappeared after the glucocorticoid therapy.

Acne: This skin manifestation often occurred.

Muscle power weakness: The muscle power often decreased when glucocorticoid was administered for a long period of time.

Oncolytic Effect

While many patients suffering from metastatic brain tumors were treated by a large dose of glucocorticoid, physicians were often aware of the scope controlling brain edema by the hormone. Glucocorticoid has two other significant effects: the inhibition of oncogenesis and oncolytic action in certain tumors. The administration of glucocorticoid inhibits the development of spontaneous and radiation-induced leukemia (Wooley and Peters, 1953; Upton and Furth, 1954; Duplan, 1962). Cortisol dramatically inhibits the development of plasma cell tumors (Takakura et al., 1966). Glucocorticoids are well known to have oncolytic effects on lymphocytic leukemia, malignant lymphoma, plasma cell tumors (Hollander et al., 1968), thymoma (Green and Forman, 1974), Ewing's sarcoma, seminoma, melanoma (Kotsilimbas et al., 1967), some breast cancer and some gliomas (Gurcay et al., 1971). Although the mechanism of the oncolytic action of glucocorticoid is not clear, it is postulated that steroid adheres to the receptor in the cytoplasm of the tumor cells and produces cytolytic action. The lack of a specific receptor protein is responsible for the resistance of tumor cells against glucocorticoid. Glucocorticoid sensitive tumors should be treated by a large dose of glucocorticoid. Standard regimens of chemosteroid therapy for the above mentioned tumors are shown in Table V-33.

Posner et al. (1977) reported on the oncolytic effects of glucocorticoid on epidural metastases of some cancers. Four patients (thymoma, seminoma, Ewing's sarcoma and malignant lymphoma) demonstrating symptoms and signs of spinal cord compression resulting from the epidural metastases were treated with glucocorticoid. Two patients were able to get prompt relief with only the administration of gluco-

Table V-33   Chemotherapy for glucocorticoid sensitive tumors.

		Chemotherapeutic schedule		Remarks
Acute lymphocytic leukemia CNS involvement	VP	Vcr Pred.	1.5 mg/m² i.v./W 40 mg/m² p.o./d	Induction therapy, 1st 4–6 Wks
	VP-D VP-L	V-P + Daunorubicin V-P + L-asparagenase	25 mg/m² i.v./W 10,000 U/m² i.v./W	Induction therapy, 2nd 2 Wks
		Mtx i.t. + radiation		CNS involvement
Malignant lymphoma (Non-Hodgkin lymphoma)	CVP	Cyc Vcr Pred.	400 mg/m² p.o. D1–5 1.4 mg/m² i.v. D1 100 mg/m² p.o. D1–5	4 Wk course, 1st
	CHOP	Cyc Adria. Vcr. Pred.	750 mg/m² i.v. D1 50 mg/m² i.v. D1 1.4 mg/m² i.v. D1 100 mg/m² p.o. D1–5	4–6 Wk course, 2nd
	BACOP	Cyc Adria. Vcr Bleo. Pred.	650 mg/m² i.v. D1 & D5 25 mg/m² i.v. D1 & D8 1.4 mg/m² i.v. D1 & D8 5 mg/m² i.v. D15 & D22 60 mg/m² p.o. D15–D28	4–6 Wk course, 2nd
Plasma cell tumor	MP	Melphalan Pred.	10 mg/m² p.o. D1–4 60 mg/m² p.o. D1–4	6 Wks
	CP	Cyc Pred.	1 mg/m² i.v. D1 60 mg/m² p.o. D1–4	6 Wks
	BP	BCNU Pred.	150 mg/m² i.v. D4 60 mg/m² p.o. D1–4	6 Wks

Cyc: cyclophosphamide, Vcr: vincristine, Pred.: prednisolone, D1: Day 1.

corticoid.   The marked shrinkage or complete disappearance of the metastasis was encountered by a direct oncolytic effect of the steroid.   For the other two patients, glucocorticoid combined with other chemotherapeutic agents caused the disappearance of the extradural tumor.   They mentioned a very important point: "Neurologists and neurosurgeons are so accustomed to attributing the beneficial effects of glucocorticoids for CNS tumors to the relief of edema that they may overlook instances in which clinical improvements result from the oncolytic action of the glucocorticoids.   Failure to fully understand the oncolytic potential of the glucocorticoid therapy may lead to an inadequate treatment, namely, an unnecessay surgical procedure."   A particularly interesting observation of Posner's thymoma case is the histological type, which was composed of a mixed epithelial and lymphoid rather than a purely lymphoid tumor.   From our experience, the tumor progression stopped in some cancer patients both in metastatic sites and primary tumors during large-dosage glucocorticoid therapy.   The oncolytic effects of glucocorticoid should be studied more extensively in the future, in the field of not only metastatic brain tumors but also gliomas.

Hormonal Control of Brain Metastases Due to Breast Cancer

The possibility of treating breast cancer by hormonal control was first suggested by Beatson in 1896, and the benefits of oophorectomy for tumor suppression was investigated. Later, Huggins and his associates established the concept of hormone dependency in the field of cancer treatment (Huggins and Hodges, 1941; Huggins, 1965). The hormone dependency has been observed in cancers of the breast, prostate, thyroid, kidney, endometrium and seminal vesicles; glucocorticoid dependency has also been noted in leukemia, lymphoma and some melanomas.

For breast cancer, oophorectomy is the most widely accepted treatment (Kennedy, 1974) for premenopausal patients. Its effectiveness is between 20 to 40 per cent. A rapidly progressing tumor in younger patients under 35 years of age cannot generally be suppressed by hormonal therapy alone, and should first be treated by chemotherapy. Patients who respond to the oophorectomy can be treated with secondary hormonal therapies, including androgen administration, adrenalectomy or hypophysectomy. This also applies to the younger patients. For patients whose age falls within five years after the menopausal period, the effects of oophorectomy and adjuvant hormonal therapy have only a limited effect. The administration of androgen was effective in about 13 per cent of the cases. Therefore, chemotherapy is the first choice. For patients in the latter part of menopause, the first choice for treatment is estrogen therapy. Androgen or anti-estrogen therapies are also recommended.

For the indication of hypophysectomy, the selection of the patients is most important. Patients who responded to other hormonal therapies, i.e., oophorectomy, androgen or estrogen therapies, are believed to also be able to respond to hypophysectomy. A rapidly growing tumor will not respond to hypophysectomy. The aggressiveness of breast cancer can be estimated from the free interval between mastectomy and the appearance of metastases (Wilson, C.B. and Saglam, 1973). Postmenopausal patients do respond better to hypophysectomy than premenopausal patients. Hypophysectomy is generally not recommended for patients having lung metastases with lymphangitis, liver metastases with jaundice, or brain metastases (Carter et al., 1977). From our experience, however, hypophysectomy, is still recommended for selected patients having brain metastases. Since the hormone dependency of breast cancer is now possible to estimate by the hormone receptor assay of each tumor, the proper hormonal treatment can be rationally selected. The following results are, however, based on our past records for nonselected cases regarding the aspects of hormone dependency.

Since the metastatic brain tumor due to breast cancer is already a pathophysiological manifestation of the advanced stage of this cancer, the general hormonal therapy for breast cancer without brain metastasis cannot be simply applied. Immediate action must be taken to reduce intracranial pressure. Removal of the tumor by surgery or radiotherapy with chemotherapy is essential in the first stage of treatment. Hormonal treatment should be considered in the second stage of treatment. Many patients often receive some form of hormonal therapy before consulting a neurosurgical clinic. Hormonal treatment for metastases to the brain is mainly the use of some type of steroid hormones. The decision for oophorectomy or hypophysectomy should be based on two main conditions. The first is the hormone dependency of the tumor. The second is the general condition of the patient, whether she will be able to tolerate the surgery and can expect to have meaningful and useful life after the operation.

Androgens

Testosterone propionate was first given to a breast cancer patient by Ulrich and Loeser in 1939, and its effects on tumor suppression were verified. The large dose of testosterone, however, caused the undesirable side effect of masculinization. As a result, other hormonal agents having less virilizing effects have been developed. Methyl-androstenediol, methyl-dihydrotestosterone, halogenated testosterone and dromostanolone are some examples. Since Segaloff and Kennedy reported on the effectiveness of orally administered fluoxymesterone (Halotestin) in 1958, it has been widely used for the treatment of breast cancers (Cooperative Breast Cancer Group, 1964; Kennedy, 1974).

Fluoxymesterone was given to 15 patients having metastatic brain tumors. A daily dose of 12 to 20 mg of fluoxymesterone was orally given every day, as long as the suppressive effects of this hormone existed. Its effectiveness was seen in about 40 per cent of the patients (Table V-34). The effectiveness was evaluated by the following two observations: first, whether the amelioration of clinical symptoms and signs could be seen after administered fluoxymesterone and second, whether the patient could survive more than six months after the onset of neurological signs. Its effectiveness was proven in 30 per cent of the cases of premenopausal patients and 60 per cent of postmenopausal patients. Of seven patients who received both oophorectomy and fluoxymesterone, four of them (57%) showed good response. Three of

Table V-34 Effect of hormonal treatment on metastatic brain tumors from breast cancer.

Hormonal treatment.	No. of patients	No. of* effective cases	Ratio of effectiveness Premenopausal patients	Ratio of effectiveness Postmenopausal patients
1) Androgen group	22	6 (27%)	3/14	3/7
Fluoxymesterone (Halotestin)	15	6 (40%)	3/10	3/5
2) Estrogen group	27	8 (30%)	3/11(9)**	5/16
Diethylstilbestrol &	11	3 (30%)	1/3(2)	2/8
stilbestrol diphosphate (Honvan)				
Hexestrol (Hexron)	6	2 (33%)	0/(2)(2)	2/4
Other estrogen group	10	3 (30%)	2/5(5)	1/5
3) CB 154 (bromocriptine)	3	2*** (76%)	1/1	1/2
4) Hypophysectomy	14	7*** (50%)	3/9	4/5
5) Oophorectomy	44	9 (20%)	6/33	3/11
Oophorectomy + Adrenalectomy	22	3 (14%)	2/14	1/8

  * Effective case: see text for the criteria of effectiveness.
  ** Number in parentheses indicates the cases received oophorectomy.
  *** Hormone-dependent tumor.

them survived more than one year, and two for more than two years. One patient was given fluoxymesterone after hypophysectomy, and she was able to survive for five years and two months. These results suggested that the combined treatment with surgical abrasion of the endocrine organ and the administration of selected steroid hormones could produce significant palliation in patients having metastatic brain tumors due to breast cancer, when the appropriate hormone dependency was present.

Although fluoxymesterone can be given to patients of any age, it is expected to be more effective for postmenopausal or oophorectomized patients. Other types of androgens failed to demonstrate any significant suppressive effects on metastatic brain tumors in our series of treatments.

Estrogens

Estrogen was first given to breast cancer patients by Haddow et al. in 1944 (Kennedy, 1974). The administration of estrogens is the first choice for postmenopausal patients, but it sometimes causes tumor progression in premenopausal patients. Therefore, caution should be taken in the use of estrogen for premenopausal patients. The sensitivity of tumors to estrogens needs further study in future.

Diethylstilbestrol (25 to 50 mg a day), stilbestrol diphosphate (Honvan, 300 to 1,200 mg a day) or hexestrol (Hexron, 30 to 90 mg a day) is given orally every day. Their collective effectiveness was seen in about 30 per cent of the metastatic brain tumor patients (Table V-34). There was no significant difference in effectiveness among these hormones. Estrogens were administered to nine out of 11 premenopausal patients receiving both oophorectomy and adrenalectomy. The beneficial effects of the combined treatment, however, could not be verified.

Prolactin Inhibitor

It is well known that prolactin causes the progression of breast cancer in prolactin dependent tumors. The use of prolactin inhibitors, L-DOPA, ergocornine, or bromocriptine (CB-154), for the treatment of breast cancers is studied elsewhere. It is also postulated that one of the suppressive effects of hypophysectomy for breast cancers is that it is able to reduce the prolactin level. We administered bromocriptine to three patients having metastatic brain tumors due to breast cancer. Two of them responded (Table V-34) and the serum prolactin level was reduced significantly. The number of patients tested is still not sufficient and further studies will be required to evaluate the effectiveness of bromocriptine.

Hypophysectomy

The effect of hypophysectomy for disseminating breast cancers has been well documented by Pearson and Ray (1959), Kjellberg et al. (1972), Zervas (1969), Rand et al. (1964), Hardy (1971), and McGuire (1974). Hypophysectomy caused the tumor to regress in 11 per cent of the unselected postmenopausal patients by the Study

Group of Breast Cancer (Witt et al., 1963). A response rate of 87 per cent for oophorectomized patients was reported by Ray (1960). Nevertheless, since the criteria of response were different for each researcher, the response rate cannot really be compared. Wilson, C.B. et al. (1966, 1967, 1969) reported that of patients who were not selected according to age or their previous response to hormonal therapy, 40 per cent responded favorably to cryohypophysectomy.

In our series, surgical hypophysectomy was performed on 14 patients having metastatic brain tumors. Seven of them (50%) responded (Table V-34) and survived for more than six months. Two patients survived for more than one year following hypophysectomy. The most effective case is described in the section titled, "The Multidisciplinary Treatment of Metastatic Brain Tumors", which appears later (p. 277). Three out of the 14 patients received both oophorectomy and hypophysectomy. They responded to oophorectomy, but not to hypophysectomy. Therefore, the hormonal treatment does not always predict the effectiveness of hypophysectomy in metastatic brain tumors due to breast cancer. Relief of pain due to pituitary gland destruction with alcohol injections were reported by Moricca (1974a, b). There is a possibility that alcohol injections cause a fine lesion in the hypothalamus and this releases endorphin and encephalin which relieve the pain.

Oophorectomy

Oophorectomy was generally performed by surgeons before the neurological manifestations of the metastatic brain tumors appeared. Therefore, oophorectomy for metastatic brain tumors, as shown in Table V-34, does not demonstrate direct effects on metastatic brain tumors. The reduction of the tumor growth rate, however, evidently succeeded in causing beneficial effects and even prolonged the life of the patients afflicted with metastatic brain tumors. Here, the effectiveness of oophorectomy was seen in approximately 20 per cent of the patients. Combined adrenalectomy did not, however, demonstrate any beneficial effects for metastatic brain tumors due to breast cancer.

Chemotherapy and Radiotherapy for Metastatic Tumors of the Brain, Meninges and Skull of Children

Fifty-nine cases of metastatic tumors of the brain, meninges and skull in children, admitted during the years from 1962 to 1975, were studied to clarify the effects of the treatment, with special emphasis on the use of chemotherapy and radiotherapy. The patients included 20 leukemias, 13 neuroblastomas, 10 retinoblastomas, 12 sarcomas, 3 malignant lymphomas and 1 embryonal carcinoma. Forty-nine patients were treated with chemotherapy and/or radiotherapy. The therapeutic methods and prognoses are summarized in Table V-35. Fourteen patients received intrathecal administration of methotrexate and radiotherapy, 12 patients received intrathecal methotrexate therapy without radiation, and 11 patients received only radiotherapy.

Table V-35 Therapy and prognosis of metastatic tumors to the brain, meninges and skull in children.

| Diagnosis | No. of cases | Therapeutic method | | | | Duration** from the onset of primary tumor to the metastasis | Median*** survival time |
		Mtx +Rad.	Mtx*	Rad.	Other chemo-therapy		
Leukemia	20	8 (8)****	9 (5)			11.8 mos	4.9 mos
Retinoblastoma	10	1 (1)	6 (2)	1 (1)		18.2	4.7
Neuroblastoma	13			5 (4)	6 (1)	5.6	5.3
Sarcoma	12	5 (3)		4 (3)	1 (0)	15.0	8.7
Malig. lymphoma				1 (1)	2 (2)	14.3	8.7
Other tumor	4						
Total	**59**	**14 (12)**	**15 (7)**	**11 (9)**	**9 (3)**	**12.3**	**6.0**

    *   Mtx: Methotrexate intrathecal administration.
   **   Duration from the onset of primary tumor to the onset of metastasis.
  ***   Survival time from the onset of symptoms due to metastasis.
****   Number in parentheses indicates the number of effective cases.

Nine other patients received chemotherapy using various chemotherapeutic agents. Radiotherapy was effective in most cases. Twelve out of 14 patients received radiation and intrathecal infusion of methotrexate. Nine out of 11 patients treated with simple radiotherapy responded to the treatment. On the other hand, only 7 out of 15 patients treated with intrathecal methotrexate therapy responded. The median survival times after the onset of symptoms due to metastasis were 4.9 months for leukemia, 4.7 months for retinoblastoma, 5.3 months for neuroblastoma and 8.7 months for sarcomas and other tumors.

Leukemia

Leptomeningeal infiltration existed in most cases. Diagnosis was verified by the presence of leukemic cells in the cerebrospinal fluid. Autopsies indicated that the typical pattern of the metastases was the diffuse infiltration of tumor cells in the leptomeninges and in the subarachnoid space. Multiple intracerebral hematomas accompanied by leukemic cells were occasionally observed. The intrathecal injection of methotrexate with or without whole brain irradiation was effective in the initial stage of metastasis.

    Case report   3-year-old girl. NCC 154896. Acute myelocytic leukemia.
    The patient noticed swelling of her forehead in November 1971. Acute myelocytic leukemia was diagnosed by biopsy. She was treated with chemotherapy using vincristine, 6-MP and prednisolone. Symptoms of meningeal irritation appeared in August 1973, and leukemic cells were detected in the cerebrospinal fluid. The symptoms subsided the intrathecal infusion of methotrexate. Remission, however, continued for only three months, and the symptoms reappeared. The second and third administration of intrathecal methotrexate were effective for less than two months, and she died in March 1974. Autopsy revealed the infiltration of leukemic cells with hemorrhagic foci in the pia and arachnoid and subarachnoid hematoma.

Retinoblastoma

Autopsies indicated that tumor cells infiltrated along the optic nerve into the intracranial subarachnoid space spread into diffuse pattern and sometimes formed solitary lesions in the hypothalamus, the cerebellum or other intracerebral regions. An intrathecal injection of methotrexate with radiotherapy was effective in some cases.

Case report 2-year-old boy. NCC 123871. Retinoblastoma.
The patient's eyeball was enucleated in October 1969, immediately after the establishment of diagnosis. Ten months after the surgery, he complained of headaches and nausea, and nuchal stiffness was noticed. Tumor cells were detected in the cerebrospinal fluid. Ommaya's reservoir was set and intraventricular administration of methotrexate with radiotherapy was initiated. All symptoms soon disappeared and the fractionated infusion of intraventricular methotrexate was continued (2 to 5 mg of methotrexate, every week). The remission continued for more than a year, but he died 14 months after the onset of the neurological symptoms. Autopsy revealed the tumor infiltration along with the optic nerve, in the hypothalamus, brain stem and cerebellum.

Neuroblastoma

Metastatic skull tumors were palpated in all 13 cases. Autopsy findings revealed that metastatic lesions existed not only in the skull but also in the meninges. Radiotherapy was given with a slight suppressive effect.

Case report 5-year-old boy. NCC 138552. Neuroblastoma.
The patient complained of pains in the abdominal region and in his lower extremities in September 1970. Two months later, a nodule, 4 cm in diameter, was found on his skull. Radiotherapy with systemic administration of vincristine and cyclophosphamide was started. The tumor completely regressed, but in March 1972, it reappeared and further chemotherapy showed no effect. He died in June 1972. Autopsy revealed that the skull tumor had invaded the dura mater and had infiltrated the cerebral cortex.

Sarcomas such as rhabdomyosarcoma or osteogenic sarcoma and malignant lymphomas showed some temporary response to some chemotherapeutic agents. A general prognostic survey showed that the effect of neurosurgical removal of the tumors was limited in most cases. Early diagnosis and care under pediatricians and neurosurgeons might bring about a better chance of recovery by intensive treatment with chemotherapy and radiotherapy. High-dose methotrexate rescue treatment with citrovorum factor is effective in some cases.

Prophylactic Chemotherapy for the CNS Involvement of Leukemia

Involvement of the central nervous system is a common fatal complication of leukemia. The clinical development of CNS leukemia ranges from 26 to 83 per cent according to various investigators. Controlled studies to clarify the effect and toxicity of two prophylactic therapies for CNS involvement of leukemia were initiated by a study group on leukemia in children in Tokyo (Ise, 1977). Two hundred sixty-seven previously nontreated children were evaluated in that study from January 1968 to September 1977. All the patients had complete remission after the treatment. The children's ages ranged from three months to 15 years (the mean age was four years and one month).

Vincristine and prednisolone were used in all cases except for 20 patients who also received 6-mercaptopurine and methotrexate (VAMP therapy). After complete remission through the treatment, the patients were randomly divided into three groups for prophylactic therapy for CNS involvement. Group A (121 patients) received no prophylactic therapy. Group B (85 patients) received intrathecal methotrexate infusion once during the period of complete remission and then once at each consolidation therapy session. Group C (61 patients) received radiotherapy throughout the whole skull with intrathecal methotrexate infusion during the period of complete remission. All patients received consolidation therapy with VAMP every two months during the first year, and then every three months after the second year. The incidence of CNS involvement of leukemia was 47.9 per cent for Group A, 21.2 per cent for Group B and 8.2 per cent for Group C, respectively. The median duration of complete remission was 12 months for Group A, 22 months for Group B, and 24 months for Group C. The ratio of patients that survived until the end of the study was 10.7 per cent for Group A, 69.4 per cent for Group B, and 70.5 per cent for Group C. The number of patients and the duration of survival in Groups B and C did not differ significantly. The temporary reduction of methotrexate was frequently necessary because of toxicity which included pancytopenia, nausea, vomiting, diarrhea, constipation, abdominal pains and stomatitis. The long-term results for such a study are not yet available, but the following conclusions can be made. (1) Periodic intrathecal administration of methotrexate combined with radiotherapy of the head were effective in preventing CNS involvement due to leukemia. (2) The irradiated group had shown a more pronounced reduction in the development of CNS involvement. (3) The median duration of continuous hematologic remission in the irradiated group was longer than that of the non-irradiated group. (4) The duration of the survival for the methotrexate group and that for the methotrexate plus the radiation group did not differ significantly. (5) Life-threatening infections occurred more frequently in the irradiated group (13.1%) than in the group treated with methotrexate alone (1.2%). The dramatic improvement in the survival time of children with acute lymphoblastic leukemia (ALL) has been demonstrated in the last decade. Without prophylactic treatment, central nervous system (CNS) leukemia develops in more than 50 per cent of the patients, and when it appears, the patient cannot be cured. Although the prevention of CNS leukemia has been widely investigated and substantial progress has been made in recent years, it is still controversial as to how to properly manage the leukemia patient in complete remission.

For preventing CNS involvement of leukemia, most investigators agree on the following points:

1) Radiotherapy is effective in reducing the development of CNS leukemia, but the suggestive total dose of radiation differs.

2) Intrathecal administration of methotrexate has a major role.

3) Systemic chemotherapy is valuable and it should be started as early as possible after the introductory treatment for primary leukemia.

4) The side effects of the treatment, such as leukoencephalopathy (a demyelinating syndrome), mineralizing microangiopathy, and the damage of late neurological functions (school performance, recent memory disturbance, etc.) should be considered when establishing the therapeutic schedule.

Progressive multifocal leukoencephalopathy often complicates leukemias and lymphomas. It was thought to be a latent viral infection, which became prevalent in immunologically suppressed patients. Prophylactic therapy of leukemias was reported to be a factor which produced leukoencephalopathy. Clinical manifestations include speech disturbance, ataxia, spasticity, dysphagia, seizures, lethargy, confusion, decerebration and coma (Price and Jamieson, 1975). It appears mainly in the cerebral white matter of the fronto-parietal region and is characterized by demyelination, reactive astrocytosis and white matter degeneration. A second complication is a mineralizing microangiopathy. Its clinical manifestations include focal seizure, poor muscular coordination, ataxia, perceptual motor disability and behavioral disorders. It is a non-inflammatory mineralizing degeneration of the microvasculature, seen mainly in the gray matter (putamen and cerebral or cerebellar cortex) and dystrophic calcification of adjacent brain tissue. The pathogenesis of this complication is supposed to be a small vessel injury due to radiation by systemic chemotherapy (Price, 1979).

Various methods of radiotherapy combined with intrathecal administration of methotrexate were reported for prophylaxis of CNS involvement from acute lymphoblastic leukemia (Simone et al., 1979; Freeman et al., 1979; Willoughby, 1979). Simone and his colleagues noted that a high cumulative dose of intrathecally administered methotrexate was essential for developing leukoencephalopathy, and therefore recommended the radiotherapy with concomitant administration of a small dose of methotrexate. They found that a total dose of radiation less than 12 Gy. failed to reduce the frequency of CNS relapse due to acute lymphoblastic leukemia, and suggested that a total dose of about 20 to 25 Gy. is the most appropriate.

It has been reported that leukoencephalopathy occurs most often when irradiation is given concomitantly with intrathecal methotrexate administration (Price and Jamieson, 1975; McIntosh et al., 1978) and also when there is a high intraventricular level of methotrexate due to blockage of ventricular pathways (Shapiro et al., 1975) or when methotrexate is given intravenously in a high dose (Allen et al., 1978).

Since radiation is responsible for development of leukoencephalopathy, it is naturally better not to use radiotherapy on the brain or spinal cord. Clarkson and his colleagues (1979) at Sloan Kettering Memorial Cancer Center carried out clinical trials to see if it is possible to prevent CNS leukemia by chemotherapy without radiotherapy. They gave extensive chemotherapies (methotrexate intrathecally, 6.25 mg/m² once a week concomitantly with vincristine, Danuomycin, cytosine arabinoside, 6-thioguanine, L-asparaginase, BCNU and prednisolone or further add to hydroxyurea and cyclophosphamide to the previous regimen) and concluded that it should be possible to prevent CNS leukemia by chemotherapy alone without cranial irradiation. The intraventricular administration of methotrexate using Ommaya's reservoir is a safe procedure without hazardous spinal cord complications, but further studies will be required to see whether it is superior to the injection by lumbar puncture.

It is also known that the risk of initial CNS relapse is greater in patients with a high initial leucocyte count. Patients with an initial leukocyte count above 20,000/ mm³ (Simone et al., 1979) or 25,000/mm³ (Clarkson et al., 1979) are at a critical level.

From an immunological point of view, Jasmin et al. (1979) in France have noted that active immunotherapy using a mixture of BCG and irradiated frozen leukemic cells along with chemo-radiotherapy may enhance the protection of the development of CNS leukemia.

Various protocols for prophylactic treatment of CNS involvement of acute lymphoblastic leukemia are precisely described in a monograph entitled, "CNS Complications of Malignant Disease," edited by Whitehouse and Kay (1979), but the problems in this field should be solved by further investigations in the future.

On the contrary, the frequency of CNS involvement from acute myelogenous leukemia (AML) is less common than acute lymphoblastic leukemia. The general prognosis of AML is poor and the overall rate of CNS leukemia is around twenty per cent of the patients. Although headache is the most common symptom, peripheral nerve root lesion, cauda equina syndrome and paraplegia are more frequently encountered in CNS involvement of AML than ALL. The presence of papilledema is comparatively rare. Although not as many studies on the schedule of prophylactic therapy for CNS involvement of AML have been carried out as for ALL, the induction chemotherapy regimen at Royal Marsden Hospital includes cytosine arabinoside, Daunorubicin, 6-thioguanine, cyclophosphamide and adjuvant immunotherapy with BCG (McElwain et al., 1979). The regimen of the Memorial Sloan Kettering Cancer Center includes Daunorubicin, cytosine arabinoside and 6-thioguanine (DAT) with radiotherapy—24 Gy. (Rees, 1979). The prognosis of patients having CNS leukemia from AML is very poor. The median survival time of the patients in whom CNS leukemia developed early was six weeks, with the longest survivor living only 11 weeks (McElwain, 1979). Although the prophylaxis of CNS leukemia from AML seems to be valuable, the outcomes of the above-mentioned studies were not definitely concluded.

In cases of chronic myeloid leukemia (CML), the terminal stage of the blast crisis is usually formed by myeloblastic leukemic cells (M-type). Recent investigations on the surface markers, however, have revealed that about 20 to 30 per cent of the patients demonstrated lymphoblast transformation, resembling acute lymphoblastic leukemia (L-type), and the cells carried Philadelphia (Ph') chromosome. The prognosis of M-type blast crisis is very poor. The median survival time of the patients was only two months, whereas the median survival time of L-type blast crisis was 10 to 14 months. Because of the short period of the M-type blast crisis, M-type CNS leukemia from CML has not been found. The prognosis of L-type meningeal involvement of CML was between 10 to 30 months (Durrant et al., 1979).

IMMUNOTHERAPY

Historical Note

The dawn of immunotherapy for cancer was brought about due to work carried out by Hericourt and Richet in 1895. They inoculated cancer cells into dogs and monkeys to produce an antibody. Regression of the tumors, however, did not result from the antisera injection (passive immunization). Leyden and Blumenthal (1902) transplanted autologous cancer cells intradermally into patients (active immunization), but no therapeutic effects were observed. Many papers regarding cancer immunotherapy have been published, but with no fruitful results. Immunological studies on brain tumors were initiated by Siris in 1936. He separated protein from an alcohol extract of glioblastoma and injected the protein into rabbits to produce an antibody, but failed to demonstrate any specific glioma antigen.

The immunological treatment of brain tumors has recently drawn much attention. In 1958, Murray reported on the effects of antisera against human breast cancer homogenate. They were injected into three patients having metastatic brain tumors. The amelioration of double vision and headaches were observed. This report is probably the first paper regarding the immunological treatment of metastatic brain tumors. Bloom et al. (1960) reported that the autologous transplantation of glioma failed to suppress tumor growth or to demonstrate any increase in the autoantibody in serum. On the other hand, Grace et al. (1961) transplanted autologous glioma to the patients. Two patients having tumor cell transplantations did not demonstrate any increase in serum antibodies to counter the tumors, but two patients who rejected the transplantation demonstrated a delayed hypersensitive skin reaction countering the nonsoluble fraction of the glioma and normal brain. These active and passive immunizations could not demonstrate any significant tumor-suppressing effects.

Mahaley and Day (1965) investigated the role of antibodies against glioma homogenate. Antisera was absorbed by normal tissue. It was then labeled with radioactive iodine and injected into the patient. Isotope uptake was observed in the glioma tissue. They suggested the possibility of internal radiotherapy using an isotope labeled antibody. This kind of therapy essentially requires a pure antibody. Mahaley et al. (1968, 1969) reported on the method for further separating the antibodies by producing an antigen-antibody complex, and then separating this by electrophoresis and density gradient techniques.

Trouillas and Lapras (1970) reported on active immunization using BCG and Freund's adjuvant. Autologous glioma cells mixed with BCG were inoculated into the thighs of the patients. Lymphocytes were separated from lymph drained out from the thoracic duct, after the PPD skin reaction turned positive. The separated lymphocytes were inoculated into the tumor. Two glioblastoma patients thus treated died within five months, and one oligodendroglioma patient survived for more than 17 months. In other treatments, glioma homogenates mixed with Freund's adjuvant were injected into 17 patients. The length of time before recurrence was 4.5 months for the controlled group, and 8.5 months for the immunized group.

The use of immunocompetent cells for treatment of glioma was initiated at our clinic. Autologous or allogeneic lymphocytes, or allogeneic bone marrow cells were transplanted to glioma patients (Takakura et al., 1972, 1975). Some long-term survivors among the glioma patients were noted, but there are problems of host-vs-graft reactions. Young et al. (1977) utilized autologous lymphocytes for the treatment of glioma and observed favorable effects in some cases. Ommaya (1977) reported that glioma cells mixed with BCG were inoculated into the host patient and PPD was infused into the dead space of the tumor through a device called Ommaya's implant. No suppressive effects on the tumor growth were observed, however.

Since the use of allogeneic lymphocytes has its limitations, recent approaches to the immunological treatment of cancer tend towards using various immunopotentiators or lymphocyte chemical factors.

The concept that infection suppresses cancer growth has existed for more than two centuries. Today BCG is one of the most widely studied immunopotentiators in the field of cancer immunotherapy. It is quite interesting to note that the relationship between tuberculosis and cancer has been discussed for more than a century. Rokitansky (1855) remarked that an antagonism prevailed between tuberculosis and cancer. McCaskey had the same view and suggested a systematic local injection of tuberculin into the cancerous tissue in properly selected inoperable cases of cancer. Dabney (1916) agreed with McCaskey and he suggested the injection of tuberculin in cancer cases. It has been proven that lymphoid cell activity is an essential factor in the immunization process and it would seem that tuberculosis stimulates lymphoid cell activity and demonstrates an inhibitory influence on cancer (Broders, 1919).

On the other hand, negative views were also presented by several investigators. Lebert (1852) and Williams (1887) found a history of tuberculosis in 47.7 per cent of 316 cancer patients. Lubarsch (1888) found carcinoma in 4.4 per cent of the tuberculous patients, and in 11.7 per cent of the nontuberculous patients. Of 569 carcinomatous cadavers, he found tuberculosis in 20.6 per cent of them. In 5,967 noncarcinomatous cadavers, tuberculosis was detected in 42.7 per cent of them. Thus, his statistics indicated that carcinoma was found more often in nontuberculous than in tuberculous patients, the ratio being about 3:1 in favor of the former.

After reviewing previous reports, Broders (1919) surveyed 20 cases of his own autopsied specimens and found that tuberculosis and cancer were associated in the same specimen in seven cases (35%). He, himself, opposed the theory that the two diseases were antagonistic.

Based on experimental trials of treatments using living tubercle bacilli and tuberculin of transplantable cancer in rats, a small number of carefully selected cases of cancer were treated with tuberculin by Shutton under the direction of and in consultation with Pearl of the Institute for Biological Research of Johns Hopkins University (Pearl and Shutton, 1929). Treatment of the first case with tuberculin began on July 10, 1928. Pearl and his colleagues (1929) summarized the favorable results of the experimental treatment of cancer with tuberculin. After treating seven cancer cases, he concluded that the clinical and histopathological data obtained were of sufficiently promising character to warrant the continuation of the investigation.

"What is the most effective method of using tuberculin in cancer therapy, or what would be the effect of tuberculin on cancer, and when it should be used in combination with surgery, radium, and other methods of cancer therapy, we are unable to either state or to predict the effects, but obviously these matters need further investigation." This remark by Pearl was made just half a century ago. In the cases that he investigated, one breast cancer patient having a metastatic brain tumor was included. Although his tuberculin therapy was not aimed at brain metastases, it is worthwhile to cite it here.

> **Case report**   62-year-old woman (Pearl et al., 1929). Adenocarcinoma.
>
> Radical removal of the left breast, Jan. 2, 1928. Radical dissection of the metastatic left supraclavicular glands, Oct. 2, 1928. Partial excision of metastatic brain tumor, Nov. 9, 1928. This last operation was undertaken for the purpose of providing an opportunity to try the tuberculin treatment, because metastatic growth was progressing rapidly, and it was felt that unless a temporary stay could be obtained, the patient would die from the brain metastasis before the tuberculin had a chance to work.
>
> **Condition at the begining of the treatment:**   General conditions were good as far as weight and blood picture were concerned. *Treatment:* Tuberculin administration began Oct. 30, 1928, and continued to the time when the paper was prepared.
>
> **The last condition:**   General nutrition was still good and the blood picture showed no particular change. Then there had been a gradual reappearance of the brain symptoms, possibly due to pressure from the edematous reaction to the residual tumorous tissue following each treatment. With this thought in mind, tuberculin was then temporarily discontinued to see whether relief of the pressure symptoms would follow.

BCG (Bacilli Calmette Guérin) was first used for experimental cancer therapy by Old et al. (1959). Using animal models, Rapp (1973) and his associates reported on a series of experiments demonstrating the suppressive effects of BCG on tumor growth, and in clinical trials, Mathé (1976) and his associates reported their extensive experiences in the treatment of leukemia. Nonspecific immunotherapy with BCG proved effective in prolonging remission and survival duration of melanoma (Morton et al., 1970; Morton et al., 1978), lung cancer (McKneally et al., 1978; Miyazawa et al., 1978), and myelogenous leukemia (Powles et al., 1973). For breast cancer, BCG or corynebacterium parvum can prolong the duration of remission and survival of chemotherapy-treated patients (Gutterman et al., 1976; Pinsky et al., 1978). BCG is considered to be a T-cell and macrophage activator (De Vita, Jr., 1977). It may require an intact T-cell system. The significant effect and limitation of BCG for cancer therapy will be clarified in the next few years.

Besides BCG, various kinds of immunopotentiators have been investigated for their cancer-suppressive effects. Among those in the bacterial group, Corynebacterium parvum was employed by Selker (1977) for the treatment of glioma. The tumor-suppressing effects of Picibanil (low virulent streptococcus hemolyticus) were reported by Koshimura et al. (1958) and Okamoto et al. (1967). Streptococcus hemolyticus is considered to be mainly a macrophage activator and probably a nonspecific lymphocyte activator. Tanimura (1974) reported on the suppressive effects of Picibanil on brain tumor growth.

Among low molecular weight adjuvants, levamisole has been widely investigated for its immunostimulatory action (Symoens, 1976). In 1966, Thienpont et al. found that tetramizole acts as a potent broad spectrum antihelminthic. Renoux, G. and Renoux, M. (1971) reported shortly afterward that this substance called levamisole (1-[-]-2, 3, 5, 6, -tetrahydro-6-phenylimidazo [1, 1–6] thiazole hydrochloride) had activating effects on cellular immunity. It stimulated the phagocytic function of macrophage, lymphocyte blastogenesis, delayed hypersensitive skin reactions, lymphocyte reproduction after chemotherapy and other functions. Double blind controlled studies of levamisole on the effects of tumor suppression were undertaken for lung cancer (Amery et al., 1975, 1977; Amery, 1978) and for breast cancer (Rojas et al., 1976, 1977). Both study groups have obtained promising results. Amery (1978) treated 211 resected lung cancer patients with levamisole. This treatment is expected to prolong both the disease-free interval and survival time without causing major side effects in a significant number of patients. The result is achieved primarily by the inhibition of hematogenous dissemination and noted especially in those patients who had more advanced tumors at the time of the resection. For breast cancer, the combination of chemotherapy and levamisole with or without BCG was investigated by Hortobagyi et al. (1977, 1978). The median survival periods were 17 months for cases treated only with chemotherapy (5-FU + Adriamycin + cyclophosphamide) and 28.6 months (p<0.01) for the chemotherapy and levamisole treated group. No conclusion was reached on the effect of the additional BCG, but the results seemed to be the best of all. Wanebo et al. (1978) treated squamous cell carcinoma of the head and neck. Decreased recurrence rates in patients with cancer of the oral cavity (stage II) receiving levamisole were demonstrated. The effects of combined treatment with levamisole and BCG are somewhat controversial. No difference in the survival rate was demonstrated in lung cancer patients treated with intrapleural BCG with or without the administration of levamisole (Wright et al., 1978). Olkowski et al. (1976, 1978) and Wright et al. noted that the administration of BCG and levamisole tended to delay the increase of various immunologic parameters in the immunotherapy group, compared with the group having no immunotherapy, but it seemed paradoxical that prognosis was better in the immunotherapy group. Levamisole has been used in our clinic as an adjuvant therapeutic regimen for malignant brain tumors (Takakura, 1976, 1977).

Interferon is well known for its inhibitory action on viruses. Various synthetic nucleotides, of which the structures are similar to double stranded DNA or RNA, were studied for their interferon inducing action. Park at New York University reported in 1968 that a synthetic nucleotide, Poly IC (Polyinosinic-polycytidylic acid) cured viral keratitis. Poly IC is a potent interferon inducer. A similar synthetic nucleotide, poly AU (polyadenylic-polyuridylic acid), also has interferon inducing action, which is weaker than that of Poly IC. Both synthetic nucleotides also have immunopotentiating actions (T-cell activation and probably B-cell activation, too). Since Poly IC has a stronger interferon inducing action, it is widely investigated for tumor therapy. Levy et al. (1969) reported that a slow growing mouse transplantable tumor was cured by Poly IC. Poly IC, however, is known to be a poor interferon inducer in man, and is not considered suitable for clinical use at any dosage. It is known that primate serum demonstrates a high level of hydrolytic activity (nuclease) against Poly IC, and thus rapid hydrolysis appears to be responsible for the absence of clinical activity (Nordl et al., 1970). Poly IC stabilized with poly-L-lysine and carboxymethyl cellulose (Poly ICLC) has been prepared.   It appears to resist hydrolysis due to the serum nuclease, and is an effective interferon inducer in subhuman primates.   In clinical studies, Poly ICLC induced significant serum interferon levels in 76 per cent of the trials.   With large doses, Poly ICLC i.v. also increased the interferon level in the cerebrospinal fluid (Levine and Levy, 1978).   Although both Poly IC and Poly ICLC show toxic pyrogenic effects, the application of Poly ICLC for the treatment of human cancer is worthy of being studied.   Our recent investigations revealed that Poly ICLC i.v. administration increased the serum interferon activities for 48 hours and suppressed tumor growth in some glioma patients.   On the other hand, various synthetic anionic polymers were noted to stimulate the interferon and antiviral activity (Merigan and Finkelstein, 1968).   Recently, polymers having structures simpler double stranded synthetic nucleotides such as Poly IC have been gaining attention and are being widely investigated.   Morehan et al. (1974) reported on the antitumor action of maleic anhydride-vinyl ether copolymer (MVE) pyran against Lewis lung carcinoma and B-16 melanoma in experimental animals.   Mohr et al. (1976) noted the specific potentiating action of a tumor vaccine by pyran copolymer.   Stolfi et al. (1978) reported on the significant tumor suppressive activity of MVE on a spontaneous solid tumor system in a true therapeutic setting with only the immunological treatment.   The antiviral and antitumor activities of the polymers are related to their molecular weights.   MVE having larger molecular weights exhibited potent antitumor and antiviral activities, but also demonstrated dose dependent toxicity (Morahan et al., 1978; Dean et al., 1978; Pavlidis et al., 1978).   Regelson (1978) summarized that pyran copolymer had consistently reproducible molecular weight-related biologic effects, associated with toxic, immunologic, antitumor and antiviral effects.   Fortunately, the antitumor action occurs with the least toxic lower molecular weight fraction.

Acid from bacterial adjuvants such as BCG, glucan, and neutral polyglucose (β1, 3-glucosidic polyglucose) derived from the cell walls of saccharomyces cerevisiae was reported to be a potent immunopotentiator.   The administration of glucan to mice or rats is associated with the induction of a hyperphagocytic state and the hypertrophy of major reticuloendothelial organs.   Glucan is effective in enhancing both humoral and cellular immune responses to unrelated antigens.   It is nonantigenic and nonvirulent, as opposed to bacterial immunopotentiators, and is thought to induce fewer toxic complications.   Glucan inhibited the growth and prolonged the survival time of four syngeneic murine tumor models (Di Luzio et al., 1978).   The suppressive effect of glucan in combination with BCNU was evaluated using disseminated AKR transplantable leukemia.   The combined treatment yielded more cures compared with the group treated by either agent separately (Stewart et al., 1978).

It has been established by the studies by Miller (1961) and Good et al. (1962) that the normal development of immunological functions requires the thymic functions to be intact.   It was also demonstrated that there was a humoral component of the thymus that could give immune competence (Osoba and Miller, 1963).   Studies aimed at purifying the humoral factor of the thymus have been undertaken.   The first preparation demonstrating the lymphocytopoietic activity was extracted and named thymosin by Goldstein et al. (1966).

Further purification of thymosin was actively investigated, and immunologically active thymic polypeptide (Thymosin fraction 5) was separated (Goldstein et al., 1977). Thymosin fraction 5 and its component parts influence a variety of lymphocyte properties, including the cyclic nucleotide levels, migration inhibitory factor production, T-dependent antibody production and expressions of certain surface markers (Marshall, Jr. et al., 1978). It activates T-cell rosettes in immunodeficient patients (Wara and Ammann, 1975). Pazmino et al. (1978) demonstrated that thymosin controlled the early differentiation of prothymocytes in bone marrow. The application of thymosin for the treatment of primary immunodeficient diseases and cancer has been studied by Goldstein et al. (1976), and Rossio and Goldstein (1977). A radiosensitive and thymic hormone-responsive suppressor cell may be present in the peripheral blood of cancer patients (Patt and Hersh, 1978). Chretien et al. (1978) suggested that cancer patients most likely to benefit from the thymosin treatment were those with relatively low initial T-cell levels and other parameters of cellular immunity. Greater understanding of the mechanism of the action of the thymosin peptides on T-cell subpopulations from patients with primary and secondary immunodeficient diseases, certain cancers, and autoimmune diseases (whose etiology is associated with an immunity imbalance) gives hope that one day thymosin may be routinely used in the treatment of these diseases (Marshall, Jr. et al., 1978).

A large number of studies on immune modulation and the control of cancer by adjuvant immunotherapy have been carried out. Some of these studies were related to metastatic brain tumors and they have suggested some future directions in which immunotherapy can be used for suppressing metastatic tumors.

Immunocompetence of Patients Having Metastatic Brain Tumors

The brain is often referred to as the "immunologic sanctuary." The immunocompetence of the brain is still controversial. Arguments for impaired immunity of the brain are based on the following facts (Harris and Sinkovics, 1976). (1) Metastases to brains from cancers of other organs are common, even after systemic tumors were suppressed as seen in leukemia patients. (2) Xenogeneic transplants of tumors in animal brains are accepted (Greene, 1951). (3) Slow virus infections of the brain are tolerated. These arguments are not acceptable due to the following reasons. (1) Chemotherapeutic agents usually cannot penetrate the blood-brain barrier, thus cannot suppress tumor growth properly as in other organs. (2) Xenogeneic transplants of tumors are usually rejected later. (3) Leukocyte infiltration immediately occurs when infection arises in the brain.

On the other hand, arguments for adequate immunity of the brain are based on the following facts. (1) Brain tumors develop their own blood supply, which is vulnerable to defense reactions of the host. (2) Lymphocytic infiltrations in brain tumors occur (Ridley and Cavanagh, 1971). (3) Labeled antibodies reach the brain tumor tissue (Day et al., 1965). (4) Sensitization against host brain tissue (i.e. allergic encephalitis) is possible. (5) Immune reactions to virus-carrier cells cause damage to the brain (Harris and Sinkovics, 1976).

Impaired immunocompetence both in primary brain tumor and metastatic brain tumor patients has now been clearly demonstrated.

Delayed Hypersensitive Skin Reaction—PPD Reaction

More than 90 per cent of all healthy adults show positive PPD (purified protein derivative of tuberculin) skin reaction in Japan, since almost all children showing negative PPD skin reaction receive BCG vaccination. The PPD skin reaction of every child is tested annually under a school health care program aimed at preventing tuberculosis. Only 15 per cent of the metastatic brain tumor patients and 18 per cent of the glioma patients, however, showed positive PPD skin reaction (Table V-36). The rate was 61 per cent in case of benign brain tumor patients. Sixty-four per cent of the metastatic brain tumor patients and 71 per cent of the malignant brain tumor patients showed negative PPD skin reactions. Thus, delayed hypersensitivity skin reaction demonstrates weak or anergic response in about 65 per cent of the metastatic brain tumor or malignant glioma patients. A comparison of reactions measured by size in the course of immunotherapy is useful in assessing the effectiveness of the treatment. The DNCB (dinitrochlorobenzene) test is also a simple technique for determining delayed hypersensitive skin reaction. The DNCB test, however, makes a large dermatitis on the test site, and no patient wants to repeat this test. Since the results of our preliminary DNCB tests were almost equivalent to the PPD skin reaction, the DNCB test is not routinely used in our clinic. A weak sensitizing reaction to the DNCB test in brain tumor patients was reported by Brooks et al. (1972) and Young (1976).

Lymphocyte Count

The lymphocyte count in peripheral blood decreases in malignant glioma and metastatic brain tumor patients. Eighty-five per cent of all healthy adults showed a lymphocyte count of more than $1,800/mm^3$. On the contrary, only 22 per cent of the malignant glioma patients and 26 per cent of the metastatic brain tumor patients showed the same lymphocyte count (Table V-37). Naturally, lymphocyte counts fluctuate in response to various treatments. It is noted, however, that all patients whose tumors are expanding demonstrate a decrease in their lymphocyte count and the negative PPD skin reaction is in an anergic state, as shown in Figure V-10. On the

Table V-36 PPD skin reaction of brain tumor patients.

Brain tumor	PPD skin reaction			Total No. of cases
	+	±	−	
Metastatic tumor	8 (15%)	11 (21%)	34 (64%)	53
Glioma	20 (18)	12 (11)	78 (71)	110
Astrocytoma	10 (26)	1 (3)	27 (71)	38
Glioblastoma	4 (13)	4 (13)	23 (74)	31
Medulloblastoma	2 (20)	0 (0)	8 (80)	10
Other glioma	4 (13)	7 (23)	20 (65)	31
Benign brain tumor	20 (61)	2 (6)	11 (33)	33
Total	**48 (24)**	**25 (13)**	**20 (65)**	**196**

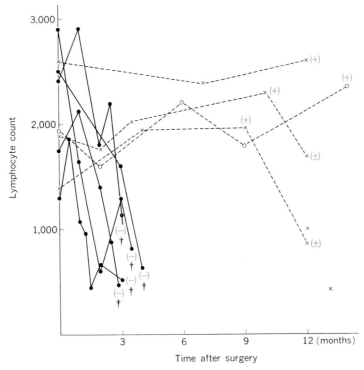

Fig. V-10 Lymphocyte count and PPD skin reaction of the patients after the surgery. Straight line: Patient whose tumor progressed and died. Dotted line: Patient whose tumor was well controlled. The signs + and − in parentheses indicate the PPD skin reaction.

contrary, stable patients in the complete remission stage have a normal lymphocyte count and a positive PPD skin reaction.

Table V-37 Peripheral lymphocyte count of brain tumor patients.

	No. of cases	Ratio of persons having lymphocyte count more than 1,800/mm³
Control (Healthy adults)	60	85%
Metastatic tumor	20	26
Malignant glioma	23	22
Benign brain tumor	39	69

Lymphocyte Blastogenesis

The method of measuring lymphocyte blastogenesis treated with PHA is a simple test to determine cellular immunity. It is measured by the method of ³H thymidine incorporation to the DNA of lymphocytes. This method, however, requires isotopes and cannot indicate the real ratio of blastoid lymphocytes against total cell count. Thus, the technique using flow cytometry has been investigated. Lymphocytes are separated from heparinized blood by centrifugation using ficol-conray. Lymphocytes are incubated in PHA containing RPMI 1640 medium supplemented with 20 per cent fetal calf serum for 72 hours. The DNA of lymphocytes is stained by ethidium bromide and measured by flowcytometry. The histogram of the DNA and cell count is analyzed by computer (Takakura, 1978; Kosugi et al., 1978).

Lymphocyte blastogenesis is determined by the ratio of the blastoid cell population (cell count in S, G_2 and M phases $\times$ 100/ total lymphocyte count). Lymphocyte blastogenesis in healthy adults and malignant brain tumor patients are 28.2 ± 7.1 per cent and 9.0 ± 4.9 per cent ($p < 0.01$), respectively. There is a significant decrease in malignant brain tumor patients (Table V-38).

Table V-38 Lymphocyte blastogenesis of brain tumor patients and effect of immunopotentiators.

	No. of cases	Lymphocyte blastogenesis
Control (Healthy adults)	8	$28.2 \pm 7.1\%$
Malignant brain tumor	19	9.0 ± 4.9 ($p < 0.01$)
After treated with { BCG	8	21.0 ± 6.9
Levamisole	5	24.3 ± 8.1
Picibanil	4	19.8 ± 6.7

*   Lymphocyte blastogenesis was measured by computer-aided flow-cytometric analysis. (Kosugi et al., 1978)

These results are in agreement with studies by Thomas et al. (1975) on the stimulation ratio of lymphocyte protein synthesis by various concentrations of PHA. They demonstrated that there was a definite impairment of PHA responsiveness in the lymphocytes of patients with malignant glioma and disseminated metastases including cerebral and spinal metastases. Cancer patients with disseminated metastases demonstrate a more marked depression in their cell-mediated immunity than glioma patients.

Cytotoxicity of Lymphocytes

A wide variety of human neoplasms have been shown to carry tumor-specific antigens and to elicit, in the host, cytotoxic cell-mediated and humoral immunity. Levy et al. (1972) demonstrated that patients with primary intracranial neoplasms possessed peripheral blood lymphocytes that were specifically cytotoxic to the cultured autologous tumor cells. With respect to antigenic cross-reactivity between glioblastoma cells from different patients, and moreover, between glioblastoma and melanoma cells, they suggested no difference in the magnitude of the cellular immune response induced by "benign" and "malignant" glial tumors. Cytotoxicity of lymphocytes in patients having metastatic brain tumors, however, has not been fully investigated.

Humoral Factors

It is difficult to clarify the role of humoral immunity in metastatic brain tumors. The serum complement (CH_{50}) was measured in various malignant brain tumors at our clinic. The normal level of serum CH_{50} ranges between 20 to 40 mg/dl. Serum CH_{50} level increases gradually at first with the progression of the tumor, and then decreases again in the terminal stage of the patients. In the case of glioma, patients

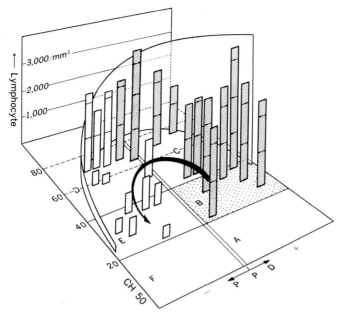

Fig. V-11 The immunological parameters (PPD skin reaction, lymphocyte count and serum CH_{50}) and the prognosis of the brain tumor patients. A white bar indicates a patient who died within three months, and a black bar indicates a patient who lived more than one year after the examination. Area B indicates the normal range. The arrow demonstrates the direction of deceasing immunosurveilance.

generally die with a higher level of serum CH_{50}, but in the case of metastatic brain tumors, the patients die with a lower level of CH_{50}. The relationship between the patient's prognosis and the three immunological parameters—PPD skin reaction, lymphocyte count and serum CH_{50} level—is illustrated in Figure V-11. The white bars indicate patients who died within three months after testing these parameters, and the shaded bars indicate the patients who lived more than a year after the test. Even these simple parameters can roughly predict the prognosis of the patients. Immunotherapy should move these parameters to the opposite direction of the arrow, indicating the deterioration of immunocompetence in Figure V-11.

There was no significant change in the immunogloblin level in patients with malignant brain tumors, including metastatic tumors. Although an increase in serum IgM level is a common biological phenomenon induced by the neoplastic process caused by tumors such as sarcoma, melanoma (Hughes, 1971) and biliary carcinoma (Beng et al., 1970), many other cancers were found to have normal or slightly suppressed levels of serum IgM level (Dostalova et al., 1970; Rowinska-Zakrewsk et al., 1970). Only meningioma has been reported to show a significant increase in serum IgM level (Tokumaru and Catalano, 1975).

The presence of the autoantibody in patients with brain tumors was investigated at our clinic using the immunoadherence hemagglutination technique (Nishioka, 1971). The technique used is one of the most sensitive methods currently available for the titration of antigens and antibodies. The brain tumor cell suspension was mixed and incubated at 37°C with the patient's serum and human erythrocytes (0-type, RH $+$), using a microplexiglass U-type plate (Shimizu et al., 1974). Human erythrocytes adhered to the tumor cell surface when the antibody against the surface antigen of the tumor cells was present in patient's serum. On the other hand, no erythrocytes adhered when the antibody was not present or when the complement became inactive by heating the patient's serum at 56°C for 30 minutes. The sera from the malignant glioma showed a strong titer of the autoantibody to counter the tumor cells. The autoantibody was not detected in the sera of the patients with meningioma or craniopharyngioma. Metastatic brain tumor patients demonstrated weak titer of the autoantibody. Three sarcoma patients, however, showed strong titer of the autoantibody. The presence of the autoantibody in the serum was thus evident in the glial tumor and sarcoma. The presence of the autoantibody in systemic cancer patients has not been confirmed. Further studies are necessary to elucidate the significance of the autoantibody on the growth of brain tumors.

Role of Immunopotentiators for Treatment of Metastatic Brain Tumors

BCG

Method of Administration

i) **Oral administration (p.o.)**
BCG (Japan BCG), 100 mg (5–8×10^7 viable cells) a day is administered once a week. Enterocoating capsules of BCG are available.

ii) **Intradermal administration (i.d.)**
BCG (Japan BCG); a total 1 to 2 mg is injected intradermally into a few separate places in the upper arm. The administration is repeated at intervals of two weeks to two months.

Presently, oral administration of BCG is being routinely used since it has no side effects such as those seen in intradermal injections. The effect of sensitization by intradermal administration is evidently more potent, but oral administration can be repeated very easily without any complications.

It was shown that animals can be well sensitized to tuberculin and immunized against virulent tuberculous infections by the oral administration of BCG (Murohashi et al., 1978; Rosenberg and da Rocha, 1970). The viable bacilli recovered from various organs revealed in experimental animals that orally administered BCG was absorbed through Peyer's patches and distributed rapidly to such remote organs as the bronchial lymph nodes (Murohashi et al., 1978; Muller-Shoop and Good, 1975).

Results

i) **Effects on immunoparameters**
Fifty-two malignant brain tumor patients (32 primary and 20 metastatic tumors) who showed negative PPD skin reactions were evaluated for the sensitizing

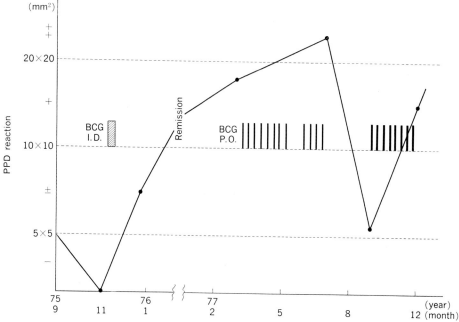

Fig. V-12   Effect of BCG administration on the PPD skin reaction of a metastatic brain tumor patient (NCC 178357, lung cancer).

effects of the intradermal administration of BCG.   In 69 per cent of all patients treated (23 out of 32 (72%) primary and 13 out of 20 (65%) metastatic tumors), PPD skin reactions were positive, while 40 per cent of the patients treated by oral administration had positive PPD skin reactions.   Thus, by repeating the administrations both intradermally or orally, more patients are sensitized against BCG.   The cessation of BCG administration often results in a decrease in cellular immunity. Figure V-12 demonstrates the relationship between the PPD skin reaction and the frequency of the BCG administration.   The effects of oral BCG administration on the peripheral lymphocyte count were evaluated in 16 cases for patients who were treated only by BCG during the test period.   The average lymphocyte count was $1,800 \pm 360/mm^3$ before, and it increased to $2,400 \pm 980/mm^3$ ($p < 0.05$) one month after oral BCG treatment.   The lymphocyte blastogenesis was tested in nine cases. It was 6.8 ± 5.1 per cent before and increased to 15.3 ± 9.2 per cent ($p < 0.05$) after oral BCG treatment.   Lymphocyte blastogenesis is related to the degree of PPD skin reaction.   The average rate of lymphocyte blastogenesis in the patients whose PPD skin reaction turned positive during oral BCG administration was 21.9 ± 5.2 per cent, whereas for the patients whose PPD skin reaction remained negative, it was 7.1 ± 5.0 per cent.

ii)   Effects on survival time

Forty-one patients (26 lung and 15 other cancers) received the adjuvant BCG treatment.   The median survival time of those patients after the onset of neurological signs was 18.7 months.   To evaluate the adjuvant therapeutic effect of BCG, 68 metastatic brain tumor patients who had received the same method of therapy were compared.   All of them had undergone craniotomy or craniectomy, and their metastatic tumors were removed either totally or partially.   Patients who received biopsy alone or simple external decompression were excluded.   All the patients received full course postoperative radiotherapy.   The primary tumor was adequately treated.   All patients received some form of chemotherapy.   Nineteen patients received the adjuvant BCG treatment, and the remaining 49 patients did not. The median survival time was 27.4 months for the BCG treated group and 13.7 months ($p<0.01$) for the non-BCG treated group.   The survival rates of both group are shown in Figure V-13.   The survival rates of the BCG treated and non-treated groups were 73.7 and 46.9 per cent ($p<0.05$) at one year after surgery, 36.8 and 10.2 per cent ($p<0.01$) at two years and 21.1 and 6.1 per cent ($p<0.05$) at three years, respectively.   There was a significant difference in the survival rates up to two and a half years after the onset of the neurological signs.   Since there was no significant difference in the survival rate before six months after the surgery, the beneficial effect of the BCG adjuvant therapy seems to be more likely.   The controlled prospective Phase-III study is now under investigation.

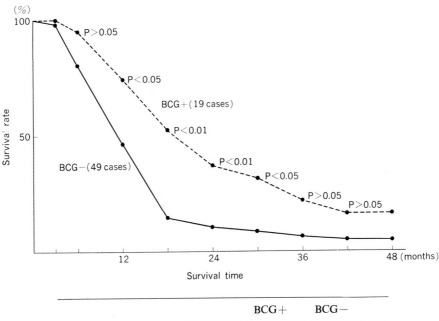

	BCG+	BCG−
No. of cases	19	49
Operation — total removal	10	24
Operation — partial removal	9	25
Radiation	+	+
Chemotherapy	+	+
Median survival time (months)	27.4	13.7 ($p < 0.01$)

Fig. V-13   Effect of adjuvant BCG treatment on the survival rate of metastatic brain tumor patients who were treated by surgery, radiation and chemotherapy.

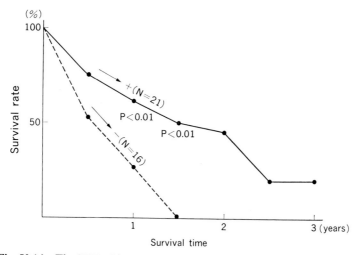

Fig. V-14 The PPD skin reaction and the survival rate of patients with metastatic brain tumors after BCG treatment. (+): The PPD skin reaction turned to positive with BCG treatment. (−): The PPD skin reaction remained negative even after BCG treatment.

It is evident that the adequate immunocompetence of the patients plays the most important role in the success of immunotherapy. Patients in an immunoparalytic state do not respond to BCG stimulation. Thirty-seven patients who received adjuvant BCG therapy were divided into two groups. The postoperative median survival time of 21 patients whose PPD skin reaction turned positive during the BCG treatment was 19.5 months, while 16 patients whose PPD skin reaction remained always negative was 7.3 months (p<0.01). The survival rates of these two groups are listed in Figure V-14. The results suggest that patients whose immunocompetence was preserved and who responded to nonspecific BCG immunotherapy showed significantly better prognosis compared with those whose immunocompetence had totally deteriorated. The following case demonstrates a patient with a metastatic brain tumor due to lung cancer who seemed to respond to the adjuvant BCG immunotherapy.

Case report 58-year-old man. NCC 178357. Lung cancer (Squamuous cell carcinoma).

A left upper lobectomy was performed to remove lung cancer on July 3, 1974. Left hemiparesis appeared in August 1975. The RI scintigram revealed a metastatic brain tumor in the right parietal lobe. Craniotomy was performed on Sept. 28, 1975, and the tumor was totally removed. Postoperative radiotherapy (30 Gy.) followed and chemotherapy with tegafur (800 mg/day) was commenced. The PPD skin reaction was negative (completely anergic). On Nov. 22, 1975, he received an intradermal injection of BCG. At that time, the lymphocyte count was 1,180/mm³; serum CH_{50}, 68 mg/dl; IgG, 1,420 mg/dl; IgA, 267 mg/dl; IgM, 181 mg/dl; CRP 5+. The lymphocyte count on Dec. 2, 1975 was 1,650/mm³, and on Jan. 28, 1976 it was 1,960/mm³. On Dec. 22, 1975, the PPD skin reaction turned pseudopositive (5 × 10 mm). He returned to work without any neurological deficit. In October 1976, he had a convulsive seizure, and a local recurrence of metastasis was suspected. Chemotherapy with tegafur and glucocorticoid was maintained. From March 30, 1976, radiotherapy (20 Gy.) was given again, and oral administration of BCG (80 mg/day/week) was started. On May 30, 1976, second craniotomy was performed and the recurrent tumor was removed.   BCG oral administration was continued 12 times until July 16, when he was discharged.   The PPD skin reaction turned positive (20 × 26 mm) and the lymphocyte blastogenesis increased from 8.2 per cent before to 20.7 per cent after the oral administration of BCG.   During the two months after his discharge, BCG administration was discontinued, and the PPD skin reaction returned to negative (5 × 5 mm).   BCG oral administration, 80 mg/d per week, was restarted and maintained.   The PPD skin reaction became positive (15 × 16 mm) again. He remained in good condition for the whole next year.   However, metastasis reappeared again in April 1978.   Although chemotherapy with tegafur with glucocorticoid and oral BCG administration was continued, the metastasis gradually progressed and he died in Novermber 1978.   He survived three years and two months after the initial craniotomy for the brain metastasis.

Side Effects

No side effects have ever been encountered in more than 1,000 oral administrations of BCG to 100 patients, for both primary and metastatic tumors.   On the other hand, an intradermal injection of BCG caused several side effects.   Local inflammatory reactions with swelling, ulcers and pain were the most common complications. Slight fever, malaise and poor appetite were less common, but did exist.   An injection of more than 8 mg of BCG at the same place usually caused a local ulcer in all of the patients.   An injection of less than 1 mg of BCG rarely caused an ulcer.   An ulcer can be cured by local application of antiseptics, or by a small amount of streptomycin or Kanamycin.   Four patients developed local lymphadenitis.   It was relieved by the administration of INAH 0.4 g/d for one to two weeks.   Three patients needed incisions to remove the abscess.   Only a few patients complained of flu-like malaise and arthritic pain.   Serum enzyme levels indicating liver functions such as GOT, GPT and LDH temporarily increased slightly in about half of the patients.   No anaphylaxic shock or stimulation of the tumor growth has ever been encountered.

Levamisole

Method of Administration

Levamisole (Jansen pharmaceutica) was administered orally, 150 mg a day, three times every day for three days.   This three-day course of administration was repeated every two to four weeks.

Results

i)   Effects on immunoparameters
Twenty-four malignant brain tumor patients were treated using the adjuvant levamisole therapy.   The peripheral lymphocyte count generally increased with the administration of levamisole.   The increase was more evident when lymphocytopenia was present.   The PPD skin reaction turned positive in 33 per cent of the patients.   Levamisole has demonstrated no effect on serum immunoglobulin nor

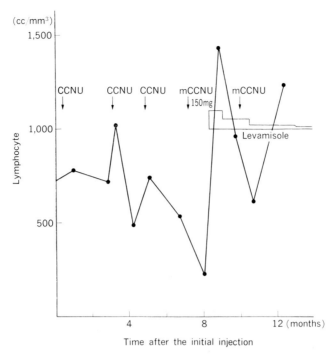

Fig. V-15 Effect of levamisole on lymphocyte count of the patient under chemotherapy with nitrosourea compound.

CH_{50} levels. These results suggest that levamisole stimulates the cellular immunity rather than the humoral immunity. The most favorable effect of levamisole in the clinical aspect is that lymphocytes increased substantially at the time of chemotherapy. Chemotherapy with nitrosourea compounds often causes severe lymphocytopenia (Fig. V-15). The concomitant use of levamisole prevents this lymphocyte depression. Therefore, chemotherapy could be continued in several cases.

ii) Effect on the survival time

It is not possible to conclude the effect of levamisole on the survival time of metastatic brain tumor patients. Preliminary results revealed that the median survival time of 11 metastatic brain tumor patients treated with the adjuvant levamisole treatment from the onset of neurological signs was 18.8 months. In cases of seven glioblastoma and six astrocytoma and oligodendroglioma patients, the median survival time was more than 26.1 months (three out of seven patients are still alive) and 26.2 months (all patients are still alive), respectively. Debois (1975) reported that the median survival time for advanced breast cancer (stage IV) patients was six months for the group treated with the ordinary method, and 20 months for the group treated with levamisole. Effects on lung cancer described by Amery (1978) are related in the historical notes.

Side Effects

Dermatitis is the most common side effect, appearing in 15 per cent of the patients. About 10 per cent of the patients complained of nausea, loss of appetite or dizziness. All these side effects disappeared soon after the administration was stopped. One patient developed severe agranulocytosis. It was properly treated by blood transfusion, antibiotics and glucocorticoid. Similar side effects of levamisole were reported by Symoens et al. (1978).

Picibanil

Method

Picibanil (Detoxicated streptococcus hemolyticus SV strain, Chugai Pharmaceutical Co.) was injected intramuscularly. The initial dose was 0.2 K.E. (Klinische Einheit, equivalent to 0.02 mg) and the dose was increased to 0.5, 1, and 2, 5 K.E. every three days. The maintenance dose was 2 to 5 K.E. three days a week.

Result

Picibanil was given to nine metastatic brain tumor patients (3 lung, 3 renal, 1 gastric, 1 breast cancer and 1 hepatoma). It has the effect of stimulating the lymphocyte blastogenesis. The PPD skin reaction was enhanced in about 25 per cent (Kimura, 1978) of the patients, and it was significant, compared with cases which were treated without Picibanil. One gastric carcinoma patient with multiple metastases to the brain survived 18 months (21 months after the onset of neurological signs) after craniectomy with radiation and chemotherapy using tegafur and Picibanil.

MULTIDISCIPLINARY TREATMENT OF METASTATIC BRAIN TUMORS

Every metastatic brain tumor has different characters in oncogenic, anatomical and physiological aspects. It cannot be properly treated by a single therapeutic procedure such as surgery, radiation or chemotherapy alone. The multidisciplinary approach is essential for controlling this pathophysiological presentation of systemic cancer. The following cases are provided as examples.

Case 1 50-year-old woman. NCC 158771. Endometrial carcinoma of the uterus.
The patient underwent a gynecological surgery for endometrial carcinoma of the uterus on April 16, 1971. She gradually complained of headaches from July 1972. Right hemiparesis soon appeared. At the time of admission, she was completely disoriented. Right hemiplegia, memory disturbance and motor aphasia with marked choked discs were noted. The RI scintigram revealed an abnormal uptake in the left frontal region (Fig. V-16). On Sept. 20, craniectomy with total removal of the tumor was performed. The tumor was round shaped, approximately 4 cm in diameter, containing necrotic bloody fluid inside. The histology revealed adenocarcinoma, partly mixed with squamous cell carcinoma. Postoperative radiotherapy (Linac 60 Gy.) and chemotherapy with Mitomycin C (25 mg) and Bleomycin (70 mg) were given. Glucocorticoid was administered for almost a year. The intradermal injection of BCG (10 mg) was administrated twice. The PPD skin reaction was negative in the beginning, but became extensively positive after the administration of BCG.

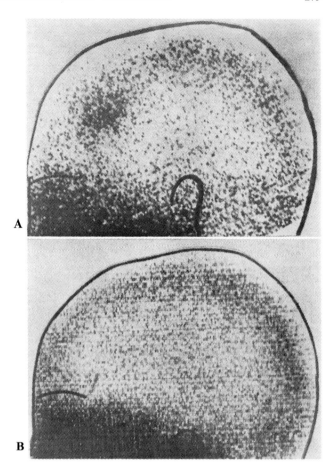

Fig. V-16 A. RI scintigram. Case 1. 50-year-old woman, uterine endometrial carcinoma. Before the craniectomy (NCC 158771).
B. RI scintigram taken two years after the craniectomy.

Her condition remained good and cranioplasty with resin was performed in January 1975. At that time, the RI scintigram showed no abnormal uptake in the isotope and there was no evidence of recurrence. She received adjuvant treatment with BCG and levamisole. The PPD skin reaction was always positive thereafter, and the lymphocyte count was always more than 2,000/mm³. She had no neurological deficits and has maintained a normal social life as a housewife. She could even enjoy a trip abroad. A recent CT scan revealed no recurrence (Fig. V-17). She has been well without any recurrence since September 1972, nine years after the removal of the metastatic brain tumor.

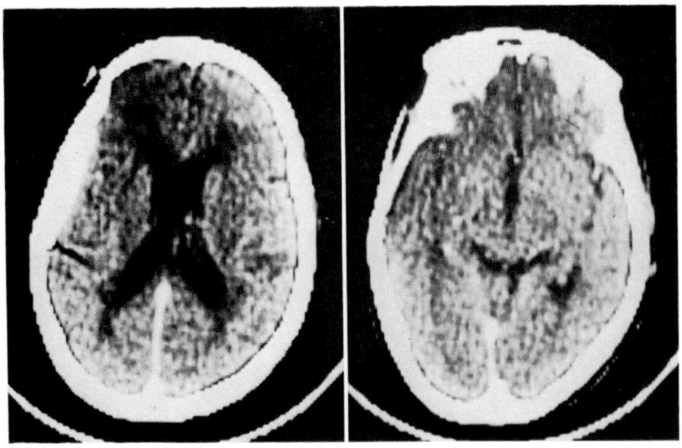

Fig. V-17 Same case as shown in Figure V-16. CT scan taken six and half years after the craniectomy. No residual tumor was present, and no neurological deficit was detected.

Case 2   40-year-old woman. TU 730084. Choriocarcinoma.

She was diagnosed to have a hydatiform mole in February 1965 and received a curettage.   Occipital headaches gradually appeared from the end of 1971.   In March 1972, she had a sudden attack of vertigo and could not walk for a few hours.   On May 16, 1972, left quadrant homonymous hemianopsia suddenly appeared, but there was no headache, nausea or vertigo.   Episodes of temporary headache, nausea, vomiting, left homonymous hemianopsia and a dizziness sometimes occurred during 1972.   In February 1973, a lumber puncture was performed.   The CSF pressure was 320 mm H_2O. CSF showed xanthochromia.   The total protein was 485 mg/dl and cell count was 2713. The RI scintigram with ^{99}Tc did not, however, demonstrate any sign of abnormality. A chest x-ray examination revealed small tumor shadows in the right lower lobe.   She was admitted to our hospital on March 26, 1973.   Left lower quadrant homonymous hemianopsia was evident.   Bilateral choked discs were noted, but there was no headache or nausea.   The right CAG revealed a right occipital mass lesion (Fig. V-18). The Friedman reaction was 10,000U.   Right occipital craniotomy and the removal of the tumor was performed on April 21, 1973.   The tumor was cystic and contained approximately 10 ml of old hematoma.   Histological examination revealed choriocarcinoma.   Postoperative radiotherapy and chemotherapy with local methotrexate (total 65 mg), systemic methotrexate, Actinomycin D, and intradermal BCG adjuvant im-

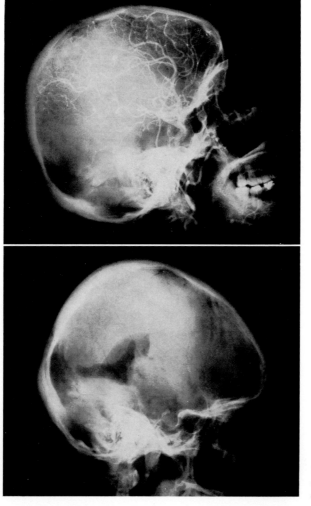

Fig. V-18 Right carotid angiogram. 40-year-old woman. Choriocarcinoma. A walnut-sized avascular mass was demonstrated in the right occipital region (UT 730084).

Fig. V-19 Chest x-ray film. Same case as shown in Figure V-18. The metastatic tumor was demonstrated in the right lower lobe.

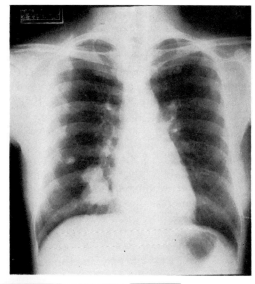

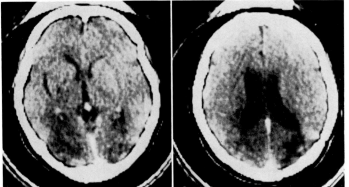

Fig. V-20 CT scan (Same case as shown in Figure V-18) taken six years after the craniotomy. No residual tumor was detected.

munotherapy were performed. On Sept. 5, 1973, a right lower lobectomy for metastatic lung carcinoma was performed (Fig. V-19). Chemotherapy with methotrexate and Actinomycin D with BCG therapy were continued. The Friedman reaction decreased and became nondetectable. A recent CT scan revealed no reappearance of the tumor (Fig. V-20). The patient returned to a normal social life and is working as a clerk (1981) without any signs of recurrence.

Case 3 59-year-old woman. NCC 167479. Breast cancer.

Radical mastectomy for right breast cancer was performed on April 1963. Ten years later, swelling developed in the left centro-parietal region of her head. Headaches soon appeared. A plain x-ray examination revealed bone destruction in the left centro-parieto-occipital region of her skull. The RI scintigram and angiography revealed that the metastatic skull tumor had invaded the brain. Craniectomy was performed on Aug. 10, 1973. The tumor had spread to the dura mater and protruded into the cortex. The tumor and the affected skull were removed. Dural plasty was performed. The defected scalp area was covered with the adjacent healthy scalp. A dermal transplantation from her thigh was performed to the healthy scalp area where the skin flap was turned. The small metastatic nodules, however, appeared on the grafted skin soon after plastic surgery was completed.   Radiotherapy was then carried out.   Mean-while, metastases to several parts of her vertebrae appeared.   Hypophysectomy was performed on June 24, 1974.   Halotestin and methotrexate were administered.   The adjuvant BCG therapy was concomitantly administered orally.   The tumor was well controlled by hormonal therapy.   The remission continued for about four years afterwards.   She was able to carry on a normal life at home during this period.   The recurrence came in the summer of 1978, and she died in October 1978, five years and two months after the craniectomy.

Case 4   51-year-old man. NCC 85163. Lung cancer (squamous cell carcinoma).
In April 1966, an abnormal shadow in the left pulmonary hylus was detected in an annual health check at his company.   Pulmonary tuberculosis was suspected and treatment was commenced.   In August 1967, the abnormal shadow in the left lung enlarged and the diagnosis of lung cancer was confirmed.   Total lobectomy of the left lung was performed on Sept. 19, 1967.   Histological examination revealed that it was squamous cell carcinoma.   Left hemiparesis with a gradual appearance of headaches started from April 1968.   The RI scintigram and CAG revealed a metastatic tumor in the right parietal lobe.   Craniotomy was performed and the tumor was totally removed on May 23, 1968.   Postoperative radiotherapy (60 Gy.) was given.   He returned to his job without any neurological deficits.   Amelioration continued until July 1976, when an ataxic gait and the narrowing of his field of vision appeared.   The recurrence of the metastatic tumor was suspected.   On Oct. 25, 1976, recraniotomy was performed and a cyst accompanied by brain atrophy was noted.   The presence of a tumor was not de-tected.   The cystic fluid was removed.   The postoperative course was excellent, but on Nov. 18, he went into a convulsion and then into a coma.   He died on Nov. 24, 1976.   He lived eight years and six months after the removal of the metastatic brain tumor.   An autopsy revealed no tumor recurrence in the brain or the lung.   His death was caused by meningoencephalitis with hematoma.

Case 5   61-year-old man. NCC 131084. Lung cancer (squamous cell carcinoma).
Lung cancer was diagnosed, and a right upper lobectomy was performed in May 1973.   From July 1974, headaches and nausea gradually appeared.   Increasing deterioration in his mental activity and a somnolent tendency were noted.   Two weeks later, he was attacked by a generalized convulsive seizure.   At the time of admission, he was delirious and disoriented.   The impairment of his left seventh and eighth nerves with marked choked discs was noted.   The RI scintigram and angiogram revealed ab-normal mass lesions in the left frontal base and the left cerebellopontine angle.   Man-nitol infusion and betamethasone treatment with an anticonvulsant relieved most of the neurological signs within a week.   Chemotherapy with tegafur (800 mg a day, orally) and betamethasone (3 mg a day) was administered for two weeks.   The dosage was reduced and a combined treatment of tegafur (500 mg a day, suppository form) and betametha-sone (2.3 mg a day) was continued for six months (the total dose of tegafur was 101.2 g).   BCG was injected intradermally (2 mg at a time).   Betamethasone was changed to hydrocortisone and a daily dose of 10 to 20 mg was maintained.   The dosage of gluco-corticoid was adjusted to the neurological signs, and when ataxia appeared, the dose of glucocorticoid was increased.   Levamisole was also administered in 1975.   The PPD skin reaction was initially negative, but after the BCG and levamisole treatments, it became positive.   He remains in good health and has returned to his work as a cook.   In March 1980, he was still in good condition.   Although the metastatic brain tumor was not verified by surgery, all the examinations suggest its presence, and he has been well controlled by chemo-immuno-glucocorticoid therapy.

The control of metastatic brain tumors should be considered as a part of the treatment for systemic cancers (Fig. V-21).   The induction therapy for brain metas-

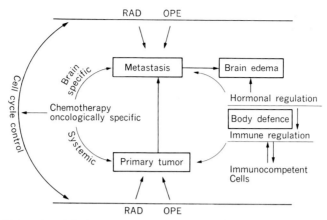

Fig. V-21 Multidisciplinary approach for treatment of metastatic brain tumors.

tases is often initiated by neurosurgery and/or radiation whenever they are applicable. When a primary tumor and brain metastases are found at the same time, the brain lesion should be treated first before control of the primary tumor is attempted, by consulting specialists concerning the primary tumor. The characteristics of both the brain and the primary tumor are important in determining the chemotherapeutic agents to be selected. Radiotherapy and chemotherapies must be applied in consideration of the cell kinetics of each tumor. Brain edema caused by metastasis should be properly controlled by using glucocorticoid. The defense mechanisms of the patient against cancer, consisting of both immunological and hormonal regulation, must be enhanced by the appropriate balancing of the homeostasis of the patient.

CONCLUSION

The results of the treatment of 616 patients having metastatic brain tumors treated at our clinic during the past 20 years were described with reviews of the historical backgrounds. Although the prognoses, even today, are extremely poor compared with other malignant brain tumors, it must be known that many of these patients were able to spend meaningful lives much longer than expected.

The implication and limitation of surgical management and radiotherapy were well realized. It is, however, noted that surgery for single and solitary metastases to brain and radiotherapy for properly selected patients brought about enormous benefits to the patients. Advancements in chemotherapy and immunotherapy in recent years have opened up many new possibilities for this type of treatment. Since the metastatic brain tumor is a part of the pathophysiological manifestation of advanced and systemic cancer, the control and management of this disease require a multidisciplinary approach to the treatment. Specific plans for treatment should be established for each patient, because the characteristics of the tumor differ in each case. Successful therapeutic results can always be expected through cooperative management by neurosurgeons, radiologists, chemotherapeutists, immunologists and specialists for each primary tumor.

VI. METASTATIC TUMORS OF THE SPINAL CANAL

Secondary malignant neoplasms affect various parts of the spinal canal and cause functional deficits of the spinal cord or spinal nerve roots. The spinal epidural tissue is most frequently involved in secondary tumors.

Spinal leptomeninges and spinal nerve roots are also infiltrated in another form of metastasis (diffuse leptomeningeal carcinomatosis). Tumor cells, spread by the flow of cerebrospinal fluid make numerous colonies, frequently in the leptomeninges of the caudal portion of the cord. Spinal leptomeninges and spinal nerve roots are sometimes solely involved, without the lesions in the cranial leptomeninges. Parsons (1972) reported three cases of the spinal form of leptomengeal carcinomatosis and reviewed 13 cases that appeared in literature. In cases of leukemia, breast cancer or adenocarcinomas of other origins, leptomeningeal metastasis should be included in differential diagnosis when symptoms or signs of the spinal cord or spinal nerve appear. Patients with leptomeningeal dissemination usually complain of headaches and show meningeal signs of acute onset. In such cases, examination of cerebrospinal fluid is essential to achieve correct diagnosis. Malignant cells are often revealed in the cerebrospinal fluid (CSF). Glucose concentration decreases and protein level increases. Myelography reveals disseminated lesions.

The spinal cord itself is also the target of tumor spread. It is not very rare to find this blood-borne metastasis. Chason et al. (1963) reported that 0.9 per cent of patients with malignant tumors had this type of metastasis, which corresponds to 5.0 per cent of all metastases to the central nervous system. Barron and his co-workers (1959) found two cases of intramedullary metastasis among 127 cases of metastasis in the spinal canal. Since patients with this form of metastasis are frequently associated with cerebral metastasis, it is sometimes difficult to clinically find the intramedullary metastasis. This form of metastasis causes rapid progression of spinal cord symptoms without pain, which is almost always present in cases of spinal epidural metastasis. Lung cancer is the most common primary lesion. Myelography is important in differentiating intramedullary metastasis from epidural metastasis.

A less frequent type of metastasis is subdural metastasis. Some authors reported cases in which spinal subdural metastasis existed without epidural involvement (Rogers, 1958; Beehler, 1960; Feiring and Hubbard Jr., 1965). Subdural extension from epidural metastasis is more frequently observed. Chandler and his co-workers (1954) reported two such cases from among 49 cases of epidural metastasis.

Other forms of clinical manifestations involving malignancies include carcinomatous neuropathy and myopathy, which are thought to be remote effects of malignancy. Side effects of therapeutic procedures such as radiation, myelopathy or neuropathy caused by chemotherapeutic agents like vincristine may also bewilder clinicians.

In the following section, the most common spinal cord lesion, spinal epidural metastasis, will be discussed.   The spinal epidural space is filled with adipose tissue and contains the rich venous network, Batson's channel.   This channel was supposed to be the route for the spread of tumor cells into the vertebrae and the epidural tissue (see pathology section).   Since the secondary neoplasm of this space may be the extension from the tumor in the vertebrae or the paravertebral lymph nodes, the bony lesion in the vertebrae accompanies epidural metastasis in most cases.   In some cases, patients with vertebral metastasis showed myelographic changes without neurological deficits (Longeval et al., 1975).

The rate of spinal epidural metastasis among patients with malignancy has been reported by several authors.   Abrams et al. (1950) found that 7.7 per cent of the patients with maligancy (4 cases in 52 cases) had spinal epidural metastasis.   Barron et al. (1959) reported the frequency of epidural metastasis as five per cent.   In our autopsy series, 140 cases of epidural metastasis were found among 3,359 cases with malignancy (see pathology section).   Certain tumors, such as carcinomas of prostate or breast, metastasize frequently to the spine and epidural tissue.

Table VI-1   Primary sites of spinal epidural metastasis.

Author	Lung	Breast	Kidney	Pros-tate	Thy-roid	Lym-phoma	Mye-loma	Others or unknown origins
Arseni et al. (1959) N = 231	17	12	4	7	1	5	—	54%
Barron et al. (1959) N = 127	24	16	9	5	2	16	7	21%
Wright (1963) N = 84	12	15	2	8	6	17	5	35%
White et al. (1971) N = 226	14	16	6	10	4	12	4	34%
Chade (1976) N = 172	16	13	15	11	12	1	—	32%
Paillas et al. (1976) N = 60	20	13	13	7	3	5	—	38%
Gilbert et al. (1978) N = 235	13	20	7	9	—	11	4	36%
Present series of Montefiore Hosp. (1980) N = 167	25	16	7	8	2	13	3	26%

Ratios of primary tumors causing epidural metastasis have been reported by many investigators (Table VI-1).   The figures varied largely with investigators.   Most investigators who reported series with a large number of cases agreed that lung and breast cancers are the most frequent causes of spinal epidural metastasis.   Kidney and prostate carcinomas are the second most frequent primary tumors, and they are followed by carcinomas of the thyroid and melanoma.   Other tumors such as carcinomas of the rectum and colon, uterine cancer and sarcoma also spread in the epidural tissue.   Lymphoma and multiple myeloma are other important neoplasms which cause spinal compression as frequently as lung and breast cancers.

Different opinions have been presented regarding the difference of frequency for epidural metastasis according to sex.   Many authors have reported that spinal metastasis is more common in men (Alexander et al., 1956; Arseni et al., 1959; Barron et al., 1959; Smith, 1965; Chade, 1976).   Other authors have suggested equal sex incidence or more frequent metastasis in woman (Toumey, 1943; Törmä, 1957; Perese, 1958).   This sex difference reflected the source of the patients in each clinic. Regarding the frequency of primary tumors in each sex, it was reported by Barron et al. (1959) that lung cancer, lymphoma and renal cancers were most frequent in men, while breast cancer, lung cancer and lymphoma were most frequent in women (see pathology section).

The age distribution of patients is in accordance with the incidence of primary tumors.   Most patients are included in the age group of 50 to 70 years.   The mean age of woman is younger than that of men because breast cancer affects a younger age group than lung cancer.

Secondary tumors of the epidural space may compress any level of the spinal cord.   There is some discrepancy between the level of cord compression and epidural lesion, especially in the caudal part of the cord.   The lesion at levels below the second lumbar vertebra does not compress the cord but causes cauda equina syndrome. Regarding the level of vertebral lesions, some authors reported that the thoracic spine was more frequently affected than other parts of the spine (Wright, 1963; Chade, 1976; Gilbert, R.W. et al., 1978).   Other authors, however, reported that the lumbar spine was also as frequently involved as the thoracic spine (Lenz and Fried, 1931; Arseni et al., 1959).   Reporting on the level of the cord compression, Wild and Porter (1963) stated that the lower thoracic segment (Th5-L1) was found to have been affected in 47 per cent of patients with epidural metastasis, the upper thoracic segment in 38 per cent, the cervical cord in two per cent and the cauda equina in 13 per cent.

The predilection of the levels may differ with the various primary tumors. Carcinomas of the kidney, prostate and rectum have predilection to the lower spine (Barron et al., 1959).   Gilbert, R.W. et al. (1978) also reported that cancer of the colon frequently metastasized to the lower spine.

SIGNS AND SYMPTOMS

Neurological deficits are produced by the compression of the spinal cord by tumor masses or the pathological fracture of vertebrae.   Ischemic or hemorrhagic processes may also be an influence on some occasions and cause acute aggravation of symptoms.   One of the characteristics of epidural metastasis is the rapid progression of symptoms.   The whole course of this manifestation can be divided into two stages, the prodromal stage and the stage of cord compression.   In the prodromal stage, patients complain of back pain and tenderness around the spine.   They also complain of pains of radicular origin.   Following this prodromal stage, the tumor grows large enough to compress the spinal cord and show symptoms of partial or complete transectional spinal syndrome.   This consists of progressive motor weakness and sensory as well as autonomic disturbances.   The cauda equina syndrome is caused by tumors below the second lumbar vertebra.   This peripheral nerve deficit may respond better to treatment than the cord syndrome.

Pain is the most prominent symptom of this tumor dissemination and it is the initial symptom in most patients.   This symptom reportedly developed in 96 per cent of the cases (Chade, 1976). Back pain is divided into two types, local and radicular pains. Local pains are caused by stimulation of the small nerve branches in the periostium or in the tissue involved by the tumor. This type of pain is usually initiated as a dull ache and is aggravated gradually until it becomes intolerable. In these instances, tenderness along the spine is noted.

Radicular pains, which radiate to each dermatome, result from compression or infiltration of nerve roots by the tumor. This symptom appears for a considerable period after the onset of a nonspecific pain. The pain radiates to limbs when the lesion is localized in the cervical or lumbar region. The pain of band-type distribution is caused by a tumor affecting the thoracic level. Root pain is frequently bilateral and is triggered by trunchal or neck movements, coughing or sneezing. The symptom is usually continuous and progressive, but in some cases, it is intermittent as is observed in cases of herniated discs.

Motor weakness, following the stage of pain, is a common symptom in many cases. The paraparesis of the lower extremities is usually a sign of motor weakness. Gilbert, R.W. et al. (1978) reported that 87 per cent of the patients showed motor weakness at the time of the initial diagnosis. In some patients, the weakness develops so rapidly that they demonstrate paraplegia by the time of diagnosis.

Although sensory disturbances, especially numbness of lower extremities, are not prominent complaints of the patients, they can be found by careful neurological examinations. These disturbances progress parallel to motor weakness. Gilbert, R.W. et al. (1978) reported that 78 per cent of the patients had sensory disturbances at the time of diagnosis. With the progression of spinal cord compression, the partial transectional syndrome grows into a complete form. The typical Brown-Séquard syndrome, which includes dissociated sensory disturbances, is rarely seen in the metastatic lesion. Arseni et al. (1959) reported that two per cent of the patients showed the Brown-Séquard syndrome. Careful neurological examinations usually reveal bilateral dysfunction, even in cases which are thought to be the hemitransection syndrome.

Sphincter dysfunction is a grievous sign and usually found in advanced stages of cord compression. But in some cases, urinary disturbances may not be associated with other cord signs (McAlhany and Netsky, 1955). Lesions of the conus and cauda equina cause sphincter dysfunctions as chief complaints. Gilbert, R.W. et al. (1978) mentioned that the lesions between Th8 and Th12 segments frequently caused urinary incontinence. They also reported that 57 per cent of the patients had autonomic dysfunctions at the time of diagnosis. The lesions, which compress the sacral cord and cauda equina, cut nerve connections between the bladder and the lower micturition center and cause the autonomous neurogenic bladder. A lesion that damages the upper cord, on the other hand, interrupts the tracts between the cortical and sacral regulatory center and results in the reflex neurogenic bladder.

Among other less frequent complaints, some patients had ataxia as a major complaint with a loss of proprioception (Gilbert et al., 1978). Herpes zoster infection may appear in the same dermatome as the level of compression (Barron et al., 1959; Mullins et al., 1971; Gilbert, R.W. et al., 1978). But judging from the fact that this viral disease frequently appears in patients with other types of malignancy, it may not be a localizing sign and only the result of the immuno-suppressive condition of the patients.

The rapid exacerbation of neurological symptoms is a characteristic of epidural metastasis. The speed of progression, however, differs in various tumors. In lung cancer, renal cancer and lymphoma, the symptoms progress rapidly. The progression of symptoms, by contrast, is slow in breast cancer (Barron et al., 1959). The interval between the time of diagnosis of the primary tumor and the development of the spinal cord compression ranges from zero to several years. Rates of patients developing spinal compression before discovery of the primary tumor were reported as 10 to 62 per cent (Rowbotham, 1955; Botterelli and Fitzgerald, 1959; Wild and Porter, 1963; Wright, 1963; Vieth and Odom, 1965b; Chade, 1976). It frequently occurs in cases of lung or renal cancer, lymphoma and multiple myeloma. The discrepancy of the rates might be attributed to the variety of primary tumors treated in each hospital. In hospitals specializing in cancer treatment, primary lesions are usually found before the patients are referred to a neurosurgical clinic. The primary lesion of breast cancer is always found before the development of cord compression. The latency before the development of spinal manifestation was longer than ten years in some patients with breast cancer.

The period of the prodromal stage between the onset of pain and the beginning of a transectional syndrome also varies with tumors. It ranges from five days to two years, the median interval being seven weeks (Gilbert, R.W. et al., 1978). Botterelli and Fitzgerald (1959) reported that the mean period of the prodromal stage was three and half months in cases with carcinoma, and nine and half months in myeloma cases. Lung cancer, renal cancer and lymphoma often developed cord signs soon after the onset of pain. In carcinomas of the breast, prostate and multiple myeloma, pain, on the other hand, precede the cord sign for a long period. The speed of progression of cord compression also differs in various kinds of tumors. Weeks or months may pass before signs of complete spinal cord transection develop. In one third of the patients, complete paraplegia appeared within one week after the onset of compressive signs (Barron et al., 1959). Gilbert, R.W. et al. (1978) reported that in nine out of 130 cases with cord compression, paraplegia was completed within 48 hours. Paraplegia of sudden onset is often observed in lung cancer, in particular. Flaccid paraplegia is observed in rapid growing tumors or in cases with pathological fractures. It is a sign of poor prognosis compared with spastic paraplegia. It was believed that the acute exacerbation of symptoms was also caused by vascular accidents, ischemia or hemorrhage. Wild and Porter (1963) reported a case of sudden exacerbation of symptoms in a patient with myeloma that bled spontaneously.

DIAGNOSTIC MEASURES

If the history of the patients includes malignant neoplasm and if their clinical features are typical of spinal epidural metastasis, it may be easy to diagnose a metastatic epidural tumor. According to neurological findings, such as the level of sensory disturbances, motor weakness and alteration of reflexes, diagnosis of tumor localization is accomplished. In some cases, however, the patients appeared at the hospital without a history of malignancy. Since the symptoms do not, in some cases, indicate the accurate level of a tumor, several diagnostic procedures are required to make a definite diagnosis.

Plain roentgenograms are positive in most cases at the level of neurological deficits. Rates of positive findings were reported to be from 50 to 90 per cent (Botterelli and Fitzgerald, 1959; Kennady and Stern, 1962; Wild and Porter, 1963; Brice and McKissock, 1965; Sellwood, 1972). Barron et al. (1959) reported that patients with lung cancer or lymphoma with cord signs frequently had negative roentgenograms. Patients with breast cancer or prostatic cancer, on the other hand, always showed positive roentgenograms. Vertebral metastasis, however, is not always accompanied by spinal compression. Lenz and Fried (1931) examined patients with bony metastasis from breast cancer and found, among 85 cases with vertebral metastasis, 15 cases that had cord signs. In autopsy findings, the frequency of vertebral metastasis from carcinomas and other malignancies was reported to be more than 30 per cent (see pathological section).

Typical radiological findings of bones affected by metastatic tumors are partial destruction or total collapse of the vertebrae. Hypertrophied bony lesions are found in osteoblastic metastasis, which is often seen in prostatic cancer. Similar findings can also be obtained in various kinds of carcinomas and lymphomas. Most cases demonstrate an osteoblastic change in the osteolytic lesion simultaneously. The vertebral bodies are the site of predilection of metastasis. The posterior arch, however, is also affected and the pedicles are often destructed. In cases with a collapsed vertebral body, the affected bone reduces its height and increases the diameter of anteroposterior or lateral projection (Fig. VI-1). The angulation and posterior protrusion

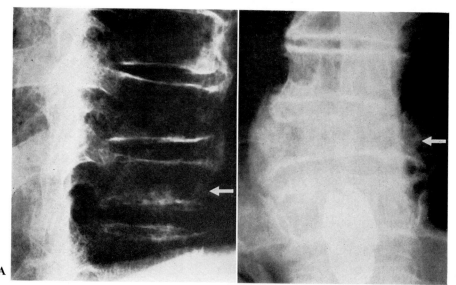

Fig. VI-1 A 72-year-old man, who had severe backache three months before admission, developed gait disturbance. One week later he became paraplegic and incontinent. A) X-ray film of the spine showed compression fracture of the 11th thoracic vertebra (arrow). B) The myelogram showed complete blockage at the same level. (Courtesy of Dr. A. Teraoka.)

of the destructed bone may cause acute transection of the cord.   Wright (1963) found
pathological fractures in 17 of 61 cases with cord signs.   Intervertebral discs are
always preserved.   X-ray films show normal distances between two adjacent vertebral
bodies.   Among other important findings are masses around the vertebral column.
An accurate estimation of this extension in the soft tissue is necessary for surgical or
radiation therapies.   Tomography of the spine is a useful method of examination,
demonstrating further details of metastatic lesions.

Radioactive isotopes are used to detect bony lesions of abnormal metabolism.
Radioisotope scintigraphy is more sensitive in the detection of wide spread metastasis than other radiological examinations.   This is performed as a screening test for
vertebral metastasis (Osmond et al., 1975; Pistenma et al., 1975).   Several radio-
nuclides, such as ^{68}Ga, ^{99m}Tc-diphosphate and ^{85}Sr, are used for this purpose.

Myelography is the most important diagnostic procedure in determining the
location of an epidural tumor.   It is essential that the extension of the mass, the upper
and lower limits of the tumor and the number of lesions should be confirmed before
the treatment.   Rates of positive myelograms among patients with cord compression
were reported to be over 90 per cent (Sellwood, 1972; Chade, 1976).   Gilbert, R.W.
et al. (1978) reported that the block of contrast media in myelography was found in
all 130 cases they treated, 97 cases of which showed complete block while the rest
showed incomplete block.   When the lower limit of neoplasms, which cause complete

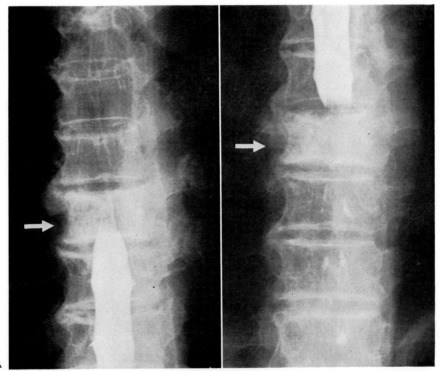

A   B

Fig. VI-2   A 64-year-old man had back pain two months before admission.   He then
developed gait disturbance and became paraplegic and incontinent within the next three
weeks.   Plain film revealed hyperostosis in his 8th thoracic vertebra.   Ascending (A) and
descending (B) myelography showed complete blockage at the same level (arrow).   This
patient was diagnosed after laminectomy to have prostatic cancer.   (TU 75107)

block, is determined by lumbar myelography, the upper limit should also be determined by the cisternal or cervical puncture (Fig. VI-2). Some authors recommended retention of the oil contrast medium in the subarachnoid space to follow the effects of therapy (Mullins et al., 1971).

Myelography is also valuable in differentiating epidural metastasis from other forms of metastases, intramedullary metastasis or leptomeningeal spread. Guyer and Westbury (1968) and Prentice et al. (1973) referred to the myelographic characteristics of leptomeningeal involvement. The spinal nerve roots showed nodular expansion. The spinal cord became wide, and in severe cases, the flow of the contrast media was blocked. In recent years, a water-soluble contrast media (Amipaque) which does not cause severe complications has become available. This contrast media excellently demonstrates the fine contours of disseminated tumors on the leptomeninges and nerve roots.

CT demonstrates its superb efficiency in determining the extension of a tumor at each segment of the cord. It was found by CT that the tumor surrounded the dural tube and extended into the vertebral bodies and para-vertebral tissue (Nakagawa et al., 1977; Lee et al., 1978) (Fig. VI-3). Reconstruction of images and computer-assisted myelography with water-soluble contrast media will become available for diagnosis of metastasis in the spinal canal.

Lymphangiography or angiography is sometimes performed to reveal characteristics of neoplasms and differentiate the metastases from the vascular lesion (Mullins et al., 1971).

Cerebrospinal fluid manometry by lumbar puncture and cytological and chemical analysis of CSF give information on the existence of CSF blockage and the type of metastasis. The opening pressure in a case with complete blockage is normal and the pressure falls rapidly when a small amount of CSF is removed. The block can also be revealed by Queckenstedt's test. Because a partial block with an opening larger than the diameter of needle does not show abnormality in Queckenstedt's test, discrepancies were noted in some cases between the findings by a manometric test and oil myelography (Poppen and Hurxthal, 1934). Rates of positive manometric tests were reported as 64 per cent by Kennady and Stern (1962) and 89 per cent by Wright (1963). The lumbar puncture should be performed cautiously since it causes some side effects and the patient's condition sometimes deteriorates after examination (Botterelli and Fitzgerald, 1959).

Cerebrospinal fluid analysis shows albuminocytological dissociation in cases with CSF block. In this condition, the cell count remains normal, whereas protein concentration increases. Chade (1976) reported increased protein concentration in 73 of 77 cases with cord compression. The value of protein concentration ranges 50 mg/100 ml to over 1,000 mg/100 ml. At such high levels of protein concentration, Froin's syndrome is observed. Cytological examination of the CSF will be helpful if meningeal spread is suspected.

Electromyogram performed in the early stages may detect subtle changes of functions of peripheral nerves (La Ban and Grant, 1971).

A needle biopsy of vertebra and the adjacent tissue was performed to facilitate histological diagnosis of the tumor and determine the method of treatment (Otto-lenghi, 1969).

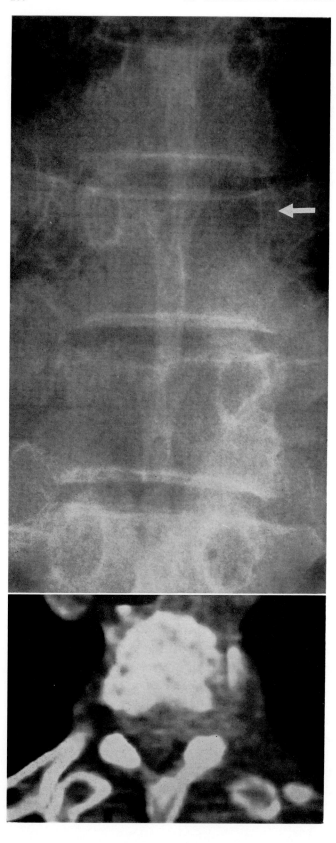

Fig. VI-3 A 70-year-old man, who was diagnosed as liver cirrhosis and revealed elevated serum alfa-fetoprotein six months before admission, suddenly developed gait disturbance. Four days later, he became paraplegic. There was destruction of pedicle of the 2nd thoracic vertebra (arrow). CT revealed a destructed vertebral body and extention of the tumor into the spinal canal and paravertebral tissue. (Courtesy of Dr. A. Teraoka.)

TREATMENT

The treatment of secondary tumors surrounding the spinal cord is an urgent task in neurosurgery. Since most patients are admitted to hospitals after the onset of definite neurological deficits, treatment should be started as soon as possible after establishment of the diagnosis.

Unfortunately, the results of treatment for spinal compression caused by metastatic tumors have not always been satisfactory. Prognosis was so poor before 1950 that many surgeons and radiologists were opposed to surgical treatment (Elsberg, 1928; Rasmussen et al., 1940; Shenkin et al., 1945; Törmä, 1957). Progress in surgery and radiation therapies in later years, however, gave impetus to our treatment of this metastasis. Since 1960 several authors have reported on increasing the effectiveness of surgical treatment, combined with radiation therapies (Wright, 1963; Wild and Porter, 1963; Chade, 1976). Some investigators recently reported that radiation had equal effectiveness even when the therapy was not combined with surgery.

The cure of widespread metastatic tumors cannot be expected at present. The goal of treatment today is limited to prolonging survival periods, giving temporal relief of neurological symptoms and preventing the rapid progression of symptoms toward complete paraplegia. Increasing the stability of affected vertebra is also an objective of therapy.

Therapeutic procedures are classified into two categories, surgical and non-surgical approaches. Surgical removal of tumors and decompression of the spinal cord have been applied for a long time. It has usually been combined with a postoperative radiation therapy. Surgical removal is considered in cases when immediate decompression is necessary. Posterior approach to the lesion is usually performed. Several laminae are to be resected for the decompression and removal of the tumor. The rostral and caudal limits of the tumor should be determined before and visualized at the time of surgery. The tumor may localize in any part of the epidural space surrounding the dural tube. Among 145 cases that underwent laminectomy as reported by Brice and McKissock (1965), the tumor grew around the cord in 52 cases, and in 27 cases, the tumor was located mainly in the posterior portion of the epidural space. In the rest of the cases, the tumor was located in the lateral or anterior portion of the cord. A tumor posteriorly extended can easily be visualized and removed. After resection of the posterior mass, the tumor localizing anterior or lateral to the dural tube should be removed as much as possible. The spinal cord should be protected from careless retraction during manipulation. Based on accurate information on the extension of a tumor around the dural tube by computed tomography, the range of surgical intervention is determined preoperatively. When enough decompression is achieved, the pulsation of the cord will be visualized. The tumor attached to the dura mater is usually scraped off from the dura easily. The dura is not incised unless the radiologic findings indicate intradural lesions, which are relatively rarely observed. Other approaches to the epidural and vertebral lesions are indicated in some cases when the tumor remains anterior to the cord and anterior fixation is necessary.

The anterior or lateral approach is performed in these conditions (Chau et al., 1973). After laminectomy is performed, procedures are required to attain stability of the vertebral column. Posterior or anterior fusion, skeletal traction or a supporting brace are required. Reports have been made on metal or plastic prosthesis used for replacement of the affected and weakened spine (Scoville et al., 1965; Ono and Tada, 1975).

The results of surgical treatment were not as rewarding as expected. The poor results can be explained in several ways. The spinal cord had been compressed long enough before surgery, and irreversible changes took place. Barron et al. (1959) reported that patients who underwent surgery after a period of more than 72 hours of paraplegia could not expect satisfactory recovery. In some cases, a residual tumor mass, located anterior to the cord or extended into the vertebral body, is left untouched. Posterior decompression with a residual tumor mass in the anterior part of the epidural spaces may cause angulation of the cord. On other occasions, the resection of the posterior arch and supporting connective tissue may increase the instability of the spinal cord, resulting in a pathological fracture or dislocation of the vertebrae. Another obstacle for surgery is a rich vascular network in the tumor, which may cause a large amount of hemorrhage during operation. Slow healing of the skin wound is sometimes encountered, resulting in contamination of the wound.

Surgical death was reported in several of the patients, and in one fifth of the cases, the neurological state grew worse after surgery (Table VI-2 and 3).

Since the 1960s, surgical removal has been combined with radiation therapies at most clinics. It is generally accepted that postoperative radiation therapies should be included in the schedule of the treatment of spinal metastasis (Wolfson, 1951; Toumay, 1943; Wild and Porter, 1963; Chade, 1976). Mones et al. (1966) and Khan

Table VI-2 Results of surgery.

Author	Total cases	Improved %	Worsen %	Mortality %
Wild and Porter (1963)	22	26	—	—
Wright (1963)	86	33	—	—
Brice and McKissock (1965)	145	50	7	6
Smith (1965)	51	25	14	4

Table VI-3 Results of surgery and radiation therapy.

Author	Total cases	Improved %	Worsen %	Mortality %
Mullan and Evans (1957)	36	22	33	—
Perese (1958)	30	20	—	—
Barron et al. (1959)	38	29	18	—
Wild and Porter (1963)	23	44	—	—
Vieth and Odom (1965b)	34	38	9	9
Chade (1968)	165	39	15	12
White et al. (1971)	226	35	10	2.5
Giannotta and Kindt (1978)	33	42	18	12
Gilbert et al. (1978)	65	45	—	—

et al. (1967) reported favorable results of radiotherapy for the patients with spinal metastasis from breast cancer or lymphomas.   Gilbert, R.W. et al. (1978) reported that radiation therapies without surgery were as effective as laminectomy followed by radiation therapies.   To attain more rapid decompression, high daily dose rapid-course irradiation was recently proposed (Millburn et al., 1968).   According to Rubin et al. (1969), a large daily dose of 5 Gy. was given to patients for three days, and this was followed by the conventional irradiation dosage, 1.5 Gy. per day.   The results of therapy by this schedule were reportedly better than the conventional method.   Gilbert, R.W. et al. (1978) also mentioned the effectiveness of radiation therapies according to similar schedules.

Radiation is given to the region between one or two segments higher than the upper limit of CSF blockage and one or two vertebrae lower than the caudal limit. Tumors in the vertebrae or in the paravertebral region should be included in the field of radiation.   Cumulative doses are set between 30 and 60 Gy.   In cases with radiosensitive tumors, an improvement is observed after irradiation of 15 Gy.

Other therapeutic procedures are combined with two main methods.   Chemo-therapy is utilized for cases of lymphomas and other tumors which are sensitive to chemotherapeutic agents.   Some patients suffering from lymphoma or leukemia with spinal epidural involvement have been satisfactorily treated with chemotherapy (Irvine and Robertson, 1964; Silverberg and Jacobs, 1971).   Hormonal therapy is applied for each hormonal dependent tumor.   Half of the breast cancers were con-sidered to be hormone dependent.   Carcinomas of the prostate or kidney are some-times recipients of hormonal therapy.

Since patients with widespread cancers are generally immunologically deterio-rated, the adjuvant immunological therapy is applied in combination with other treatments.

Radiation therapy, using radioactive iodine, is applied to patients with metastatic thyroid cancer.

Glucocorticoid is administered in the acute phase of spinal compression to reduce edema of the spinal cord and to decrease the pressure in the spinal canal (Wilson and Fewer, 1971; Ushio et al., 1977d; Posner et al., 1977; Cantu, 1968). Dehydrating agents such as mannitol, glycerol and isosorbide are also given for the same purpose.

Some surgical procedures for relief of pain are performed for patients with severe pain which cannot be controlled by medical treatment.   Rhizotomy, cordo-otomy and other kinds of tractotomy are performed for this purpose (Arseni et al., 1959; Mullan and Evans, 1957; Chade, 1976).   New methods of percutaneous ir-regular electrical nerve stimulation have brought the best relief of pain without the destruction of any nervous functions (Takakura et al., 1979).

There has been no prospective study of treatment for this form of metastasis.   It is difficult to compare the effects of different kinds of treatment since various thera-peutic schedules and different evaluation systems were applied.   Rates of improve-ment as a result of the therapies varied from 13 to 61 per cent (Table VI-2, 3 and 4). Discrepancies of the rates may depend on the types of therapy used and the selection of patients.   Two major factors which affect the results are the origin of the tumor and the stage of cord compression.   Parameters to determine the severity of cord compres-

Table VI-4   Results of radiation therapy.

Author	Total No. of cases	Improved %
Mones et al. (1966)	41	34
Khan et al. (1967)	82	41
Rubin et al. (1969)	12	75
Gilbert et al. (1978)	170	49

sion are (1) severity and duration of symptoms, (2) speed of cord compression, (3) duration of the prodromal stage before the appearance of definite signs of cord compression, and (4) extension of the tumor in the spinal canal. The level of compression has also been suggested by some investigators as another factor.

Although it is difficult to evaluate the results of a therapy, Barron et al. (1959) reported twofold prolonged survival in patients who were surgically treated. The mean survival time after surgery was reported as five months by Botterell and Fitzgerald (1959) and six months by Arseni et al. (1959). Nevertheless, one year survival was observed in about one third of the patients without cord compression, and in one quarter of the patients with cord compression. The rate of one-year survival of patients who underwent some kind of therapy was reported to be the same as that for patients who did not undergo treatment.

The survival periods for various types of tumors are varied. Gilbert, H. et al. (1978) reported that the mean survival time was short in patients with lung cancer (41 days) but long for lymphoma cases (360 days). Patients with breast cancer showed a moderate survival time of 150 days. Long survivors of over five years were reported in cases with Hodgkin's disease, multiple myeloma and prostatic cancer. A few patients with breast cancer and cancer of the bladder were also among those who survived for a long time (Jamieson, 1974).

Since the results of the treatment largely differ depending on the type of tumor and stage of cord compression, the selection of treatment may be determined on the bases of an analysis of many factors. The three most important factors are (1) type of primary tumor, (2) character of the metastatic spinal lesion and (3) general condition. The type of primary tumor determines the natural course of patient and the sensitivity to radiation therapy or chemotherapy. The factor of local lesion includes extension of the tumor, multiplicity of the lesion and the stage of spinal compression. The general condition of patient is affected by primary or metastatic spread of the tumor to vital organs.

Indication for surgery or other types of therapy is a controversial subject at the present time. Surgical treatment is indicated for patients with progressing cord signs. It is also indicated for patients with recurrent epidural growth after considerable doses of irradiation. Surgery may also be indicated in special cases where histological diagnosis is not made at the time of diagnosis. Complete dysfunction of the spinal cord at the site of compression, e.g., complete paraplegia with autonomic dysfunctions, may be cured by prompt treatment. After 72 hours of complete spinal cord transection symptoms, no improvement can be expected by surgery or any other treatment. Only immediate treatment can save the nervous functions of the patients, and thus provide both relief and hope.

If the patient shows only mild symptoms and is thought to have enough time before attaining decompression, radiotherapy is indicated. Patients who are known to have radiosensitive tumors, even if they have severe symptoms, are indicated to radiation therapy. Among other indications to radiation therapy are cases with multiple lesions in the spinal canal or patients who are generally in poor condition.

Chemotherapy should be added to surgical or radiation therapy. Some types of tumors, which are especially sensitive to chemotherapeutic agents such as lymphoma, can be treated by chemotherapy. Hormonal therapy should be combined in cases of hormone-dependent tumors.

SOME CHARACTERISTICS OF COMMON SOURCES OF SPINAL EPIDURAL METASTASIS

Lung Cancer

Case report 63-year-old man. TU 74058.

The patient began to complain of high back pain, which radiated to the band-form area of the left chest wall. Two weeks later he began to experience dysesthesia in both lower extremities. This was followed by muscle weakness of the lower extremities, which progressed to complete paraplegia within 24 hours. On admission, he had sensory disturbance below the level of the seventh segment of the thoracic cord, and had urinary incontinence. Myelography revealed blockage at the sixth and seventh thoracic vertebrae. He was operated on immediately. Posterior arches of the fifth to seventh thoracic vertebrae were removed. The tumor, which occupied mainly the posterior part of the spinal canal, was removed. Neurological symptoms improved markedly within several days. Since the chest x-ray films revealed multiple lesions of the lungs. Postoperative radiation was given to the spine and lungs.

Lung cancer is the most common origin of spinal epidural metastasis. According to Barron et al. (1959) one third of spinal metastases in male patients was metastasis from lung cancer. In this condition, a large number of the patients were seen at the hospital before the primary tumor was disclosed. Clinical signs usually progressed acutely. Some patients did not have a prodromal stage of pain and developed complete transectional symptoms as initial symptoms. Kennady and Stern (1962) reported that the period from the onset of the primary tumor to the development of nonspecific pain was shortest for lung cancer. The clinical course after the onset of pain was also rapid. Prognosis was poor in most of the cases. Barron et al. (1959) reported that none of his nine cases of lung cancer showed any improvement after surgery. The low frequency of improvement after therapy were reported as 16 per cent by Chade (1976), and seven per cent by Smith (1965) and Brice and McKissock (1965). The mean survival time after treatment was reported as 41 days by Gilbert, H. et al. (1978).

Breast Cancer

Case report   63-year-old woman. MH 14206.

The patient had received a radical mastectomy for breast cancer four years before the onset of severe backache.   She received radiation therapy to the spine and was relieved of the pain.   Two years later, however, she developed paraparesis and became paraplegic within one month.   Emergent laminectomy was performed.   She lived for five months after surgery with temporary palliation of symptoms.

Breast cancer is as common a cause of spinal epidural metastasis as lung cancer.   In half of the female patients with spinal epidural metastasis, breast cancer is the primary neoplasm.   Lenz and Fried (1931) analyzed 168 cases of breast cancer and found that 48 per cent of the cases had bony metastasis and in half of the bony metastatic cases, the vertebrae were the site of metastasis.   They also found that 8.7 per cent of the cases with breast cancer had the symptoms of cord compression. Primary tumors were detected before the onset of spinal symptoms in most of the cases.   Nevertheless, Chade (1976) reported that the primary tumor was not diagnosed preoperatively in one third of his cases.   Symptoms usually progress slowly and pain increases before cord compression develops.   Spinal metastasis from breast cancer frequently responds to therapy.   Chade (1976) found improvement in 11 of 23 cases who underwent surgery.   Survival after diagnosis was reported as 11 months by Toumey (1943) and 150 days by Gilbert et al. (1978b).

Other Carcinomas

Renal carcinoma is an important source of the spinal epidural metastasis.   The clinical characteristics resemble those of lung cancer.   The primary tumor had not been diagnosed before the onset of spinal symptoms in most of the cases.   Chade (1976) found 22 such cases among 24 patients.   Prognosis is poor.   White et al. (1971) reported that only 15 per cent of the patients responded to therapy.

Carcinoma of the prostate is another important source of spinal epidural metastasis, which frequently originates from the occult tumor of the prostate.   Chade (1976) described 15 such cases among 19 patients.   This neoplasm responds well to therapy.   Smith (1965) reported all of his cases responding to surgical treatment.   One third of the cases reported by White et al. (1971) became ambulatory after treatment.

Lymphoma

Case report   26-year-old man. TU 66146.

The patient had been treated for Hodgkin's lymphoma two years prior to the present illness.   He began to complain of shoulder pain two months before admission.   One month later a progressing gait disturbance was developed.   On admission, he was paraplegic and had sensory disturbance below the level of the 4th segment of the thoracic cord. Myelography revealed complete blockage of the fourth thoracic vertebra. Laminectomy of the third to seventh thoracic vertebrae was performed immediately. Chemotherapy with Endoxan (100 mg × 26) and methotrexate (10 mg × 4) was given. Radiation of 60 Gy. was given to the spine. When he was discharged two weeks later, the neurological signs had improved slightly.

Lymphoma is one of the most common types of tumors which causes spinal epidural spread. Williams et al. (1959) reported that three per cent of the patients with malignant lymphoma had spinal epidural metastasis. Muggia (1971) found spinal lesions in nine per cent of the patients with reticulum cell sarcoma. Mullins et al. (1971) reported the frequency of spinal epidural lesions as 4.3 per cent of Hodgkin's lymphoma and a lower frequency in non-Hodgkin's lymphoma. This neoplasm responds well to surgery, radiation and chemotherapy. Williams et al. (1959) described a favorable response to therapy in 66 per cent of Hodgkin's lymphoma and 29 per cent of non-Hodgkin's lymphoma cases. Advantageous results were also reported by Browder and de Veer (1939), Chandler et al. (1954), Irvine and Robertson (1964), Khan et al. (1967), Muggia (1971) and Mullins et al. (1971). Gilbert, H. et al. (1976) reported the mean survival time as 360 days.

Multiple myeloma is also an important disease which involves the spinal cord. Clarke (1956) reviewed literature and found cord compression in five to 20 per cent of the cases. Plain films of the spine usually reveal punched out lesions. Some special laboratory tests such as Bence-Jones protein in urine and abnormal immunogloblins in serum are positive. This neoplasm is radiosensitive. Chemotherapy is also effective. But if the patients had specific neurological deficits, immediate decompression by laminectomy is indicated. Some patients survive more than ten years (Onofrio and Svien, 1976).

Leukemia is sometimes complicated with chloroma of the spinal epidural space. Williams et al. (1959) reported that 0.7 per cent of leukemia patients had chloroma, noticed as an initial symptom of leukemia in two thirds of those patients (Wilhyde et al., 1963). Mason et al. (1973) and Stefansson and Rask (1973) reported spinal chloroma in children.

VII. ANIMAL MODELS FOR METASTATIC TUMORS OF THE CENTRAL NERVOUS SYSTEM

An experimental animal model for metastatic tumors of the central nervous system is needed for clarifying the mechanisms of pathophysiological changes on nervous functions due to metastasis and for developing new clinical approaches to the treatment. Animal experiments have been initiated to study the CNS involvement of leukemia, since leukemia in the animals is often studied in cancer investigations.

Such animal models were first reported by Thomas and his colleagues (1962, 1964) in cases of CNS involvement of leukemia. The pathology, the mode of spread of L1210 leukemia in the central nervous system of mice, as well as the suppressive effects of cyclophosphamide and methotrexate on the tumor cells, were reported. Perk et al. (1974) injected L2C leukemia cells (1×10^7) subcutaneously into strain-2 guinea pigs. On the 11th day, all inoculated guinea pigs showed tumors measuring 10 to 19 mm at the site of leukemic cell injection. Autopsies performed at this stage revealed generalized leukemia characterized by massive metastatic involvement of various organs except the central nervous system, and all animals succumbed to leukemia within 12 to 14 days. Administration of 20 mg/kg of cyclophosphamide on the 11th day resulted in the slow disappearance of the tumor as well as the return of the leukocyte count and peripheral blood picture to normal levels. The survival time of the guinea pigs treated with cyclophosphamide was extended by two to four times compared with control animals. All drug-treated animals, however, developed CNS leukemia, a phenomenon not observed in the untreated control group. These observations, both in the clinical course and in histopathological studies, were similar to those of human leukemia. Children suffering from acute lymphoblastic leukemia (ALL) with prolonged drug-induced remissions frequently develop leukemic involvement of the central nervous system, and it is more difficult to control the disease once CNS involvement occurs. Two reasons were postulated as to why CNS involvement was not seen in untreated control animals: 1) The tumor-bearing animals die from generalized leukemia very rapidly, with no time for progression to the leptomeninges; 2) The blood-brain barrier, which is located at the capillary-neural interface, has blocked the penetration of cyclophosphamide to the brain. Therefore, even though the disseminated leukemic cells are destroyed by the drug, the tumor cells remaining in the intracranial cavity further develop and grow. A similar model of murine CNS leukemia was reported by Lynch and his co-workers (1975). The treatment of a transplantable leukemia in AKR mice with both Amphotericin B and BCNU cured a significant percentage of animals with advanced diseases. Some long-term survivors developed paralysis and they invariably demonstrated CNS leukemia. Some of these animals had a systemic relapse of their leukemia and the CNS appeared to act as a focus for systemic dissemination. The patterns of occurrence and histopathologic features of the CNS leukemia in long-term survivors were similar to those observed in humans with acute lymphoblastic leukemia. Extensive and fundamental research on metastatic tumors of the central nervous system in experimental animals was carried out by Ushio, Posner and Shapiro at the Memorial Sloan-Kettering Cancer Center, New York.

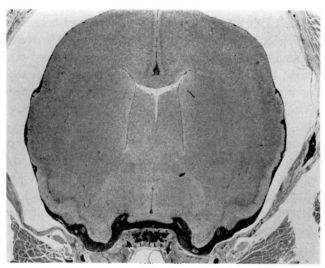

Fig. VII-1 Experimental meningeal carcinomatosis. The cell suspension of Walker 256 carcinoma was injected percutaneously into the cisterna magna of Wistar rats. The tumor grew over the leptomeninges. (Courtesy of Dr. Y. Ushio.)

Animal models of meningeal spread of a solid tumor (meningeal carcinomatosis) were initially reported by Ushio, Chernik et al. (1977a) (Fig. VII-1). The tumor (Walker 256 carcinoma) was minced in Earle's basic medium and passed through 40 and 80 mesh stainless steel screens. A concentration of $1–2 \times 10^7$ viable cells per ml of Earle's medium was obtained. Cell suspension was injected percutaneously into the cisterna magna of Wistar rats. The tumor grew rapidly and proved fatal in about 15 days if 10^6 tumor cells were inoculated. The model was histopathologically and symptomatically similar to meningeal carcinomatosis as it occurs in humans. Signs of the illness included loss of weight and paralysis of the hind legs. Spontaneous horizontal nystagmus and convulsive twitchings of limbs occurred in some animals. Severe spasticity of the limbs was observed and the rats lay with their backs hyperflexed and hind limbs extended. The most consistent gross pathological finding was thickening and opacity of the leptomeninges along the rostral portion of the longitudinal fissure and the cisterns at the base of the brain. Diffuse leptomeningeal and craniospinal nerve root infiltration was also noted. The tumor cells proliferated and blocked the subarachnoid cerebrospinal fluid pathways. They infiltrated the brain, spinal cord and nerve roots, and produced hydrocephalus. Chemotherapy on experimental meningeal carcinomatosis was studied using this animal model (Ushio et al., 1977e). An attempt was made to give chemotherapy by a single intravenous dose on the fifth, eighth or 11th day after tumor inoculation. Cyclophosphamide,

without involvement of the parenchyma, secondary to carcinoma of the lung. Am.J.Cancer 32: 361–366.

Alpinis and Purin (1973): Japan-Soviet Joint Conference on FT-207. Riga. Soviet.

Altrocchi, P.A., Reinhardt, P.H. and Eckman, P.B. (1972): Blindness and meningeal carcinomatosis. Arch. Ophthalmol. 88: 508–512.

Ambiavagar, P.C. and Sher, J. (1978): Subdural hematoma secondary to metastatic neoplasm: Report of two cases and a review of the literature. Cancer 42: 2015–2018.

Ambrose, J., Gooding, M.R. and Richardson, A.E. (1975a): Sodium iothalamate as an aid to diagnosis of intracranial lesions by computerized transverse axial scanning. Lancet 2: 669–674.

Ambrose, J., Gooding, M.R. and Richardson, A.E. (1975b): An assessment of the accuracy of computerized transverse axial scanning (EMI scanner) in the diagnosis of intracranial tumour. A review of 366 patients. Brain 98: 569–582.

American Cancer Society (1978): Cancer facts and figures. New York.

Amery, W.K. and Study Group for Bronchogenic Carcinoma (1975): Immunopotentiation with levamisole in resectable bronchogenic carcinoma: A double-blind placebo-controlled trial. Br. Med. J. 3: 461–464.

Amery, W.K. (1977): Double blind placebo controlled clinical trials of levamisole in resectable bronchogenic carcinoma. In Chirigos, M.A. (ed.): Control of Neoplasia by Modulation of the Immune System. Raven Press, New York, pp. 197–203.

Amery, W.K., Spreafico, F., Rojas, A.F., Denissen, E. and Chirigos, M.A. (1977): Adjuvant treatment with levamisole in cancer: a review of experimental and clinical data. Cancer Treat. Rev. 4: 167–194.

Amery, W.K. (1978): A placebo-controlled levamisole study in resectable lung cancer. In Terry, W.D. and Windhorst, D. (eds.): Immunotherapy of Cancer: Present Status of Trials in Man (Progress in Cancer Research and Therapy, Vol.6). Raven Press, New York, p. 198.

Ancri, D. (1971): La cinégammagraphie cérébrale. Rev. Neurol. (Paris) 125: 131–154.

Ancri, D. (1972): La cinégammagraphie cérébrale. Evolution dans l'exploration gammagraphique. Nouv. Presse Méd. 1: 231–232.

Anderson, R. (1951): Diodrast studies of the vertebral and cranial venous systems: To show their probable role in cerebral metastases. J. Neurosurg. 8: 411–422.

Aoyagi, M., Ohta, T. and Handa, H. (1971): Intra-tumor irrigation of the anticancer agents for the treatment of brain tumors. Neurol. Med. Chir. (Tokyo) 11: 259–261.

Ariel, I.M., Avery, E.E., Kanter, L., Head, J.R. and Langston, H.T. (1950): Primary carcinoma of the lung. A clinical study of 1,205 cases. Cancer 3: 229–239.

Arkin, A. and Wagner, D.H. (1936): Primary carcinoma of the lung. A diagnostic study of one hundred and thirty-five cases in four years. JAMA 106: 587–591.

Armentrout, S.A. and Ulrich, R.F. (1974): Neurological manifestation of acute granulocytic leukemia. West.J.Med. 121: 1–5.

Aronson, S.M., Garcia, J.H. and Aronson, B.E. (1964): Metastatic neoplasms of the brain; their frequency in relation to age. Cancer 17: 558–563.

Arseni, C., Simionescu, M. and Oprescu, I. (1956): Tumoule cerebrale metastatice de origine mélanica. Neurol. Psychiatr. Neurochir. 1/2: 12–21.

Arseni, C.N., Simionescu, M.D. and Horwath, L. (1959): Tumors of the spine. A follow-up study of 350 patients with neurosurgical considerations. Acta Psychiatr. Neurol. Scand. 34: 398–410.

Arseni, C. and Constantinescu, A.I. (1975): Considerations on the metastatic tumours of the brain with reference to statistics of 1,217 cases. Schweiz. Arch. Neurol. Neurochir. Psychiatr. 117: 179–195.

Ashkenazy, M., LeRoy, G.V., Fields, T. and Davis, L. (1949): The detection of intracranial tumors by the use of di-iodo[131]-flourescein. J. Lab. Clin. Med. 34: 1580–1581.

Ashkenazy M., Davis L. and Martin J. (1951): An evaluation of the technic and results of the radioactive di-iodo-fluorescein test for the localization of intracranial lesions. J. Neurosurg. 8: 300–314.

Ask-Upmark, E. (1956): Metastatic tumours of the brain and their localization. Acta Med. Scand. 154: 1–9.

Assmann, H. (1924): Zur Frage der Pathogenese und zur Klinik des Bronchialkarzinoms. Med. Klin. 20: 1757–1760; 20: 1796–1799.

Babcin, I.S. and Coltman, E.M. (1949): On cerebral metastases from malignant tumors. Probl. Neurosurg. (Moskva) 13: 48–52. (in Russian)

Bagshaw, M.A. (1963): Approaches for combined radiation and chemotherapy. Laval Medical 34: 124–133.

Bailey, P., Buchanan, D.N. and Bucy, P.C. (1939): Intracranial Tumors of Infancy and Childhood. University of Chicago Press, Chicago, pp. 396–415.

Bailey, P. (1948): Intracranial Tumors, 2nd ed. C. C. Thomas, Springfield, Ill., pp. 367–368.

Bakay, L. (1958): Results of surgical treatment of intracranial metastasis from pulmonary cancer. Report of a case with five-year survival. J. Neurosurg. 15: 338–341.

Baker, A.B. (1938): Subdural hematoma. Arch. Pathol. 26: 535–559.

Baker, A.B. (1942): Metastatic tumors of the nervous system. Arch. Pathol. 34: 495–537.

Baker, G.S., Kernohan, J.W. and Kiefer, E.J. (1951): Metastatic tumors of the brain. Surg. Clin. North Am. 31: 1143–1145.

Baker, L.H., Matter, R., Talley, R. and Vaitbevicius, V. (1975): 5-FU vs. 5-FU and Me-CCNU in gastrointestinal cancer. A phase III study of the Southwest Oncology Group. Proc. Am. Assoc. Cancer

Res. 16: 229. (Abstract)

Bannayan, G.A., Huvos, A.G. and D'Angio, G.J. (1971): Effect of irradiation on the maturation of Wilms' tumor. Cancer 27: 812–818.

Bardfield, P.A., Passalaqua, A.M., Braunstein, P., Raghavendra, B.N., Leeds, N.E. and Kricheff, I. (1977): A comparison of radionuclide scanning and computed tomography in metastatic lesions of the brain. J. Comput. Assist. Tomogr. 1: 315–318.

Barnard, R.O. and Scott, T. (1975): Patterns of proliferation in cerebral lymphoreticular tumours. Acta Neuropathol. (Berl.) [Suppl. 6]: 125–130.

Barron, K.D., Hirano, A., Araki, S. and Terry, R.D. (1959): Experiences with metastatic neoplasms involving the spinal cord. Neurology (Minneap.) 9: 91–106.

Batson, O.V. (1940): The function of the vertebral veins and their role in the spread of metastases. Ann. Surg. 112: 138–149.

Batson, O.V. (1942): The vertebral vein system as a mechanism for the spread of metastases. Am. J. Roentgenol. Radium Ther. 48: 714–718.

Beatson, G.T. (1896): On treatment of inoperable cases of carcinoma of mamma: Suggestions for new method of treatment, with illustrative cases. Lancet 2: 104–107, 2: 162–165.

Bedrossian, C.W., Weilbaecher, D.G., Bentinck, D.C. and Greenberg, S.D. (1975): Ultrastructure of human bronchiolo-alveolar cell carcinoma. Cancer 36: 1399–1413.

Beehler, E. (1960): Metastasis to spinal subdural space: Report of case. Bull. Los Angeles Neurol. Soc. 25: 44–47.

Beeler, T.T., Jr. and Irey, N.S. (1950): Bronchogenic carcinoma. A clinicopathologic study of fifty autopsied cases. Dis. Chest 18: 60–80.

Beerman, W.F. (1912): Meningeal carcinomatosis. JAMA 58: 1437–1439.

Beng, K.C., Yu, M., and Wee, R. (1970): Immunoglobulin (IgA, G, M) levels in primary carcinoma of the liver and cirrhosis of the liver in Singapore. Med. J. Aust. 57: 18–21.

Benson, D.F. (1960): Intramedullary spinal cord metastasis. Neurology (Minneap.) 10: 281–287.

Berardi, R.S. (1973): Bronchogenic carcinoma with cerebral metastases. Int. Surg. 58: 385–388.

Beresford, H.R. (1969): Melanoma of the nervous system: Treatment with corticosteroids and radiation. Neurology (Minneap.) 19: 59–65.

Berg, J.W. and Robbins, G.F. (1966): Factors influencing short and long term survival of breast cancer patients. Surg. Gynecol. Obstet. 122: 1311–1316.

Bering, E.A., Jr., Wilson, C.B. and Norrell, H.A., Jr. (1967): The Kentucky Conference on Brain Tumor Chemotherapy. J. Neurosurg. 27: 1–10.

Berkson, J.M.D. and Gage, R.P.M.S. (1950): Calculation of survival rates for cancer. Proc. Staff Meet. Mayo Clin. 25: 270–286.

Bhagwati, S.N. and McKissock, W. (1961): Spinal cord compression in Hodgkin's disease. A review of 10 cases. Br. J. Surg. 48: 672–676.

Biran, S. and Herishianu, Y. (1972): Brain involvement in Hodgkin's disease: Report of a case. Eur. Neurol. 8: 352–358.

Blatt, B. and Højgaard, K. (1963): Cancer metastaticus cerebri. Acta Neurol. Scand. 39: 356–368.

Blau, M. and Bender, M.A. (1959): Radiomercury (Hg^{203}) labeled neohydrin: A new agent for brain tumor localization. J. Nucl. Med. [convention issue] p. 35.

Blinkof, S.M. and Glezer, I.I. (1968): The Human Brain in Figures and Tables. A Quantitative Handbook, (translated by Haigh, B.) Basic Books, New York.

Blokhina, N.G., Vozny, E.K. and Garin, A.M. (1972): Results of treatment of malignant tumors with ftorafur. Cancer 30: 390–392.

Bloom, W.H., Carstairs, K.C., Crompton, M.R. and McKissock, W. (1960): Autologous glioma transplantation. Lancet 2: 77–78.

Blotner, H. (1958): Primary or idiopathic diabetes insipidus: A system disease. Metabolism 7: 191–200.

Blythe, J.G., Ptacek, J., Buchbaum, H.J. and Latourette, H.B. (1975): Bony metastases from carcinoma of cervix. Occurrence, diagnosis and treatment. Cancer 36: 475–484.

Bonica, J.J. (ed.) (1974a): International Symposium on Pain (Advances in Neurology, Vol. 4). Raven Press, New York.

Borsos, T. and Rapp, H.J. (eds.) (1973): Conference on the Use of BCG in Therapy of Cancer (National Cancer Institute Monograph, Vol. 39). National Institute of Health, Bethesda.

Botterell, E.H. and Fitzgerald, G.W. (1959): Spinal cord compression produced by extradural malignant tumors; early recognition, treatment and result. Can. Med. Assoc. J. 80: 791–794.

Boucot, K.R., Horie, V. and Sokoloff, M.J. (1959): Survival in lung cancer. N. Engl. J. Med. 260: 742–746.

Bowsher, D. (1957): Pathways of absorption of protein from the cerebrospinal fluid: An autoradiographic study in the cat. Anat. Rec. 128: 23–39.

Brain, W.R., Daniel, P.M. and Greenfield, J.G. (1951): Subacute cortical cerebellar degeneration and its relation to carcinoma. J. Neurol. Neurosurg. Psychiatry 14: 59–75.

Brain, W.R. and Henson, R.A. (1958): Neurological syndromes associated with carcinoma. The carcinomatous neuromyopathies. Lancet 2: 971–974.

Bramlet, D., Giliberti, J. and Bender, J. (1976): Meningeal carcinomatosis: Case report and review of the literature. Neurology (Minneap.) 26: 287–290.

Braun, E.M., Burger, L.J. and Schlang, H.A. (1973): Subdural hematoma from metastatic malignant disease. Cancer 32: 1370–1373.

Braun, W. (1974): Regulatory factors in the immune response; Analysis and perspective. In Braun, W., Lichtenstein, L.M. and Parker, C.W. (eds.): Cyclic AMP, Cell Growth, and the Immune Response. Springer-Verlag, Berlin, pp. 4–23.

Brazinsky, J.H. (1973): Metastatic intracerebral and intracerebellar Hodgkin's disease: Case report. J. Neurosurg. 38: 635–637.

Brennan, J.J. and Vaitkevicius, V.N. (1960): 5-Fluorouracil in clinical cancer experience with 155 patients. Cancer Chemother. Rep. 6: 8–11.

Brice, J. and McKissock, W. (1965): Surgical treatment of malignant extradural spinal tumors. Br. Med. J. 1: 1341–1344.

Brihaye, J., and Martin, J. (1961): Analyse de 172 tumeurs métastatiques du système nerveux. Neurochirurgie (Paris) 7: 147–151.

Brihaye, J. (1963): Les tumeurs métastatiques du système nerveux central. A propos de 239 observations. Acta Chir. Belgica 1: 43–61.

Broders, A.C. (1919): Tuberculosis associated with malignant neoplasia. Report of twenty cases. JAMA 72: 390–394.

Brooks, W.H., Netsky, M.G., Normansell, D.E. and Horwitz, D.A. (1972): Depressed cell-mediated immunity in patients with primary intracranial tumors. J. Exp. Med. 136: 1631–1647.

Browder, J. and de Veer, J.A. (1939): Lymphomatoid disease involving the spinal epidural space. A pathologic and therapeutic consideration. Arch. Neurol. Psychiatry 41: 328–347.

Bruley-Rosset, M., Florentin, I., Kiger, N., Davigny, M. and Mathé, G. (1978): Effects of Bacillus calmette-guérin and levamisole on immune responses in young adult and age-immunodepressed mice. Cancer Treat. Rep. 62: 1641–1650.

Bryson, C.C. and Spencer, H. (1951): Carcinoma of the bronchus: a clinical and pathological survey of 866 cases. Q. J. Med. 20: 173–186.

Bucholz (1898): Casuistischer Beitrag zur Kenntnis der Carzinome des Centralnervensystems. Monatsschr. Psychiatr. Neurol. 4: 183.

Bucy, P.C. and Stilp, T.J. (1972): Metastatic choriocarcinoma of the brain. Its recognition, treatment and cure; and other matters. Arch. Swisses de Neurologie, Neurochirurgie et de Psychiatrie 3: 237–242.

Bureau-Paillas, M. and Poncet, M. (1974): Les tumeurs métastatiques de l'encéphale. Etude électroencéphalographique. Neurochirurgie (Paris) 20 [Suppl. 2]: 106–113.

Burford, R.W. (1950): Radiation therapy of diseases of the nervous system. In Pohle, E.A. (ed.): Clinical Radiation Therapy, 2nd ed. Lea & Febiger, Philadelphia, pp. 515–548.

Burger, P.C. and Vogel, F.S. (1976): Surgical Pathology of the Nervous System and its Coverings. John Wiley & Sons, Inc., New York.

Byfield, J.E. (1972): Ionizing radiation and vincristine; possible neurotoxic synergism. Radiol. Clin. Biol. 41: 129–138.

Cala, L.A. and Mastaglia, F.L. (1976): Computed tomography in multiple sclerosis. Lancet 1: 689.

Canellos, G.P., Pocock, S.J., Taylor, S.G. III, Sears, M.E., Klaasen, D.J. and Band, P.R. (1976): Combination chemotherapy for metastatic breast carcinoma. Cancer 38: 1882–1886.

Cantu, R.C. (1968): Corticosteroids for spinal metastases. Lancet 2: 912.

Cappelen, C.Jr., Efskind, L. and Poppe, E. (1961): Bronchial carcinoma with special reference to prognosis. Acta Pathol. Microbiol. Scand. 148 [Suppl.]: 23–33.

Carbajal, U.M. (1959): Metastasis in retinoblastoma. Am. J. Ophthalmol. 48: 47–69.

Carbone, P.P., Frost, J.K., Feinstein, A.R., Higgins, G.A., Jr., and Selawry, O.S. (1970): Lung cancer: perspectives and prospects. Ann. Intern. Med. 73: 1003–1024.

Carter, S.K. (1974): The chemical therapy of breast cancer. Semin. Oncol. 1: 131–144.

Carter, S.K. (1976): Integration of chemotherapy into combined modality treatment of solid tumors. VII. Adenocarcinoma of the breast. Cancer Treat. Rev. 3: 141–174.

Carter, S.K. Bakowski, M.T. and Hellmann, K. (1977): Chemotherapy of Cancer. John Wiley & Sons, Inc., New York.

Carter, T.L., Gabrielsen, T.O. and Abell, M.R. (1968): Mechanism of split sutures in metastatic neuroblastoma. Radiology 91: 467–470.

Cashion, E.L. and Young, J.M. (1973): Intramedullary spinal cord metastasis. South. Med. J. 66: 1266; 66: 1297.

Castaigne, P., Escourolle, R. and Hauw, J.J. (1972): Les lesions du systeme nerveux en rapport avec les cancers visceraux. Rev. Med. (Liege) 27: 1–12.

Castelli, A., Paoletti, P. and Villanti, R. (1968): Brain scan for neurosurgical purposes: Analysis of 217 verified tumours. Neurochirurgia (Stuttg.) 11: 234–245.

Catane, R., Kaufman, J., West, C., Merrin, C., Tsukada, Y. and Murphy, G.P. (1976): Brain metastasis from prostatic carcinoma. Cancer 38: 2583–2587.

Cervos-Navarro, J., Betz, E., Matakas, F. and Wüllenweber, R. (eds.) (1976): The Cerebral Vessel Wall. Raven Press, New York.

Chade, H.O. (1968): Metastasen der Wirbelsäule und des Rückenmarks. Schweiz. Arch. Neurol. Neurochir.

Psychiatr. 102: 257–287.

Chade, H.O. (1976): Metastatic tumours of the spine and spinal cord. In Vinken, P.J. and Bruyn, G.W. (eds.): Handbook of Clinical Neurology, Vol. 20. North-Holland Publishing Co., Amsterdam, pp. 415–433.

Chan, P.Y.M., Byfield, J.E., Campbell, T., Sadoff, L. and Rao, A.R. (1980): Combined chemotherapy and irradiation in the treatment of brain metastases from lung cancer. In Weiss, L.W., Gilbert, H.A. and Posner, J.B. (eds.): Brain Metastasis. G.K. Hall & Co., Boston, Mass., pp. 364–379.

Chandler, H.C., French, L.A. and Peyton, Wm.T. (1954): Surgical treatment of metastatic tumors of the spine. Ann. Surg. 140: 197–199.

Chao, J., Phillips, R. and Nickson, J.J. (1954): Roentgen-ray therapy of cerebral metastases. Cancer 7: 682–689.

Chason, J.L., Walker, F.B. and Landers, J.W. (1963): Metastatic carcinoma in the central nervous system and dorsal root ganglia: A prospective autopsy study. Cancer 16: 781–787.

Chirigos, M. (ed.) (1976): Control of Neoplasia by Modulation of the Immune System (Progress in Cancer Research and Therapy, Vol.2). Raven Press, New York.

Chous, S.N. and Seljeskog, E.L. (1973): Alternate surgical approaches to the thoracic spine. Clin. Neurosurg. 20: 306–321.

Chretien, P.B., Lipson, S.D., Makuch, R., Kenady, D.E., Cohen, M.H. and Minna, J.D. (1978): Thymosin in cancer patients: In vitro effects and correlations with clinical response to thymosin immunotherapy. Cancer Treat. Rep. 62: 1787–1790.

Christensen, E. (1949): Intracranial carcinomatous metastases in a neurosurgical clinic. Acta Psychiatr. Neurol. 24: 353–361.

Chu, F.C.H. and Hilaris, B.B. (1961): Value of radiation therapy in the management of intracranial metastasis. Cancer 14: 577–581.

Ciembroniewicz, J. and Kolar, O. (1969): Tissue culture study of glioblastoma cells with addition of autologous lymphocytes. Acta Cytol. 13: 42–47.

Clarke, E. (1954): Cranial and intracranial myelomas. Brain 77: 61–81.

Clarke, E. (1956): Spinal cord involvement in multiple myelomatosis. Brain 79: 332–348.

Clarkson, B.D., Haghbin, M., Murphy, M.L., Gee, T.S., Dowling, M.D., Arlin, Z.A., Kempin, S., Posner, J., Shapiro, W., Galicich, J., Dufour, P., Passe, S. and Burchenal, J.H. (1979): Prevention of central nervous system leukaemia in acute lymphoblastic leukaemia with prophylactic chemotherapy alone. In Whitehouse, J.M.A. and Kay, H.E.M. (eds.): CNS Complications of Malignant Disease. MacMillan Press, Ltd., London, pp. 36–58.

Clarysse, A., Kenis, Y. and Mathé, G. (1976): Cancer Chemotherapy (Recent Results in Cancer Research, Vol. 53). Springer-Verlag, Berlin.

Clausen, R.E., Jr., Lincoln, A.F. and Silberman, H.K. (1956): Diffuse lymphosarcomatosis of the central nervous system simulating infectious polyneuritis. Am. J. Med. 20: 292–300.

Clemente, C.D. and Holst, E.A. (1954): Pathological changes in neurons, neuroglia, and blood-brain barrier induced by X-irradiation of heads of monkeys. Arch. Neurol. Psychiatry 71: 66–79.

Clemmesen, J., Nielsen, A. and Jensen, E. (1953): The increase in incidence of carcinoma of the lung in Denmark, 1931 to 1950. Br. J. Cancer 7: 1–9.

Clifford, J.R., Kirgis, H.D. and Connolly, E.S. (1975): Metastatic melanoma of the brain presenting as subarachnoid hemorrhage. South. Med. J. 68: 206–208.

Coats, J. (1888): Primary carcinoma of brain. Br. Med. J. 1: 959.

Coman, D.R. and DeLong, R.P. (1951): The role of the vertebral venous system in the metastasis of cancer to the spinal cord: Experiments with tumor-cell suspension in rats and rabbits. Cancer 4: 610–618.

Comis, R.L. and Carter, S.K. (1974a): A review of chemotherapy in gastric cancer. Cancer 34: 1576–1586.

Comis, R.L. and Carter, S.K. (1974b): Integration of chemotherapy into combined modality treatment of solid tumors, III: Gastric cancer. Cancer Treat. Rev. 1: 221–238.

Committee for Radiation Oncology Studies, Radiation Sensitizers. (1976): In Committee for Radiation Oncology Studies Research Plan for Radiation Oncology. Cancer 37 (Suppl.): 2062–2070.

Constans, J.P., Askienazy, S., Renou, G., Chodkiewicz, J.P. and Schlienger, M. (1973a): Surveillance gamma encéphalographique de l'évolution des tumeurs cérébrales malignes traitées. Neurochirurgia (Stuttg.) 16: 41–50.

Constans, J.P., Rouesse, J., Roujeau, J. and Schlienger, M. (1973b): Indications thérapeutiques dans les métastases cérébrales. Bull du Cancer 60(3): 301–326.

Constans, J.P. and Cioloca, C. (1974): Chimiothérapie des métastases cérébrales. Neurochirurgie (Paris) 20 [Suppl. 2]: 212–219.

Constans, J.P., Roujeau, J., Schlienger, M., Askienazy, S. and Védrenne, C. (1974): Les indications de la neurochirurgie en cancérologie. Sem. Hôp. Paris 50: 1009–1017.

Cooper, R. (1969): Combination chemotherapy in hormone resistant breast cancer. Proc. Am. Assoc. Cancer Res. 10: 15 (abstr.).

Cooperative Breast Cancer Group (1964): Testosterone propionate therapy in breast cancer. JAMA 188: 1069–1072.

Copeland, D., Stewart, T. and Harris, J. (1974): Effect of levamisole (NSC-177023) on in vitro human lymphocyte transformation. Cancer Chemother. Rep. 58: 167–170.

Correa, P. and O'Connor, G.T. (1973): Geographic pathology of lymphoreticular tumors: Summary of survey from the Geographic Pathology Committee of the International Union Against Cancer. J. Natl. Cancer Inst. 50: 1609–1617.

Cortes, E.P., Takita, H. and Holland, J.F. (1974): Adriamycin in advanced bronchogenic carcinoma. Cancer 34: 518–525.

Courville, C.B. (1945): Pathology of the Central Nervous System; A study based upon a survey of lesions found in a series of thirty thousand autopsies, 2nd ed. Pacific Press Publishing Assn., Mountain View, Calif., pp. 406–410.

Courville, C.B. and Abbott, K.H. (1945): Note on the pathology of cranial tumors. 2. Metastatic tumors of the calvalium with incidental reference to their occurrence in American aborigines. Bull. Los Angeles Neurol. Soc. 10: 129–154.

Courville, C.B. (1948): Note on the pathology of cranial tumors. Tumors originating in the marrow of the diploe. Bull. Los Angeles Neurol. Soc. 13: 19–41.

Courville, C.B. (1950): Pathology of the Central Nervous System; A study based upon a survey of lesions found in a series of forty thousand autopsies, 3rd ed. Pacific Press Publishing Assn., Mountain View, Calif., p. 367.

Cowen, R., Siqueira, E. and George, E. (1970): Angiographic demonstration of a glioma involving the wall of the anterior cerebral artery. Radiology 97: 577–578.

Craig, W.M., Woltman, H.W. and Kernohan, J.W. (1939): Metastasis to the central nervous system from carcinoma of the lung. Am. J. Cancer 36: 12–24.

Crock, H.V., Yoshizawa, H. and Kame, S.K. (1973): Observation on the venous drainage of the human vertebral body. J. Bone Joint Surg. 55-B: 528–533.

Croll M.N., Brady L.W., Faust D.S., Kazem I., Antoniades J. and Tatem, H.R. (1968): Comparison brain scanning with mercury 203 and technetium 99m. Radiology 90: 747–749.

Cuneo, H.M. and Rand, C.W. (1952): Brain Tumors of Childhood. C.C. Thomas, Springfield, Ill., pp. 144 156.

Cushing, H. (1932): Intracranial tumors; Notes upon a series of two thousand verified cases with surgical-mortality percentages pertaining thereto. C. C. Thomas, Springfield, Ill., p. 8.

Cushing, H. (1937): Tumeurs Intracraniennes. Étude analytique de 2,000 tumeurs vérifiées et de leur mortalité opératoire. Masson & Cie, Paris.

Dabney, W.M. (1916): Tuberculosis and cancer: A possible explanation of the long-discussed question of their mutual antagonism with the suggestion of the use of tuberculin for the prevention of recurrence of cancer. Med. Rec. 90: 804–805.

Dahmen, Z. (1905): Pachimeningitis carcinomatosa. Ztschr. Krebsforsch. 3: 300.

D'Andrea, F. and de Divitiis, E. (1966): Neoplasie metastatiche dell'encefalo. Ed. Glaux, Napoli.

Dandy, W.E. (1932): Brain tumors—General diagnosis and treatment. In Lewis (ed.): Practice of Surgery, Vol. 12. Prior/Harper & Row, Publishers, New York, pp. 443–674.

Daniel, P.M. (1964): The management of metastases in the central nervous system. Proc. Royal Soc. Med. 57: 1151–1153.

Das Gupta, T. and Brasfield, R. (1964): Metastatic melanoma: A clinicopathological study. Cancer 17: 1323–1339.

Davis, L. (1946): The Principles of Neurological Surgery. Lea & Febiger, Philadelphia.

Davis, L. and Craigmile, T. (1954): Results of radioactive isotope encephalography in patients with verified intracranial tumors. J. Neurosurg. 11: 262–267.

Davis, P.L. and Shumway, M.H. (1961): Thio-TEPA in treatment of metastatic cerebral malignancy. JAMA 175: 714–715.

Davison, C. and Horwitz, W.A. (1930): Primary carcinoma of the lungs with metastases to the central nervous system. Arch. Intern. Med. 46: 680–704.

Davison, C. and Spiegel, L.A. (1945): The syndrome of the posterior inferior cerebellar artery resulting from a metastatic neoplasm. J. Neuropathol. Exp. Neurol. 4: 172–177.

Day, E.D., Lassiter, S., Woodhall, B., Mahaley, J.L. and Mahaley, M.S., Jr. (1965): The localization of radioantibodies in human brain tumors. Cancer Res. 25: 773–778.

Dayes, L.A., Rouhe, S.A. and Barnes, R.W. (1977): Excision of multiple intracranial metastatic hypernephroma: Report of a case with a 7-year survival. J. Neurosurg. 46: 533–535.

Dean, J.H., Padarathsingh, M.L. and Keys, L. (1978): Response of murine leukemia to combined BCNU-maleic anhydride-vinyl ether (MVE) adjuvant therapy and correlation with macrophage activation by MVE in the in vitro growth inhibition assay. Cancer Treat. Rep. 62: 1807–1816.

Debois, J.M. et al. (1975): Preliminary experience with Levamisole in cancer patients, and particularly in breast cancer. Second Conference on Modulation of Host Resistance in the Prevention or Treatment of Induced Neoplasias. N.I.H. The John E. Fogarty International Center and N.C.I., Bethesda, Maryland.

Deck, M.D.F., Messina, A.V. and Sacket, J.F. (1976): Computed tomography in metastatic disease of the brain. Radiology 119: 115–120.

Deck, M.D.F. (1980): Computed tomography of metastatic disease of the brain. In Weiss, L., Gilbert, H.A. and Posner, J.B. (eds.): Brain Metastasis. G.K. Hall & Co., Boston, Mass., pp. 208–241.

Deeley, T.J. and Rice Edwards, J.M. (1968): Radiotherapy in the management of cerebral secondaries from bronchial carcinoma. Lancet 1: 1209–1212.

De Lena, M., Brambilla, C., Morabito, A. and Bonadonna, G. (1975): Adriamycin plus vincristine compared to and combined with cyclophosphamide, methotrexate and 5-fluorouracil for advanced breast cancer. Cancer 35: 1108–1115.

Denny-Brown, D. (1948): Primary sensory neuropathy with muscular changes associated with carcinoma. J. Neurol. Neurosurg. Psychiatry 11: 73–87.

Derby, B.M. and Guiang, R.L. (1975): Spectrum of symptomatic brain stem metastasis. J. Neurol. Neurosurg. Psychiatry 38: 888–895.

Deutsch, M., Parsons, J.A. and Mercado, R. (1974): Radiotherapy for intracranial metastases. Cancer 34: 1607–1611.

De Vita, V.T., Jr. (1977): Adjuvant theraphy; an overview. In Salmon, S.E. and Jones, S.E. (eds.): Adjuvant Therapy of Cancer. Elsevier/North-Holland Biomedical Press, Amsterdam, pp. 613–641.

Dewey, W.C. and Humphrey, R.M. (1972): Relative radiosensitivity of different phases in the life cycle of L-P 59 mouse fibroblasts and ascites tumour cells. Radiat. Res. 16: 503.

Digby, K.H., Fook, W.M.L. and Che, Y.T. (1941): Nasopharyngeal carcinoma. Br. J. Surg. 28: 517–537.

Di Luzio, N.R., McNamee, R., Browder, W.I. and Williams, D. (1978): Glucan inhibition of tumor growth and enhancement of survival in four syngeneic murine tumor models. Cancer Treat. Rep. 62: 1857–1866.

Dionne, L. (1965): The pattern of blood-borne metastasis from carcinoma of rectum. Cancer 18: 775–781.

Dische, S., Saunders, M.I., Lee, M.E., Adams, G.E. and Flockhart, I.R. (1977): Clinical testing of the radiosensitizer Ro 07–0582: Experience with multiple doses. Br. J. Cancer 35: 567–579.

Djordjevic, B. and Szybalski, W. (1960): Genetics of human cell lines. III. Incorporation of 5-bromo- and 5-iododeoxyuridine into the deoxyribonucleic acid of human cells and its effects on radiation sensitivity. J. Exp. Med. 112: 509–513.

Dommisse, G.F. (1975): The Arteries and Veins of the Human Spinal Cord from Birth. Churchill Livingstone, Edinburgh, pp. 81–96.

Doppman, J.L., Ramsey, R. and Thies, R.J., II. (1973): A percutaneous technique for producing intraspinal mass lesions in experimental animals. J. Neurosurg. 38: 438–447.

Dostalova, O., Schon, E., Kubelka, V. and Holik, F. (1970): Observation of immunoglobulins in the course of a tumor disease. Neoplasma 17: 231–240.

Drury, R.A.B., Palmer, P.H. and Highman, W.J. (1964): Carcinomatous metastasis to the vertebral bodies. J. Clin. Pathol. 17: 448–457.

Duchen, L.W. (1966): Metastatic carcinoma in the pituitary gland and hypothalamus. J. Pathol. Bacteriol. 91: 347–355.

Du Four, M.H. (1904): Méningite sarcomateuse diffuse avec encahissement de la moelle et des racines: Cytologie positive et special du liquide céphalorachidien. Rev. Neurol. (Paris) 12: 104–106.

Dunlap, H.F. (1932): Metastatic malignant tumors of the brain. Ann. Intern. Med. 5: 1274–1288.

Duplan, J.F. (1962): Effets de l'hydrocortisone et de l'irradiation X sur la leucémogénèse spontanée des Souris AkR. Compt. Rend. Soc. Biol. (Paris) 156: 779–782.

Durrant, J., Janossy, G. and Woodruff, P.K. (1979): CNS leukemia in blast cell crisis in CML and Philadelphia (Ph') positive acute lymphoid leukaemia. In Whitehouse, J.M.A. and Kay, H.E.M. (eds.): CNS Complications of Malignant Disease. MacMillan Press, Ltd., London, pp. 100–109.

Durrant, K.R., Berry, R.T., Ellis, F., Ridehalgh, F.R., Black, J.M. and Hamilton, W.S. (1971): Comparison of treatment policies in inoperable bronchial carcinoma. Lancet 1: 715–719.

Dyke, C.G. and Davidoff, L.M. (1942): Roentgen Treatment of Diseases of the Nervous System. Henry Kimpton, London.

Earle, K.M. (1954): Metastatic and primary intracranial tumors of the adult male. J. Neuropathol. Exp. Neurol. 13: 448–454.

Eason, E.H. (1950): A case of cerebral infarction due to neoplastic embolism. J. Pathol. Bacteriol. 62: 454–457.

Eberth, C.J. (1870): Zur Entwicklung des Epithelioms (Cholesteatoms) der Pia und der Lunge. Virchows Arch. 49: 51–63.

Edelson, R.N., Deck, M.D.F. and Posner, J.B. (1972): Intramedullary spinal cord metastases: Clinical and radiographic findings in nine cases. Neurology (Minneap.) 22: 1222–1231.

Ederer, F., Cutler, S.J., Goldenberg, I.R. and Eisenberg. H. (1963): Cause of death among long-term survivors from breast cancer in Connecticut. J. Natl. Cancer Inst. 30: 933–947.

Edmonson, J.H. and Lagakos, S.W. (1974): Combination chemotherapy for metastatic lung cancer. Proc. Am. Assoc. Cancer Res. 15: 180 (abstr.).

Effler, D.B. and Barr, D. (1960): Five year survival after surgery for bronchogenic carcinoma. Dis. Chest 38: 417–422.

El-Batata, M. (1968): Cytology of cerebrospinal fluid in the diagnosis of malignancy. J. Neurosurg. 28: 317–326.

Elkington, J.StC. (1935): Metastatic tumors of the brain. Proc. R. Soc. Med. 28: 1080–1096.

Ellingson, R.J. and Lundy, B.W. (1962): Electroencephalograms of patients suspected of having metastatic lesions of the brain. Cancer 15: 1138–1141.

Ellis, F. (1969): Dose, time and fractionation: a clinical hypothesis. Clin. Radiol. 20: 1–7.

Elsaesser, K.H. (1949): Zur Klinik der metastatischen Hirngeschwülste. Zentralbl. Neurochir. 9: 150–183.

Elsberg, C.A. (1928): Extradural spinal tumors; primary, secondary, metastatic. Surg. Gynecol. Obstet. 46: 1–20.

Elvidge, A.R. and Baldwin, M. (1949): Clinical analysis of eighty-eight cases of metastatic carcinoma involving the central nervous system with an outline of therapeutic principles. J. Neurosurg. 6: 495–502.

Engelman, R.M. and McNamara, W.L. (1954): Bronchogenic carcinoma. A statistical review of two hundred and thirty-four cases. J. Thorac. Cardiovasc. Surg. 27: 227.

Epstein, S., Ranchod, M. and Goldswain, P.R.T. (1973): Pituitary insufficiency, inappropriate antidiuretic hormone (ADH) secretion, and carcinoma of the bronchus. Cancer 32: 476–481.

Erikson, R.L. and Szybalski, W. (1963): Molecular radiobiology of human cell lines. V. Comparative radio-sensitizing properties of 5-halodeoxycytidines and 5-halodeoxyuridines. Radiat. Res. 20: 252–262.

Evans, A.E., Gilbert, E.S. and Zandstra, R. (1970): The increasing incidence of central nervous system leukemia in children: Children's cancer study group A. Cancer 26: 404–409.

Everson, T.C. and Cole, W.H. (1956): Spontaneous Regression of Cancer: Preliminary Report. Ann. Surg. 144: 366–383.

Falk, R.E., Mann, P. and Langer, B. (1973): Cell-mediated immunity to human tumors; abrogation by serum factors and nonspecific effects of oral BCG therapy. Arch. Surg. 107: 261–265.

Feiring, E.H. and Hubbard, J.H., Jr. (1965): Spinal cord compression resulting from intradural carcinoma: Report of 2 cases. J. Neurosurg. 23: 635–638.

Fenoglio, C.M., Ferenczy, A. and Richart, R.M. (1975): Mucinous tumors of the ovary. Ultrastructural studies of mucinous cystadenomas with hostogenetic considerations. Cancer 36: 1709–1722.

Fewer, D., Wilson, C.B., Boldrey, E.B., Enot, K.J. and Powel, M.R. (1972): The chemotherapy of brain tumors. Clinical experience with carmustine (BCNU) and vincristine. JAMA 222: 549–552.

Field, E.J. and Brierly, J.B. (1948): The lymphatic connections of the subarachnoid space: An experimental study of the dispersion of particulate matter in the cerebrospinal fluid, with special reference to the pathogenesis of poliomyelitis. Br. Med. J. 1: 1167–1171.

Filson, E.J. and Rodriguez-Antunez, A. (1968): Isotope scanning of brain tumors using [99m] Tc. Acta Radiol. [Diagn.] 7: 380–384.

Fink, M.A. (1974): Tumor immunotherapy: Current trials and future developments. Semin. Oncol. 1: 425–427.

Fisher, B., Ravdin, R.G., Ausman, R.K., Slack, N.H., Moore, G.E. and Noer, R.J. (1968): Surgical adjuvant chemotherapy in cancer of the breast: Results of a decade of cooperative investigation. Ann. Surg. 168: 337–356.

Fisher, B., Slack, N.H., Bross, I.D.J. and Cooperating Investigators (1969): Cancer of the breast: Size of neoplasm and prognosis. Cancer 24: 1071–1080.

Fischer-Defoy, W. (1905): Vier Fälle von osteoplastischem Prostatacarcinom. Zugleich eine Uebersicht über 20 andere in Dresden beobachtete Knochencarcinome. Ztschr. Krebsforsch. 3: 195–217.

Fischer-Williams, M., Bosanquet, F.D. and Daniel, P.M. (1955): Carcinomatosis of the meninges: A report of three cases. Brain 78: 42–58.

Fitzpatrick, P.J. and Keen, C.W. (1980): The Princess Margaret and Ontario Cancer Foundation experience. In Weiss, L., Gilbert, H.A. and Posner, J.B. (eds.): Brain Metastasis. G.K. Hall & Co., Boston, Mass., pp. 281–302.

Flavell, G. (1949): Solitary cerebral metastases from bronchial carcinomata. Their incidence and a case of successful removal. Br. Med. J. 2: 736–737.

Fleming, I., Simone, J., Jackson, R., Johnson, W., Walters, T. and Mason, C. (1974): Splenectomy and chemotherapy in acute myelocytic leukemia of childhood. Cancer 33: 427–434.

Folkman, J., Merier, E., Abernathy, C. and Williams, G. (1971): Isolation of a tumor factor responsible for angiogenesis. J. Exp. Med. 133: 275–288.

Folkman, J. and Cotran, R. (1976): Relation of vascular proliferation to tumor growth. Int. Rev. Exp. Pathol. 16: 207–245.

Folkman, J. and Tyler, K. (1977): Tumor angiogenesis: Its role in metastasis and invasion. In Day, S.B., Myers, W.P.L., Stansly, P., Garattini, S. and Lewis, M.G. (eds.): Cancer Invasion and Metastasis: Biologic Mechanisms and Therapy (Progress in Cancer Research and Therapy, Vol. 5). Raven Press, New York, pp. 95–103.

Fornasier, V.L. and Horne, J.G. (1975): Metastases to the vertebral column. Cancer 36: 590–594.

France, L.H. (1975): Contribution to the study of 150 cases of cerebral metastases: II. Neuropathological study. J. Neurosurg. Sci. 19: 189–210.

Freeman, A.I., Wang, J.J. and Sinks, L.F. (1979): The treatment of primary childhood acute lymphocytic leukaemia (ALL) with intermediate dose methotrexate (IDM). In Whitehouse, J.M.A. and Kay, H.E.M. (eds.): CNS Complications of Malignant Disease. MacMillan Press, Ltd., London, pp. 59–68.

French, J.D., West, P.M., von Amerongen, F.K. and Magoun, H.W. (1952): Effects of intracarotid administration of nitrogen mustard on normal brain and brain tumors. J. Neurosurg. 9: 378–389.

French, L.A. (1948): Brain tumors in children. Minn. Med. 31: 867–874.

Fried, B.M. (1927): Primary carcinoma of the lungs. Further study, with particular attention to incidence, diagoosis and metasteses to the central nervous system. Arch. Intern. Med. 40: 340–363.

Fried, B.M. (1930): Primary carcinoma of the lung. Bronchiogenic cancer—a clinical and pathological study. Medicine (Baltimore) 10: 375–508.

Fried, B.M. and Buckley R.C. (1930): Primary carcinoma of the lungs. IV. Intracranial metastases. Arch. Pathol. 9: 483–527.

Friedell, G.H. and Parsons, L. (1961): The spread of cancer of the uterine cervix as seen in giant histological sections. Cancer 14: 42–54.

Friedman, H.H. (1943): So-called "benign metastasizing goiter"; Report of two cases with intracranial metastasis. Arch. Surg. 46: 377–385.

Fu, Y.S., Kaye, G.I. and Lattes, R. (1975): Primary malignant melanocytic tumors of the sympathetic ganglia with an ultrastructural study of one. Cancer 36: 2029–2041.

Fujita, H., Ogawa, K., Akimoto, H., Taira, K., Fukunaga, Y., Takakura, K., Kohno, T. and Kimura, K. (1976): Distribution of FT-207 and its active substances into the brain and cerebrospinal fluid. Cancer and Chemotherapy (Tokyo) 3: 551–555. (in Japanese with English abstract)

Fusek, I. and Kunc, Z. (eds.) (1972): Present Limits of Neurosurgery. Avicenum Czechoslovak Medical Press, Prague.

Galicich, J.H. and French, L.A. (1961): Use of dexamethasone in the treatment of cerebral edema resulting from brain tumors and brain surgery. Am. Practit. 12: 169–174.

Galicich, J.H., French, L.A. and Melby, J.C. (1961): Use of dexamethasone in treatment of cerebral edema associated with brain tumors. J. Lancet (Minneap.) 81: 46–53.

Gallavardin, L. and Varay, F. (1903): Etude sur le cancer secondaire du cerveau, du cervelet et de la moelle. Rev. Méd. (Paris) 23: 441–449.

Galluzzi, S. and Payne, P.M. (1955): Bronchial carcinoma: a statistical study of 741 necropsies with special reference to the distribution of blood-borne metastases. Br. J. Cancer 9: 511–527.

Galluzzi, S. and Payne, P.M. (1956): Brain metastases from primary bronchial carcinoma: A statistical study of 741 necropsies. Br. J. Cancer 10: 408–414.

Gamache, F.W., Jr., Galicich, J.H. and Posner, J.B. (1980): Treatment of brain metastases by surgical extirpation. In Weiss, L., Gilbert, H.A. and Posner, J.B. (eds.): Brain Metastasis, G.K. Hall & Co., Boston, Mass., pp. 390–414.

Gamble, H.J. (1976): Spinal and cranial nerve roots. In Landon, D.N. (ed.): The Peripheral Nerve. Chapman and Hall, London, pp. 330–354.

Garde, A., Tommasi, M. and Aimard, G. (1958): Les complications neurologiques des néoplasmes viscéraux. C.R. du Congrès de Psych. et de Neurol. de langue française. 56e session, Strasbourg. Masson & Cie, Paris, pp. 255–392.

Garfield, J. and Anthony, D. (1973): Postoperative intracavitary chemotherapy of malignant gliomas. A preliminary study using methotrexate. J. Neurosurg. 39: 315–322.

Garin, C., Plauchu, M. and Masson, P. (1932): Naevo-carcinome de la joue avec métastases cérébrales se traduisant par un tableau d'hémorragie méningée à allure paroxystique. Lyon Méd. 149: 803.

Gastaut, H., Roger, A. and Chatrian, G.E. (1954a): Etude électro-encéphalique des sujets porteurs d'un poumon avec ou sans métastase. Rev. Neurol. (Paris) 90: 321–323.

Gastaut, H., Roger, A. and Chatrian, G.E. (1954b): Electroencephalographic findings in cases of lung cancer. Electroencephalogr. Clin. Neurophysiol. 6: 525.

Gate, J. and Boyer, C.E. (1932): Néoplasme cutané avec généralisation à caractères mélaniques. Lyon Méd. 149: 330.

Gates, G.F., Dore, E.K. and Taplin, G.V. (1971): Interval brain scanning with sodium pertechnetate Tc 99m for tumor detectability. JAMA 215: 85–88.

Gedge-Latham, (1869): Primary carcinoma of brain. Br. Med. J. 1: 284.

Geist, R.M. and Portmann, U.V. (1952): Primary malignant tumors of the nasopharynx. Am. J. Roentgenol. Radium Ther. Nucl. Med. 68: 262–271.

Gendelman, S., Rizzo, F. and Mones, R.J. (1969): Central nervous system complications of leukemic conversion of the lymphomas. Cancer 24: 676–682.

Gercovich, F.G., Luna, M.A. and Gottlieb, J.A. (1975): Increased incidence of cerebral metastases in sarcoma patients with prolonged survival from chemotherapy: Report of cases of leiomyosarcoma and chondrosarcoma. Cancer 36: 1843–1851.

German, W.J. (1938): Carcinomatous metastases to the brain. Ann. Surg. 108: 980–991.

Ghatak, N.R. (1975): Unusual infections of the nervous system in malignant lymphomas. Acta Neuropathol. (Berlin) [Suppl. 6]: 261–265.

Giannotta, S.L. and Kindt, G.W. (1978): Metastatic spinal cord tumors. Clin. Neurosurg. 25: 495–503.

Gilbert, H., Apuzzo, M., Marshall, L., Kagan, A.R., Wagner, J., Fuchs, K., Push, J., Rao, A., Nusshaum, H. and Chan, P. (1978): Neoplastic epidural spinal cord compression. A current perspective. JAMA 240: 2771–2773.

Gilbert, R.W., Kim, J. and Posner, J.B. (1978): Epidural spinal cord compression from metastatic tumors: Diagnosis and treatment. Ann. Neurol. 3: 40–51.

Glasgow, L.A., Crane, J.L., Jr., Kern, E.R. and Youngner, J.S. (1978): Antitumor activity of interferon against murine osteogenic sarcoma *in vitro* and *in vivo*. Cancer Treat. Rep. 62: 1881–1888.

Glass, J.P., Melamed, M., Chernik, N.L. and Posner, J.B. (1979): Malignant cells in cerebrospinal fluid (CSF): The meaning of a positive CSF cytology. Neurology (Minneap.) 29: 1369–1375.

Glenn, W.V., Jr., Johnston, R.J., Morton, P.E., et al. (1975a): Further investigation and initial clinical use of advanced CT display capability. Invest. Radiol. 10: 479–489.

Glenn, W.V., Jr., Johnston, R.J., Morton, P.E., et al. (1975b): Image generation and display techniques for CT scan data. Thin transverse and reconstructed coronal and sagittal planes. Invest. Radiol. 10: 403–416.

Globus, J.H. and Selinsky, H. (1927): Metastatic tumors of the brain. A clinical study of twelve cases with necropsy. Arch. Neurol. Psychiatry. 17: 481–513.

Globus, J.H. and Meltzer, T. (1942): Metastatic tumors of the brain. Arch. Neurol. Psychiatry. 48: 163–226.

Globus, J.H. (1944): Metastatic brain tumor with bronchogenic carcinoma as the primary source. J. Mount Sinai Hosp. 12: 533–564.

Gold, L.H.A. and Loken, M.K. (1969): Retrospective evaluation of isotope images of the brain in 852 patients. Radiology 92: 1473–1476.

Gold, P. and Freedman, S.O. (1965): Demonstration of tumor specific antigens in human colonic carcinomata by immunological tolerance and absorption techniques. J. Exp. Med. 121: 439–462.

Goldstein, A.L., Slater, F.D. and White, A. (1966): Preparation, assay and partial purification of a thymic lymphocytopoietic factor (thymosin). Proc. Natl. Acad. Sci. USA 56: 1010–1017.

Goldstein, A.L., Cohen, G.H., Rossio, J.L., Thurman, G.B., Brown, C.N. and Ulrich, J.T. (1976): Use of thymosin in the treatment of primary immunodeficiency diseases and cancer. Med. Clin. North Am. 60: 591–606.

Goldstein, A.L., Low, T.L.K., McAdoo, M., McClure, J., Thurman, G.B., Rossio, J., Lai, C.Y., Chang, D., Wang, S.S., Harvey, C., Ramel, A.H. and Meienhofer, J. (1977): Thymosin α_1 isolation and sequence analysis of an immunologically active thymic polypeptide. Proc. Natl. Acad. Sci. USA 74: 725–729.

Gonzalez-Vitale, J.C. and Garcia-Bunuel, R. (1976): Meningeal carcinomatosis. Cancer 37: 2906–2911.

Good, R.A., Dalmasso, A.P., Martinez, C., Archer, O.K., Pierce, J.C. and Papermaster, B.W. (1962): The role of the thymus in development of immunologic capacity in rabbits and mice. J. Exp. Med. 116: 773–784.

Goodrich, J.K. and Tutor, F.T. (1965): The isotope encephalogram in brain tumor diagnosis. J. Nucl. Med. 6: 541–548.

Gottlieb, J.A., Frei, E., III and Luce, J.K. (1972): An evaluation of the management of patients with cerebral metastases from malignant melanoma. Cancer 29: 701–705.

Gough, J. (1940): The structure of the blood vessels in cerebral tumours. J. Pathol. Bacteriol. 51: 23–28.

Grace, J.T., Parese, D.M., Metzgar, R.S., Sasabe, T. and Holdridge, B. (1961): Tumor autograft responses in patients with glioblastoma multiforme. J. Neurosurg. 18: 159–167.

Graham, E.A. (1950a): Primary carcinoma of the lung. Dis. Chest 18: 1–9.

Graham, E.A. (1950b): Considerations of bronchiogenic carcinoma. Ann. Surg. 132: 176–188.

Grain, G.O. and Karr, J.P. (1955): Diffuse leptomeningeal carcinomatosis; Clinical and pathologic characteristics. Neurology (Minneap.) 5: 706–722.

Grant, F.C. (1926): Concerning intracranial malignant metastases; their frequency and the value of surgery in their treatment. Ann. Surg. 84: 635–646.

Grant, F.C. and Sayers, M.P. (1951): Notes on a series of brain tumors. J. Neurosurg. 8: 510–514.

Green, J.D. (1951): The comparative anatomy of the hypophysis, with special reference to its blood supply and innervation. Am. J. Anat. 88: 225–311.

Green, J.D. and Forman, W.H. (1974): Response of thymoma to steroids. Chest 65: 114–116.

Green, R.A., Humphrey, E., Close, H. and Patno, M.E. (1969): Alkylating agents in bronchogenic carcinoma. Am. J. Med. 46: 516–525.

Greene, H.S.N. (1951): The transplantation of tumors to the brains of heterologous species. Cancer Res. 11: 529–534.

Greenspan, E. (1963): Response of advanced breast cancer to the combination of antimetabolite, methotrexate, and the alkylating agent thio-TEPA. J. Mount Sinai Hosp. 30: 246–267.

Greenspan, E. (1966): Combination cytotoxic chemotherapy in advanced disseminated breast cancer. J. Mount Sinai Hosp. 33: 1–27.

Griffin, J.W., Thompson, R.W., Mitchinson, M.J., de Kiewiet, J.C. and Welland, F.H. (1971): Lymphomatous leptomeningitis. Am. J. Med. 51: 200–208.

Gurcay, O., Wilson, C., Barker, M. and Eliason, J. (1971): Corticosteroid effect on transplantable rat glioma. Arch. Neurol. 24: 266–269.

Gurling, K.J., Scott, G.B.D. and Baron, D.N. (1957): Metastases in pituitary tissue removed at hypophysectomy in women with mammary carcinoma. Br. J. Cancer 11: 519–523.

Gutmann, C. (1904): Zur Kenntnis der metastatischen Geschwulste im Gehirn. Fortschr. Med. 22: 141–145.

Gutterman, J.U., Hersh, E.M., Rodriguez, V., McCredie, K.B., Mavligit, G., Reed, R., Burgess, M.A.,

Smith, J., Gehan, E., Bodey, G.P., Sr. and Freireich, E.J. (1974): Chemoimmunotherapy of adult acute leukemia. Lancet 2: 1405–1409.

Gutterman, J.U., Cardenas, J.O., Blumenschein, G.R., Hortobagyi, G., Burgess, M.A., Livingstone, R.B., Mavligit, G.M., Freireich, E.J., Gottlieb, J.A. and Hersh, E.M. (1976): Chemoimmunotherapy of disseminated breast cancer; prolongation of remission and survival. Br. Med. J. 2: 1222–1225.

Gurwitt, L.J., Long, J.M. and Clark, R.E. (1975): Cerebral metastatic choriocarcinoma: A postpartum cause of "stroke". Obstet. Gynecol. 45: 583–588.

Guyer, P.B. and Westbury, H. (1968): The myelographic appearance of spinal cord metastases. Br.J. Radiol. 41: 615–619.

Gyori, E. (1976): Metastatic carcinoma in meningioma. South. Med. J. 69: 514–517.

Haar, F. and Patterson, R.H., Jr. (1972): Surgery for metastatic intracranial neoplasm. Cancer 30: 1241–1245.

Hägerstrand, I. (1961): Vascular changes in cerebral metastases. Acta Pathol. Microbiol. 51: 63–71.

Hägerstrand, I. and Schonebeck, J. (1969): Metastases to the pituitary gland. Acta Pathol. Microbiol. Scand. 75: 64–70.

Hakansson, C.H. (1967): Effect of irradiation of brain tumours on ventricular fluid pressure. Acta Radiol. [Ther. Phys. Biol.] (Stockh.) 6: 22–32.

Hålpert, B., Fields, W.S. and DeBakey, M. (1954): Intracranial metastasis from carcinoma of the lung. Surgery 35: 346–349.

Hålpert, B., Erickson, E.E. and Fields, W.S. (1960): Intracranial involvement from carcinoma of the lung. Arch. Pathol. 69: 93–103.

Hammond, C.B., Hertz, R., Ross, G.T., Lipsett, M.B. and Odell, W.D. (1967): Primary chemotherapy for nonmetastatic gestational trophoblastic neoplasms. Am. J. Obstet. Gynecol. 98: 71–78.

Hammond, C.B., Borchert, L.G., Tyrey, L., Creasman, W.T. and Parker, R.T. (1973): Treatment of metastatic trophoblastic disease: good and poor prognosis. Am. J. Obstet. Gynecol. 115: 451–457.

Hansen, H.H., Selawry, O.S., Muggia, F.M. and Walker, M.D. (1971): Clinical studies with 1-(2-chloroethyl)-3-cyclohexyl-1-nitrosourea (NSC 79037). Cancer Res. 31: 223–227.

Hansen, H.H. (1972): Intensive combined chemotherapy and radiotherapy in patients with nonresectable bronchogenic carcinoma. Cancer 30: 315–324.

Hansen, H.H., Selawry, O.S., Simon, R., Carr, D.T., van Wyk, C.E., Tucker, R.D. and Sealy, R. (1976): Combination chemotherapy of advanced lung cancer: A randomized trial. Cancer 38: 2201–2207.

Hara, M., Hojo, S., Inoue, K. and Hirano, A. (1979): Metastatic brain tumor—Macroscopic examination with methylene blue stain. Neurological Medicine (Tokyo) 11: 93–94. (in Japanese.)

Hardisty, R.M. and Norman, P.M. (1967): Meningeal leukaemia. Arch. Dis. Child. 42: 441–447.

Hardy, J. (1971): Transsphenoidal hypophysectomy. J. Neurosurg. 34: 582–594.

Hare C.C. and Schwarz G.A. (1939): Intracerebral carcinomatous metastasis. Arch. Intern. Med. 64: 542–565.

Hare, H.E. and Crew, Q.E., Jr. (1963): Nasopharyngeal tumors: Three to five year survivals. Am. J. Roentgenol. Radium Ther. Nucl. Med. 89: 35–40.

Harper, P.V., Strandjord, N., Paloyan, E., Moseley, R.D., Warner, N.E. and Lathrop, K.A. (1964): Destruction of the hypophysis with a Sr 90-Y 90 needle. Ann. Surg. 160: 743–751.

Harper, P.V., Fink, R.A., Charleston, D.B., Beck, R.N., Lathrop, K.A. and Evans, J.P. (1966): Rapid brain scanning with technetium-99m. Acta Radiol. [Diagn.] (Stockh.) 5: 819–831.

Harris, J.E. and Sinkovics, J.G. (1976): The Immunology of Malignant Disease. The C.V. Mosby Co., Saint Louis, pp. 469–471.

Harwood, A.R. and Simpson, W.F. (1977): Radiation therapy of cerebral metastases. A randomized prospective clinical trial. Int. J. Radiat. Oncol. Biol. Phys. 2: 1091–1094.

Hassin, G.B. (1919): Histopathology of carcinoma of the cerebral meninges. Arch. Neurol. Psychiatry 1: 705–716.

Hassin, G.B. and Singer, H.D. (1922): Histopathology of cerebral carcinoma. Arch. Neurol. Psychiatry 8: 155–171.

Hatiboglu, I. and Owens, G. (1961): Results of intermittent, prolonged infusion of nitrogen mustard into the carotid artery in twelve patients with cerebral gliomas. Surg. Forum 12: 396–398.

Hawley, P.R., Westerholm, P. and Marson, B.C. (1970): Pathology and prognosis of carcinoma of the stomach. Br. J. Surg. 57: 877–880.

Hayward, R.D. (1976): Secondary malignant melanoma of the brain. Clin. Oncol. 2: 227–232.

Hazra, T., Mullins, G.M. and Lott, S. (1972): Management of cerebral metastasis from bronchogenic carcinoma. Johns Hopkins Med. J. 130: 377–383.

Heathfield, K.W.G. and Williams, J.R.B. (1956): Carcinomatosis of the meninges; Some clinical and pathological aspects. Br. Med. J. 1: 328–330.

Hendricks, G.L., Jr., Barnes, W.T. and Hood, H.L. (1972): Seven-year "cure" of lung cancer with metastasis to the brain. JAMA 220: 127 (Letters).

Hendrickson, F.R. (1975): Radiation therapy of metastatic tumors. Semin. Oncol. 2: 43–46.

Hendrickson, F.R. (1977): The optimum schedule for palliative radiotherapy of metastatic brian cancer. Int. J. Radiat. Oncol. Biol. Phys. 2: 165–168.

Henriques, C.Q. (1962): The veins of the vertebral column and their role in the spread of cancer. Arch. Roy. Coll. Surg. Engl. 31: 1–22.

Heppner, F. (1952): Die Erkennung und Behandlung von neoplastischen Hirnmetastasen. Zentralbl. Neurochir. 12: 129–145.

Hericourt, J. and Richet, C. (1895): Remarques á propos de la note de M. Boureau sur la sérotherapie des neoplasms. Compt. Rend. Acad. Sci. 21: 600–601.

Herlihy, W. (1947): Revision of the venous system: The role of the vertebral veins. Med. J. Aust. 1: 661–672.

Hertz, R., Lewis, J.L. and Lipsett, M.B. (1961): Five years' experience with chemotherapy of metastatic choriocarcinoma and related trophoblastic tumors in women. Am. J. Obstet. Gynecol. 82: 631–640.

Hindo, W.A., DeTrana, F.A., III, Lee, M.S. and Hendrickson, F.R. (1970): Large dose increment irradiation in treatment of cerebral metastases. Cancer 26: 138–141.

Hirano, A., Zimmerman, H.M. and Levine, S. (1967): Fine structure of cerebral fluid accumulation. A review of experimental edema in white matter. In Klatzo, I. and Seitelberger, F. (eds.): Brain Edema. Springer-Verlag, Wien, pp. 569–589.

Hirano, A. (1969): The fine structure of brain edema. In Bourne, G.H. (ed.): The Structure and Function Nervous Tissue, Vol. 2. Academic Press, New York, pp. 69–135.

Hirano, A. and Zimmerman, H.M. (1972): Fenestrated blood vessels in a metastatic renal carcinoma in the brain. Lab. Invest. 26: 465–468.

Hirano, A., Ghatak, N.R., Becker, N.H. and Zimmerman, H.M. (1964): A comparison of the fine structure of small blood vessels in intracranial and retroperitoneal malignant lymphomas. Acta Neuropathol. (Berl.) 27: 93–104.

Hirano, A. and Matsui, T. (1975): Vascular structures in brain tumors. Hum. Pathol. 6: 611–621.

Hirano, A. (1976a): Further observations of the fine structure of pathological reaction in cerebral blood vessels. In Cervós-Navarro, J., Betz, E., Matakas, F. and Wüllenweber, R. (eds.): The Cerebral Vessel Wall. Raven Press, New York, pp. 41–49.

Hirano, A. (1976b): An Outline of Neuropathology. Igaku-Shoin, Tokyo. (in Japanese)

Hirano, A. and Matsui, T. (1978): Brain edema. Neurol. Surg. (Tokyo) 6: 211–219. (in Japanese)

Hirshaut, T., Kesselheim, H., Pinsky, C.M., Braun, D., Jr., Wanebo, H.J. and Oettgen, H.F. (1978): Levamisole as an immunoadjuvant: Phase I study and application in breast cancer. Cancer Treat. Rep. 62: 1693–1701.

Hockley, A.D. (1975): Metastatic carcinoma in a spinal meningioma. J. Neurol. Neurosurg. Psychiatry 38: 695–697.

Hojo, S., Llena, J., Hirano, A. and Zimmerman, H.M. (1978): Metastatic tumors in the central nervous system. Presented at VIIIth International Congress of the International Society of Neuropathology.

Holcomb, T., Haggard, M. and Windmiller, J. (1964): Cyclophosphamide (MSC 26271) in uncommon malignant neoplasms in children. Cancer Chemother. Rep. 36: 73.

Holland, J.M. (1973): Cancer of the kidney—Natural history and staging. Cancer 32: 1030–1042.

Holland, J.F. and Frei, E. (eds.): Cancer Medicine. Lea and Febiger, Philadelphia.

Hollander, V.P., Takakura, K. and Yamada, H. (1968): Endocrine factors in the pathogenesis of plasma cell tumors. Recent Prog. Horm. Res. 24: 81–137.

Holmes, G.W. and Schulz, M.D. (1950): Therapeutic Radiology. Lea & Febiger, Philadelphia.

Holness, R.O. and Sangalang, V.E. (1976): Myelomatous metastasis to the pineal body. Surg. Neurol. 5: 97–100.

Holzer, H. (1925): Zur Frage der Fäufigkeit des Bronchialkrebses. Med. Klin. 21: 1235–1237.

Hortobagyi, G.N., Gutterman, J.U., Richman, S.P., Snyder, R.D. and Hersh, E.M. (1978a): Pseudomonas vaccine; a phase I evaluation for cancer immunotherapy. Cancer Immunol. Immunother. 4: 201–207.

Hortobagyi, G.N., Yap, H.Y., Blumenschein, G.R., Gutterman, J.U., Buzdar, A.U., Tashima, C.K. and Hersh, E.M. (1978b): Response of disseminated breast cancer to combined modality treatment with chemotherapy and levamisole with or without bacillus Calmette-Guérin. Cancer Treat. Rep. 62: 1685–1692.

Horton, J., Baxter, D.H., Olson, K.B. and The Eastern Cooperative Oncology Group (1971): The management of metastases to the brain by irradiation and corticosteroids. Am. J. Roentgenol. Radium Ther. Nucl. Med. 111: 334–336.

Hoshino, T. (1968): The treatment of malignant brain tumors by BAR therapy. Brain and Nerve (Tokyo) 20: 601–611. (in Japanese with English abstract)

Hoshino, T. and Sano, K. (1969): Radiosensitization of malignant brain tumours with bromouridine (thymidine analogue). Acta Radiol. [Ther.] (Stockh.) 8: 15–26.

Hoshino, T., Barker, M. and Wilson, C.B. (1972): Cell kinetics of human gliomas. J. Neurosurg. 37: 15–26.

Hoshino, T., Wilson, C.B., Rosenblum, M.L. and Barker, M. (1975): Growth fraction and cell cycle time in glioblastoma. J. Neurosurg. 43: 127–135.

Hou, P.C. and Pang, S.C. (1956): Chorionepithelioma: An analytical study of 28 necropsied cases, with special reference to the possibility of spontaneous regression. J. Pathol. Bacteriol. 72: 95–104.

Houck, W.A., Olson, K.B. and Horton, J. (1970): Clinical features of tumor metastasis to the pituitary. Cancer 26: 656–659.

Huggins, C.B. and Hodges, C.V. (1941): Studies on prostatic cancer: I. The effect of castration, of estrogen and androgen injection on serum phosphatases in metastatic carcinoma of the prostate. Cancer Res. 1: 293–297.

Huggins, C.B. (1965): Propositions in hormonal treatment of advanced cancer. JAMA 192: 1141–1145.

Huguenin, R. (1935): Les syndromes metastatiques aigus. Cancer (Bruxelles) 12: 213–226.

Hughes, J.T. (1978): Pathology of the Spinal Cord, 2nd ed. W.B. Saunders Co., Philadelphia, pp. 230–238.

Hughes, N.R. (1971): Serum concentrations of IgG, A and M immunoglobulins in patients with carcinoma, melanoma, and sarcoma. J. Natl. Cancer Inst. 46: 1015–1027.

Hunt, T.R., Jr., Poser, C.M. and Williamson, W.P. (1960): Lymphoma of spinal nerve root. J. Neurosurg. 17: 342–346.

Hunter, K.M.F. and Rewcastle, N.B. (1968): Metastatic neoplasms of the brain stem. Can. Med. Assoc. J. 98: 1–7.

Hyde, L., Yee, J., Wilson, R. and Patno, M.E. (1965): Cell type and the natural history of lung cancer. JAMA 193: 52–54.

Hyman, C.B., Bogle, J.M., Brubakers, C., Sonley, M., Williams, K. and Hammond, D. (1962): Recongnition of CNS involvement in acute leukemia in children and response to therapy. Proc. Am. Assoc. Cancer Res. 3: 330.

Inoue, K. (1978): Personal communication.

Irvine, R.A. and Robertson, W.B. (1964): Spinal cord compression in the malignant lymphomas. Br. Med. J. 1: 1354–1356.

Ise, T. (1977): Personal communications.

Ishii, M. (1977): Studies on new fetal protein, basic protein in malignant tumors. Igaku no Ayumi (Tokyo) 100: 344–346. (in Japanese)

Jacobsen, H.H. and Lester, J. (1970): A myelographic manifestation of diffuse spinal leptomeningeal melanomatosis. Neuroradiology 1: 30–31.

Jameson, R.M. (1974): Prolonged survival in paraplegia due to metastatic spinal tumours. Lancet 1: 1209–1211.

Janota, I. (1966): Involvement of the nervous system in malignant lymphoma in Nigeria. Br. J. Cancer 20: 47–61.

Jasmin, C., Mathé, G., Gouveia, J., Larnicol, N., de Vassal, F. and Misset, J.L. (1979): A study of the prognostic factors of central nervous system leukaemia in acute lymphoid leukaemia patients. In Whitehouse, J.M.A. and Kay, H.E.M. (eds.): CNS Complications of Malignant Disease. MacMillan Press, Ltd., London, pp. 80–90.

Jellinger, K. and Radaszkiewicz, Th. (1976): Involvement of the central nervous system in malignant lymphomas. Virchows Arch. (Pathol. Anat.) 370: 345–362.

Jelsma, R. and Bucy, P.C. (1967): The treatment of glioblastoma multiforme of the brain. J. Neurosurg. 27: 388–400.

Jinnai, D. Mogami, H., Higashi, H., Hayakawa, T., Kuroda, R., Kanai, N. and Yamada, R. (1967): Chemotherapy of brain tumor. Studies on selection of cytostatic agents for intrathecal administration and distributions of cytostatic agents by intravenous, intracarotid and intrathecal administrations. Brain and Nerve (Tokyo) 19: 333–337. (in Japanese with English abstract)

Jones, G.M. (1944): Diabetes insipidus. Arch. Intern. Med. 74: 81–93.

Jones, R. (1959): Mitomycin C. A preliminary report of studies of human pharmacology and initial therapeutic trial. Cancer Chemother. Rep. 2: 3–7.

Jones, S.E., Durie, B.G. and Salmon, S.E. (1975): Combination chemotherapy with Adriamycin and cyclophosphamide for advanced breast cancer. Cancer 36: 90–97.

Joseph, M.C. and Levin, S.E. (1956): Leukaemia and diabetes insipidus: Case report, with unexpected effect of cortisone. Br. Med. J. 1: 1328–1331.

Kaplan, H.S., Smith, K.C. and Tomlin, P.A. (1962): Effect of halogenated pyrimidines on radiosensitivity of E. coli. Radiat. Res. 16: 98–113.

Kaufman, E. (1906): Beitrag zur Statiskik und Casuistik metastatischer Tumoren, besonders der Carcinommetastasen im Zentralnervensystem. Cor. -Bl. f. Schweiz. Aerzte 36: 255–261.

Kaung, D.T., Wolf, J., Hyde, L. and Zelen, M. (1974): Preliminary report on the treatment of nonresectable cancer of the lung. Cancer Chemother. Rep. 58: 359–364.

Kazua, O., Kurita, S. and Nishimura, M. (1972): Combination therapy with Mitomycin C, 5-fluorouracil and cytosine arabinoside for advanced cancer in man. Cancer Chemother. Rep. 56: 373–385.

Kennady, J.C. and Stern, W.E. (1962): Metastatic neoplasms of the vertebral column producing compression of the spinal cord. Am. J. Surg. 104: 155–168.

Kennedy, B.J. (1974): Hormonal therapies in breast cancer. Semin. Oncol. 1: 119–130.

Khan, F.R., Glicksman, A.S., Chu, C.H. and Nickson, J.J. (1967): Treatment by radiotherapy of spinal cord compression due to extradural metastases. Radiology 89: 495–500.

Kiefer, E.T. (1947): Metastatic brain tumors. (Thesis), University of Minnesota.

Kimura, I. (1978): Studies on cancer immunotherapy with streptococcal agent, OK-432. Jap. J. Cancer Clin. (Tokyo) 24: 428–433. (in Japanese)

Kincaid, O.W., Hodgson, J.R. and Dockerty, M.B. (1957): Neuroblastoma: A roentgenologic and pathologic study. Am. J. Roentgenol. Radium Ther. Nucl. Med. 78: 420–436.

Kindt, G.W. (1964): The pattern of location of cerebral metastatic tumors. J. Neurosurg. 21: 54–57.

King, A.B. and Ford, F.R. (1942): A clinical and anatomical study of neurological conditions resulting from
metastases in the central nervous system due to carcinoma of the lung. Johns Hopk. Hosp. Bull.
70: 124–156.

Kirsch, M.W. (1972): L'association du 5 Fluoro-uracil et de la warfarine sodique dans le traitment du cancer
cerébral. Méd. mondiale 101: 11.

Kirsch, M.W., Paoletti, E.G. and Paoletti, P. (eds.) (1972): The Experimental Biology of Brain Tumors.
C.C. Thomas, Springfield, Ill.

Kistler, M. and Pribram, H.W. (1975): Metastatic disease of the sella turcica. Am. J. Roentgenol. Radium
Ther. Nucl. Med. 123: 13–21.

Kjellberg, R.N., Nguyen, N.C. and Kliman, B. (1972): Le Bragg peak protonique en neurochirurgie stéréo-
taxique. Neurochirurgie (Paris) 18: 235–264.

Klass, D.W. and Bickford, R.G. (1958): The electroencephalogram in metastatic tumors of the brain.
Neurology (Minneap.) 8: 333–337.

Klass, D.W. and Daly, D.D. (1960): Electroencephalography in patients with brain tumor. Med. Clin.
North Am. 44: 1041–1051.

Klatzo, I., Miguel, J. and Otenasek, R. (1962): The application of fluorescein labeled serum proteins (FLSP)
to the study of vascular permeability in the brain. Acta Neuropathol. (Berl.) 2: 144–160.

Klatzo, I. and Seitelberger, F. (eds.) (1967): Brain Edema. Springer-Verlag, Wien.

Klopp, C.T., Alford, T.C., Bateman, J., Berry, G.N. and Winship, T. (1950): Fractionated intra-arterial
cancer chemotherapy with methyl-bis-amine hydrochloride: preliminary report. Ann. Surg. 132:
811–832.

Knierim, G. (1908): Über diffuse Meningealkarcinose mit Amaurose und Taubheit bei Magenkrebs. Beitr.
Pathol. Anat. 44: 409–429.

Knights, E.M., Jr. (1954a): Metastatic tumors of the brain and their relation to primary and secondary
pulmonary cancer. Cancer 7: 259–265.

Knights, E.M., Jr. (1954b): The increasing importance of lung cancer as related to metastatic brain tumors.
J. Neurosurg. 11: 306–309.

Kofman, S., Garvin, J.S., Nagamachi, D. and Taylor, S.G. (1957): Treatment of cerebral metastases from
breast carcinoma with prednisolone. JAMA. 163: 1473–1476.

Kofman, S. and Einsenstein, R. (1963): Mithramycin in the treatment of disseminated cancer. Cancer
Chemother Rep. 32: 77–96.

Kohno, T., Shitara, N., Takakura, K., Miki, Y. and Sano, K. (1976a): Statistical Analysis of long term
survival rate of brain tumors treated by chemotherapy. Neurol. Med. Chir. (Tokyo) Suppl. 16:
68–69. (in Japanese)

Kohno, T., Matsutani, M., Hoshino, T., Sano, K., Shitara, N. and Takakura, K. (1976b): Scheduled
combination chemotherapy of Adriamycin and BCNU to malignant brain tumors. Neurol. Med.
Chir. (Tokyo) 16: 545–553.

Kohno, T., Shitara, N., Takakura, K. and Fujita, H. (1976c): Role of FT-207 in the treatment of metastatic
brain tumors. Cancer and Chemotherapy (Tokyo) 3: 729–734. (in Japanese with English abstract)

Koletsky, S. (1938): Primary carcinoma of the lung. A clinical and pathologic study of 100 cases. Arch.
Intern. Med. 62: 636–651.

Korenman, G. and Mones, R.J. (1970): Carcinomatous involvement of the superior sagittal sinus. Trans.
Am. Neurol. Assoc. 95: 271–272.

Koshimura, S., Suzuki, R., Masuzaki, T., Ohta, T. and Kishi, G. (1958): On the formation of streptolysin S
by hemolytic streptococci acting on tumor cells. Jap. J. Microbiol. 2: 23–28.

Koss, L.G. (1979): Cerebrospinal fluid, miscellaneous fluids, the eye, and the skin. In: Diagnostic Cytology,
and Its Histopathological Bases, 3rd ed. J.B. Lippincott Co., Philadelphia, pp. 971–988.

Kosugi, Y., Ikebe, J., Sekine, M., Musha, T., Shitara, N., Kohno, T. and Takakura, K. (1978): Computer
aided analysis of cell-cycle phase from cytophotometric histogram. IEE Transactions on biomedical
engineering. Biomed. Eng. 25: 429–434.

Kotsilimbas, D.G., Karpf, R., Meredith, S. and Scheinberg, L.C. (1966): Evaluation of parenteral 5-FU
on experimental brain tumors. Neurology (Minneap.) 16: 916–918.

Kotsilimbas, D.G., Meyer, L., Berson, M., Taylor, J.M. and Scheinberg, L.C. (1967): Corticosteroid effect
on intracerebral melanomata and associated cerebral edema: Some unexpected findings. Neurology
(Minneap.) 17: 223–274.

Kovach, J.S., Moertel, C.G., Schutt, A.J., Hahn, R.G. and Reitemeier R.J. (1974): A controlled study of
combined 1, 3-bis-(2-chloroethyl)-1-nitrosourea and 5-fluorouracil therapy for advanced gastric and
pancreatic cancer. Cancer 33: 563–567.

Kovacs, A. (1973): Metastatic cancer of the pituitary gland. Oncology 27: 533–542.

Koyama, Y. and Takakura, K. (1969): Intracranial invasion of malignant neoplasms—Studies on autopsy
cases. Adv. Neurol. Sciences (Tokyo) 13: 188–197. (in Japanese with English abstract)

Krasting, K. (1906): Beitrag zur Statistik und Kasuistik metastatischer Tumoren, besonders der Carcinommetastasen im Zentralnervensystem. (Auf Grund von 12,730 Sektionen der pathologisch-anatomischen

Anstalt, Basel). Z. Krebsforsch. 4: 315–379.

Krause (1903): Diskussion, Demonstration einiger interessanter Krebsfälle. Dtsch. Med. Wochenschr. [Vereins-Beilage] No. 46: 361.

Krause, F. (1908): Chirurgie des Gehirns. Urban & Schwarzenberg, München.

Kriss, J.P. and Revesz, L. (1962): The distribution and fate of bromodeoxyuridine and bromodeoxycytidine in the mouse and rat. Cancer Res. 22: 254–265.

Kriss, J.P., Maruyama Y., Tung, L.A., Bond, S.B. and Révésez, L. (1963): The fate of 5-bromodeoxyuridine, 5-bromodeoxycytidine and 5-iododeoxycytidine in man. Cancer Res. 23: 260–268.

Kuhn, C. (1972): Fine structure of bronchiolo-alveolar cell carcinoma. Cancer 30: 1107–1118.

Kumanishi, T., Koga, M., Ogawa, H., Nakamura, N., Ikuta, F., Oyake, Y. and Ueki, K. (1975): Malignant lymphoma in the central nervous system. Brain and Nerve 27: 21–34. (in Japanese with English abstract)

Kumar, A.R.V., Renaudin, J., Wilson, C.B., Boldrey, E.B., Enot, K.J. and Levin, V.A. (1974): Procarbazine hydrochloride in the treatment of brain tumors. Phase 2 study. J. Neurosurg. 40: 365–371.

La Ban, M.M. and Grant, A.E. (1971): Occult spinal metastases. Early electro-myographic manifestation. Arch. Phys. Med. Rehabil. 52: 223–226.

Labet R. (1965): Contribution à l'étude des métastases cérébrales. Statistique de 154 cas. (Thesis), Paris.

Landon, D.N. (ed.) (1976): The peripheral Nerve. Chapman & Hall, London.

Lang, E.F., Jr. and Slater, J. (1964): Metastatic brain tumors. Results of surgical and nonsurgical treatment. Surg. Clin. North Am. 44: 865–872.

Lang, E.F., Jr. (1967): Neurosurgical management of intracranial malignancy. Surg. Clin. North Am. 47: 737–742.

Larson, D.L., Rodin, A.E., Roberts, D.K., D'Steen, W.K., Rapperport, A.S. and Lewis, S.R. (1966): Perineural lymphatics: Myth or fact. Am. J. Surg. 112: 488–492.

Lascu, F., Minculescu, C. and Simionescu, M. (1959): La stase papillaire hémorragique. L'aspect ophtalmoscopique des métastases cérébrales. Arch. Ophtalmol. (Paris) 19: 165–169.

Law, I.P., Dick, F.R., Blom, J. and Bergevin, P.R. (1975): Involvement of the central nervous system in non-Hodgkin's lymphoma. Cancer 36: 225–231.

Lebert, H. (1852): Beitrage zur Kenntniss des Gallertkrebses. Virchows Arch. 4: 214–215.

Lee, B.C.P., Kazam, E. and Newman, A.D. (1978): Computed tomography of the spine and spinal cord. Radiology 128: 95–102.

Leech, R.W., Welch, F.T. and Ojemann, G.A. (1974): Subdural hematoma secondary to metastatic dural carinomatosis: Case report. J. Neurosurg. 41: 610–613.

Leeds, N.E., Rosenblatt, R. and Zimmerman, H.M. (1971): Focal angiographic changes of cerebral lymphoma with pathologic correlation: A report of two cases. Radiology 99: 595–599.

Leeds, N.E. and Rosenblatt, R. (1972): Arterial wall irregular arities in intracranial neoplasm. The shaggy vessel brought into focus. Radiology 103: 121–124.

Legha, S.S. and Carter, S.K. (1976): Antiestrogens in the treatment of breast cancer. Cancer Treat. Rev. 3: 205–216.

Leiden, E. von and Blumenthal. F. (1902): Attempts to immunize humans by inoculation of their own cancer. Dtsch Med. Wockenschr. 28: 637.

Leitholf, O. and Kuhlendahl, H. (1957): Metastatische Hirngeschwülste. Die Medizinische No. 52: 1929–1934.

Lemon, H.M. (1957): Cortisone-thyroid therapy of metastatic mammary cancer. Ann. Intern. Med. 46: 457–484.

Lenz, M. and Freid, J.R. (1931): Metastases to the skeleton, brain and spinal cord from cancer of the breast and the effect of radiotherapy. Ann. Surg. 93: 278–293.

Lesse, S. and Netsky, M.G. (1954): Metastasis of neoplasms to the central nervous system and meninges. Arch. Neurol. Psychiatry 72: 133–153.

Levine, A.S. and Levy, H.B. (1978): Phase I-II trials of Poly IC stabilized with poly-L-Lysine. Cancer Treat. Rep. 62: 1907–1913.

Levy, H.B., Law L.W. and Rabson, A.S. (1969): Inhibition of tumor growth by poly inosinic-polycytidylic acid. Proc. Natl. Acad. Sci. USA 62: 357–361.

Levy, N.L., Mahaley, M.S.,Jr. and Day, E.D. (1972): In vitro demonstration of cell-mediated immunity to human brain tumors. Cancer Res. 32: 477–482.

Levy, N.L. (1973): Use of an in vitro microcytotoxicity test to assess human tumor-specific cell-mediated immunity and its serum mediated abrogation. Natl. Cancer Inst. Monogr. 37: 85–92.

Lewis, I. and Johnson, I.M. (1968): Chorea: An unusual manifestation of cerebral metastases. Neurology (Minneap.) 18: 948–952.

Lewis, J.L. (1976): Current status of treatment of gestational trophoblastic disease. Cancer 38: 620–626.

Lilienfeld and Benda, C. (1901): Ueber einen Fall von multipler metastatischer Carcinose der Nerven und Hirnhäute. Berlin Klin. Wochenschrift 38: 729–730.

Lindgren, E. (1954): Röntgenologie einschliesslich Kontrastmethoden. In Krenken, W., Olivecrona, H. and Tönnis, W. (eds.): Handbuch der Neurochirurgie, Bd.2. Springer-Verlag, Berlin.

Line, D.H. and Deeley, T.J. (1971): The necropsy findings in carcinoma of the bronchus. Br. J. Dis. Chest 65: 238–242.

Lipin, T. and Davison, C. (1947): Metastasis of uterine carcinoma to the central nervous system. A clinicopathologic study. Arch. Neurol. Psychiatry 57: 186–198.

Lissauer, M. (1911): Zur Kenntnis der Meningitis Carcinomatosa. Dtsch. Med. Wochenschr. 17: 16.

Little, R.R., Dale, A.J.D. and Okazaki, H. (1974): Meningeal carcinomatosis; clinical manifestations. Arch. Neurol. 30: 138–143.

Liu, K., Mittelman, A., Sproul, E.E. and Elias, E.G. (1971): Renal toxicity in man treated with Mitomycin C. Cancer 28: 1314–1320.

Livingston, K.E., Horrax, G. and Sachs, E., Jr. (1948): Metastatic brain tumors. Surg. Clin. North Am. 28: 805–810.

Livingston, R.B. and Carter, S.K. (1970): Single Agent in Cancer Chemotherapy. IFI/Plenum Publ. Corp., New York.

Llena, J.F., Kawamoto, K., Hirano, A. and Feiring, E.H. (1978): Granulocytic sarcoma of the central nervous system: Initial presentation of leukemia. Acta Neuropathol. (Berl.) 42: 145–147.

Locksley, H.B., Sahs, A.L. and Sandler, R. (1966): Report on the cooperative study of intracranial aneurysms and subarachnoid hemorrhage. Section III, Subarachnoid hemorrhage unrelated to intracranial aneurysm and A-V malformation: A study of associated diseases and prognosis. J. Neurosurg. 24: 1034–1056.

Lokich, J.J. (1975): The management of cerebral metastasis. JAMA 234: 748–751.

Long, D.M., Hartmann, J.F. and French, L.A. (1966a): The response of experimental cerebral edema to glucosteroid administration. J. Neurosurg. 24: 843–854.

Long, D.M., Hartmann, J.F. and French, L.A. (1966b): The response of human cerebral edema to glucosteroid administration. Neurology (Minneap.) 16: 521–528.

Long, D.M., Hartmann, J.F. and French, L.A. (1967): The ultrastructural substrates of experimental cerebral edema. In Klatzo, I. and Seitelberger, F. (eds.): Brain Edema. Springer-Verlag, Wien, pp. 419–444.

Longeval, E., Hildebrand, J. and Vollont, G.H. (1975): Early diagnosis of metastases in the epidural space. Acta Neurochir. (Wien) 31: 177–184.

Low, F.N. (1976): The perineurium and connective tissue of peripheral nerve. In Landon, D.N. (ed.): The Peripheral Nerve. Chapman and Hall, London, pp. 159–187.

Lubarsch, O. (1888): Ueber den primären Krebs des Ileum nebst Bemerkungen über das gleichzeitige Vorkommen von Krebs und Tuberculose. Virchows Arch. (Pathol. Anat.) 111: 280–317.

Lynch, R.G., Medoff, G. and Valeriote, F. (1975): A murine model for central nervous system leukemia and its possible relevance to human leukemia. J. Natl. Cancer Inst. 55: 611–617.

MacGee, E.E. (1971): Surgical treatment of cerebral metastases from lung cancer. The effect on quality and duration of survival. J. Neurosurg. 35: 416–420.

MacGregor, A.B., Falk, R.E., Landi, S., Ambus, U. and Langer, B. (1975): Oral Bacille Calmette Guérin immunostimulation in malignant melanoma. Surg. Gynecol. Obstet. 141: 747–754.

Madonick, M.J. and Savitsky, N. (1951): Subarachnoid hemorrhage in melanoma of the brain. Arch. Neurol. Psychiatry 65: 628–636.

Madow, L. and Alpers, B.J. (1951): Encephalitic form of metastatic carcinoma. Arch. Neurol. Psychiatry 65: 161–173.

Magilligan, D.J., Jr., Rogers, J.S., Knighton, R.S. and Davila, J.C. (1976): Pulmonary neoplasm with solitary cerebral metastasis. Results of combined excision. J. Thorac Cardiovasc. Surg. 72: 690–696.

Mahaley, M.S., Jr. and Day, E.D. (1965): Immunological studies of human gliomas. J. Neurosurg. 23: 363–370.

Mahaley, M.S., Jr., Day, E.D., Anderson, N., Wilfon, R.F. and Brater, C. (1968): Zonal centrifugation of brain—adult, fetal, and malignant. Cancer Res. 28: 1783–1789.

Mahaley, M.S., Jr., Day, E.D. and Bigner, D. (1969): Problems inherent to the in vivo localization of anti-brain tumor antibodies. Ann. N.Y. Acad. Sci. 147: 451–460.

Mahaley, M.S., Jr. (1972): Immunologic aspects of the growth and development of human and experimental brain tumors. In Kirsch, W.M., Paoletti, E.G. and Paoletti, P. (eds.): The Experimental Biology of Brain Tumors. C.C. Thomas, Springfield, Ill., pp. 561–573.

Mahaley, M.S., Jr., Gentry, R.E. and Bigner, D.D. (1977): Immunobiology of primary intracranial tumors, Part 2: The evaluation of chemotherapy and immunotherapy protocols using the avian sarcoma virus glioma model. J. Neurosurg. 47: 35–43.

Manaka, S. and Sano, K. (1979): Stationary potential of the brain: Part I. Basic studies. Neurol. Med. Chir. (Tokyo) 19: 643–653.

Mandybur, T.I. (1977): Intracranial hemorrhage caused by metastatic tumors. Neurology (Minneap.) 27: 650–655.

Mansuy, L., Lapras, U., Thierry, A. and Dechaume, J.P. (1964): L'évolution des métastases cérébrales opérées (métastases présumées uniques). A propos d'une série de 87 observations. Neurochirurgie (Paris) 10: 57–67.

Marsa, G.W. and Johnson, R.F. (1971): Altered patterns of metastasis following treatment of Ewing's sarcoma with radiotherapy and adjuvant chemotherapy. Cancer 27: 1051–1054.

Marshall, G., Roessmann, U. and van den Noort, S. (1968): Invasive Hodgkin's disease of brain: Report of two new cases and review of American and European literature with clinical-pathologic correlations. Cancer 22: 621–630.

Marshall, G.D., Jr., Low, T.L.K., Thurman, G.B., Hu, S.K., Rossio, J.L., Trivers, G. and Goldstein, A.L. (1978): Overview of thymosin activity. Cancer Treat. Rep. 62: 1731–1737.

Mason, G.A. (1949): Cancer of the lung. Review of a thousand cases. Lancet 2: 587–591.

Mason, T.E., Demaree, R.S., Jr. and Margolis, C.I. (1973): Granulocytic sarcoma (chloroma), two years preceding myelogenous leukemia. Cancer 31: 423–432.

Masse, S.R., Wolk, R.W. and Conklin, R.H. (1973): Peripituitary gland involvement in aute leukemia in adults. Arch. Pathol. 96: 141–142.

Mastaglia, F.L. and Kakulas, B.A. (1970): Intramedullary spinal cord metastasis from mammary carcinoma. Paraplegia 8: 14–18.

Mathé, G., Amiel, J.L., Schwarzenberg, L., Schneider, M., Cattan, A., Schlumberger, J.R., Hayat, M. and de Vassal, F. (1969): Active immunotherapy for acute lumphoblastic leukemia. Lancet 1: 697–699.

Mathé, G. (1976): Cancer active immunotherapy; Immunoprophylaxis and immunorestorations. An Introduction. (Recent Result in Cancer Research, Vol. 55). Springer-Verlag, Berlin.

Matsutani, M., Takakura, K., Hashizume, K., Nagai, M. and Sano, K. (1972): BCNU (1, 3-Bis(2-chloro-ethyl)-1-nitrosourea; NSC-409962) in the treatment of malignant brain tumors. Brain and Nerve (Tokyo) 24: 757–762. (in Japanese with English abstract)

Matsutani, M., Kohno, T., Takakura, K. and Ise, Y. (1976): Secondary tumors of the skull, the meninges and the brain in children. Neurol. med chir. (Tokyo) 16: 145–153.

Mattsson, W., Arwidi, A., von Eyben, F. and Lindholm, C. (1977): Phase II study of combined vincristine, Adriamycin, cycloposphamide, and methotrexate with citrovorum factor rescue in metastatic breast cancer. Cancer Treat. Rep. 61: 1527–1531.

Mayer, R.J., Berkowitz, R.S. and Griffiths, C.T. (1978): Central nervous system involvement by ovarian carcinoma. A complication of prolonged survival with metastatic disease. Cancer 41: 776–783.

Maynard, C.D., Witcofski, R.L., Janeway, R. and Cowan, R.J. (1969): "Radioisotope arteriography" as an adjunct to the brain scan. Radiology 92: 908–912.

McAlhany, H.J. and Netsky, M.G. (1955): Compression of the spinal by extramedullary neoplasms. A clinical and pathologic study. J. Neuropathol. Exp. Neurol. 14: 276–287.

McCabe, J.S. and Low, F.N. (1969): The subarachnoid angle: An area of transition in peripheral nerve. Anat. Rec. 164: 15–34.

McCann, W.P., Weir, B.K.A. and Elvidge, A.R. (1968): Long-term survival after removal of metastatic malignant melanoma of the brain—Report of two cases. J. Neurosurg. 28: 483–487.

McCarthy, W.D. (1955): Palliation and remission of cancer with combined corticosteroid and nitrogen mustard therapy; report of 100 cases. N. Engl. J. Med. 252: 467–476.

McCaskey, G.W. (1902): The clinical association of cancer and tuberculosis, with report of a case. Am. J. Med. Sci. 124: 97–105.

McDonald, J.V. and Burton, R. (1966): Subdural effusion in Hodgkin's disease. Arch. Neurol. 15: 649–652.

McElwain, T.J., Clink, H.M., Janeson, B., Kay, H.E.M. and Powles, R.L. (1979): Central nervous system involvement in acute myelogenous leukaemia. In Whitehouse, J.M.A. and Kay, H.E.M. (eds.): CNS Complications of Malignant Disease. MacMillan Press, Ltd., London, pp. 91–96.

McFarland, H.R. and Truscott, B.L. (1961): A brain stem lesion of unusual etiology: A case report. Neurology (Minnep.) 11: 597–600.

McGuire, W.L. (1974): A new approach for selecting patients with metastatic breast cancer for hypophysectomy. Clin. Neurosurg. 21: 39–59.

McIntosh, S., Rothman, S., Rosenfield, N., Fisher, D., Ritchey, K. and Pearson, H. (1978): Systemic methotrexate and chronic neurotoxicity in childhood leukemia—a preliminary report. Proc. Am. Assoc. Cancer Res. 19: 362.

McKneally, M.F., Maver, C.M. and Kaccsel, H.W. (1978): Regional immunotherapy of lung cancer using post-operative intrapleural BCG. In Terry, W.D. and Windhorst, D. (eds.): Immunotherapy of Cancer; Present Status of Trials in Man (Progress in Cancer Research and Treatment, Vol. 6). Raven Press, New York, pp. 161–172.

McMillan J.A. (1962): Meningitis due to carcinomatosis. Case with free carcinoma cells in cerebrospinal fluid. Br. Med. J. 2: 1452–1453.

McNeel, D.P. and Leavens, M.E. (1968): Long-term survival with recurrent metastatic intracranial melanoma: Case report. J. Neurosurg. 29: 91–93.

Meagher, R. and Eisenhardt, L. (1931): Intracranial carcinomatous metastases. With note on relation of carcinoma and tubercle. Ann. Surg. 93: 132–140.

Mehta, Y. and Hendrickson, F.R. (1974): CNS involvement in Ewing's sarcoma. Cancer 33: 859–862.

Meissner, G.F. (1953): Carcinoma of the stomach with meningeal carcinosis: Report of four cases. Cancer 6: 313–318.

Merigan, T.C. and Finkelstein, M.S. (1968a): Induction of circulating interferon by synthetic anionic polymers of known composition. Nature 214: 416–417.

Merigan, T.C. and Finkelstein, M.S. (1968b): Interferon stimulating and in vivo antiviral effects of various synthetic anionic polymers. Virology 35: 363–374.

Meyer, P.C. and Reah, T.G. (1953): Secondary neoplasms of the central nervous system and meninges. Br. J. Cancer 7: 438–448.

Meyerson, S.B. and Reynolds, D.H. (1967): Solitary metastatic brain tumors: evaluation of surgical therapy and factors influencing prognosis. Med. Times 95: 49–57.

Mikhael, M.A. (1978): Radiation necrosis of the brain; correlation between computed tomography, pathology and dose distribution. J. Comput. Assist. Tomogr. 2: 71–80.

Miki, Y. (1978): Bromouridine-antimetabolite-continuous intra-arterial infusion-radiation therapy (BAR therapy) for malignant brain tumors. Adv. Neurol. Sciences (Tokyo) 22: 111–118. (in Japanese with English abstract)

Millburn, L., Hibbs, G.G. and Hendrickson, F.R. (1968): Treatment of spinal cord compression from metastatic carcinoma. Review of the literature and presentation of a new method. Cancer 21: 447–452.

Miller, A.B., Fox, W. and Toll, R. (1969): Five year follow-up of the Medical Research Council comparative trial to surgery and radiotherapy for the primary treatment of small-celled or oat celled carcinoma of the bronchus. Lancet 2: 501–505.

Miller, D. and Constance, J. (1952): Intraventricular rupture of a secondary carcinoma of the thyroid with probable seeding into the spinal meninges. Br. J. Surg. 40: 64–68.

Miller, J.F.A.P. (1961): Immunological function of the thymus. Lancet 2: 748.

Minckler, D.S., Meligro, C.H. and Norris, H.T. (1970): Carcinoma of the larynx. Case report with metastases of epidermoid and sarcomatous elements. Cancer 26: 195–200.

Minckler, J. (ed.) (1971): Pathology of the Nervous System. McGraw-Hill, New York.

Misset, J.C. (1973): Combinaisons chimiothérapiques basées sur la notion de recrutement cellulaire par synchronisation partielle. (Thèse), Paris-Sud.

Miyazawa, N., Yoneyama, T., Naruke, T., Suemasu, K., Ogata, T. and Tsuchiya, R. (1978): Protocol study of BCG immunotherapy as an adjuvant to surgery for the resectable lung cancer. J. of the study group on the immunotherapy using BCG 2: 44–50. (in Japanese)

Moberg, A. and Reis, G.V. (1961): Carcinosis meningum. Acta Med. Scand. 170: 747–755.

Modesti, L.M. and Feldman, R.A. (1975): Solitary cerebral metastasis from pulmonary cancer. Prolonged survival after surgery. JAMA 231: 1064.

Moersch, F.P., Love, J.G. and Kernohan, J.W. (1940): Melanoma of the central nervous system. Report of thirty-four cases, in which the diagnosis was verified by operation and necropsy. JAMA 115: 2148–2155.

Moertel, C.G. and Reitemeier, R.J. (1967): Chemotherapy of gastrointestinal cancer. Surg. Clin. North Am. 47: 929–953.

Moertel, C.G. (1973): Therapy of advanced gastrointestinal cancer with the nitrosoureas. Cancer Chemother. Rep. 4: 27–34.

Moertel, C.G. (1975): Clinical management of advanced gastrointestinal cancer. Cancer 36: 675–682.

Moertel, C.G., Mittelman, J.A., Bakemeier, R.F., Engstrom, P. and Hanley, J. (1976): Sequential and combination chemotherapy of advanced gastric cancer. Cancer 38: 678–682.

Mohr, S.J., Chirigos, M.A., Smith, G.T. and Furkman, F.S. (1976): Specific potentiation of L 1210 vaccine pyran copolymer. Cancer Res. 36: 2035–2039.

Mones, R.J. (1965): Increased intracranial pressure due to metastatic disease of venous sinuses: A report of six cases. Neurology (Minneap.) 15: 1000–1007.

Mones, R.J., Dozier, D. and Berrett, A. (1966): Analysis of medical treatment of malignant extradural spinal tumors. Cancer 19: 1842–1853.

Montana, G.S., Meacham, W.F. and Caldwell, W.L. (1972): Brain irradiation for metastatic disease of lung origin. Cancer 29: 1477–1480.

Moody, R.A., Olsen, J.O., Gottschalk, A. and Hoffer, P.B. (1972): Brain scans of the posterior fossa. J. Neurosurg. 36: 148–152.

Moolten, S.E. (1972): Syndrome of profound apathy (akinetic mutism) secondary to thalamic metastasis of unrecognized lung cancer. Mt. Sinai J. Med. N.Y. 39: 76–81.

Moore, E.W., Thomas, L.B., Shaw, R.K. and Freireich, E.J. (1960): The central nervous system in acute leukemia: A post-mortem study of 117 consecutive cases, with particular reference to hemorrhages, leukemic infiltrations, and the syndrome of meningeal leukemia. Arch. Intern. Med. 105: 451–468.

Moore, G.E. (1948): Use of radioactive di-iodo-fluorescein in the diagnosis and localization of brain tumors. Science 107: 569.

Moore, G.E., Perese, D.M. and Staubitz, W.J. (1965): Survival following removal of multiple brain and lung metastases from teratocarcinoma of testis. Surgery 39: 997–1002.

Morahan, P.S., Munson, J.A., Baird, L.G., Kaplan, A.M. and Regelson, W. (1974): Antitumor action of pyran copolymer and tilorone against Lewis lung carcinoma and B-16 melanoma. Cancer Res. 34: 506–511.

Morahan, P.S., Barnes, D.W. and Munson, A.E. (1978): Relationship of molecular weight to antiviral and antitumor activities and toxic effects of maleic anhydride-divinyl ether (MVE) polyanions. Cancer Treat. Rep. 62: 1797–1805.

Morariu, M.A. and Serban, M. (1974): Intramedullary cervical cord metastasis from a nasopharynx carcinoma. Eur. Neurol. 11: 317–322.

Moricca, G. (1974a): Chemical hypophysectomy for cancer pain. In Bonica, J.J. (ed.): International Symposium on Pain (Advances in Neurology, Vol. 4). Raven Press, New York, pp. 707–714.

Moricca, G. (1974b): Neuroadenolysis for the analgegic treatment of advanced cancer patients. In Procacci, P. and Pagni, C.A. (eds.): Recent Advances on Pain. C.C. Thomas, Springfield, Ill., pp. 313–328.

Morton, D.L., Eilber, F.R., Malmgren, R.A. and Wood, W.C. (1970): Immunological factors which influence response to immunotherapy in malignant melanoma. Surgery 68: 158–164.

Morton, D.L., Holmes, E.C., Eilber, F.R., Sparks, F.C. and Ramming, K.P. (1978): Adjuvant immunotherapy of malignant melanoma: Preliminary results of a randomized trial in patients with lymph nodes metastasis. In Terry, W.D. and Windhorst, D. (eds.): Immunotherapy of Cancer; Present Status of Trials. Raven Press, New York, pp. 57–64.

Mosberg, W.H., Jr. (1976): Twelve-year "cure" of lung cancer with metastasis to the brain. JAMA 235: 2745–2746.

Mountain, C.F., Carr, D.T. and Anderson, W.A.D. (1974): A system for the clinical staging of lung cancer. Am. J. Roentgenol. Radium Ther. Nucl. Med. 120: 130–138.

Muggia, F.M. (1971): Reticulum cell sarcoma of the spinal epidural space. Ann. Intern. Med. 75: 477–478.

Mullan, J. and Evans, J.P. (1957): Neoplastic disease of the spinal extradural space. A review of fifty cases. Arch. Surg. 74: 900–907.

Müller-Schoop, J.W. and Good, R.A. (1975): Functional studies of Peyer's patches: Evidence for their participation in intestinal immune response. J. Immunol. 114: 1757–1760.

Mullins, G., Flynn, J.P.G., El-Mahdi, A.M., McQueen, J.D. and Owens, A.H. (1971): Malignant lymphoma of the spinal epidural space. Ann. Intern. Med. 74: 416–423.

Murohashi, T., Miura, K., Takahashi, H. and Kinomoto, M. (1978): Anti-tuberculosis immunity of guinea pigs inoculated BCG orally. Kekkaku 53: 465–470. (in Japanese with English abstract)

Murphy, J.T., Gloor, P., Yamamoto, Y.L. and Feindel, W. (1969): A comparison of electroencephalography and brain scan in supratentorial tumor. N. Engl. J. Med. 276: 309–313.

Murray, G. (1958): Experiments in immunity in cancer. Can. Med. Assoc. J. 79: 249–259.

Nakagawa, H., Huang, Y.P., Malis, L.I. and Wolf, B.S. (1979): Computed tomography of intraspinal and paraspinal neoplasms. J. Comput. Assist. Tomogr. 1: 377–390.

Nakahara, T., Nonaka, N., Kinoshita, K. and Matsukado, Y. (1975): Subarachnoid hemorrhage and aneurysmal change of cerebral arteries due to metastases of chorioepithelioma. Neurol. Surg. (Tokyo) 3: 777–782. (in Japanese with English abstract)

Nersesyants, S.I. (1951): The problem of metastatic brain cancer and the routes for metastatic spread. Vop. Neirokhir. [Probl. Neurosurg.] (Mosk.) 3: 25–30. (in Russian)

Netsky, M.G. and Strobos, R.R.J. (1952): Neoplasms within the midbrain. Arch. Neurol. Psychiatry 68: 116–129.

Neustaedter, M. (1944): Incidence of metastases to the nervous system. Arch. Neurol. Psychiatry 51: 423–425.

New, P.F.J. and Scott, W.R. (1975): Computed Tomography of the Brain and Orbit (EMI Scanning). Williams & Wilkins Co., Baltimore, pp. 234–257.

Newman, S.J. and Hansen, H.H. (1974): Frequency, diagnosis, and treatment of brain metastases in 247 consecutive patients with bronchogenic carcinoma. Cancer 33: 492–496.

Newton, T.H. and Potts, D.G. (1974): Radiology of the Skull and Brain, Vol.2; Angiography. The C.V. Mosby Co., Saint Louis.

Newton, W.A.,Jr. and Sayers, M.P. (1965): Intrathecal methotrexate therapy of brain tumors of childhood. Proc. Am. Assoc. Cancer Res. 6: 48.

Nisce, L.Z., Hilaris, B.S. and Chu, F.C.H. (1971): A review of experience with irradiation of brain metastasis. Am. J. Roentgenol. Radium Ther. Nucl Med. 3: 329–333.

Nishioka, K. (1971): Complement and tumor immunology. Adv. Cancer Res. 14: 231–293.

Nonne, M. (1900): In der Discussion vom 9-Januar im ärztlichen Verein zu Hamburg. Neurol. Centralbl. 19: 187.

Nonne, M. (1902): Ueber diffuse Sarkomatose der Pia mater des ganzen Zentralnervensystems. Dtsche. Ztschr. f. Nervenk. 21: 396–420.

Nordlund, J., Wolff, S. and Levy, H.B. (1970): Inhibition of biological activity of polyinosinic-polycytidylic acid by human plasma. Proc. Soc. Exp. Biol. Med. 133: 439–444.

Nyström, S. (1960): Pathological changes in blood vessels of human glioblastoma multiforme. Comparative studies using plastic casting angiography, light microscopy and electron microscopy with reference to some other brain tumors. Acta Pathol. Microbiol. Scand. 49 [Suppl. 137]: 1–83.

Obiditsch-Mayer, I. and Breitfellner, G. (1968): Electron microscopy in cancer of the lung. Cancer 21: 945–951.

O'Brien, P.H., Carlson, R., Steubner, E.A., Jr. and Staley, C.T. (1971): Distant metastases in epidermoid cell carcinoma of the head and neck. Cancer 27: 304–307.

Obrist, W.D., Thompson, H.K., King, C.H. and Wang, H.S. (1967): Determination of regional cerebral blood flow by inhalation of 133-xenon. Circ. Res. 20: 124–135.

Obrist, W.D., Thompson, H.K., Wang, H.S. and Wilkinson, W.E. (1975): Regional cerebral blood flow estimated by 133-xenon inhalation. Stroke 6: 245–256.

Ochsner, A. and DeBakey, M. (1941): Carcinoma of the lung. Arch. Surg. 42: 209–258.

O'Connel, J.E.A. (1964): The place of surgey in intracranial metastatic malignant disease. Proc. R. Soc. Med. 57: 1159–1164.

Ogawa, M., Yamanouchi, H., Tohgi, H., Asanaga, M. and Kameyama, M. (1977): A case of Wallenberg syndrome caused by metastatic lung carcinoma in the medulla oblongata. Clin. Neurol. (Tokyo) 17: 25–29. (in Japanese with English abstract)

Ohta, K., Nishimura, M., Morita, K. and Karasawa, K. (1980): Combination modality treatment of lung cancer. Cancer and Chemotherapy (Tokyo) 7 [Suppl. 1]: 96–112. (in Japanese with English abstract)

Oi, S., Ciric, I. and Mayer, T.K. (1978): Metastatic breast carcinoma in the pituitary gland. Brain and Nerve (Tokyo) 30: 69–73. (in Japanese with English abstract)

Ojima, Y., Grimaidi, R.A. and Sullivan, R.D. (1966): Distribution, retention, and excretion of tritium-labelled methotrexate in the management of brain tumor. In 9th Int. Cancer Cong., Tokyo. (Abstr.) p. 561.

Okamoto, H., Shoin, S., Koshimura, S. and Shimizu, R. (1967): Studies on the anticancer and streptolysin S-forming abilities of hemolytic streptococci. Jap. J. Microbiol. 11: 323–336.

Okei, A. (1977): Solid tumor. In Saito, T., Niitani, H. and Kanagami, H. (eds.): Chemotherapeutic Agents for Cancer. Clinic Magazine Co., Tokyo, pp. 234–248. (in Japanese)

Old, J.L., Clarke, D.A. and Benacerraf, B. (1959): Effect of Bacillus calmette-guérin infection on transplanted tumors in the mouse. Nature 184: 291–292.

Old, L.J., Benacerraf, B., Clark, D.A., Carswell, E.A. and Stockert, E. (1961): The role of the reticulo-endothelial system in the host reaction to neoplasia. Cancer Res. 21: 1281–1300.

Oldberg, E. (1933): Surgical considerations of carcinomatous metastases to the brain. JAMA 101: 1458–1461.

Olivecrona, H. (1967): The metastatic tumors. In Olivecrona, H. and Tönnis, W. (eds.): Handbuch der Neurochirurgie, Bd. 4 Tl. 4. Springer-Verlag, Berlin, pp. 292–298.

Olkowski, Z.L., McLaren, J.R. and Mansour, K. (1976): Immunocompetence of patients with bronchogenic carcinoma. Ann. Thorac. Surg. 21: 546–551.

Olkowski, Z.L., McLaren, J.R. and Skeen, M.J. (1978): Effect of combined immunotherapy with levamisole and Bacillus calmette-guérin on limmunocompetence of patients with squamous cell carcinoma of the cervix, head and neck, and lung undergoing radiation therapy. Cancer Treat. Rep. 62: 1651–1661.

Olson, K.B. (1935): Primary carcinoma of the lung. A pathological study. Am. J. Pathol. 11: 449–468.

Olson, M.E., Chernik, N.L. and Posner, J.B. (1971): Leptomeningeal metastasis from systemic cancer: A report of 47 cases. Trans. Am. Neurol. Assoc. 96: 291–293.

Olson, M.E., Chernik, N.L. and Posner, J.B. (1974): Infiltration of the leptomeninges by systemic cancer. A clinical and pathologic study. Arch. Neurol. 30: 122–137.

Ommaya, A. (1977a): Combined chemotherapy and immunotherapy for malignant gliomas. Brain Tumor Immunotherapy Conference, Durham, North Carolina.

Ommaya, A. (1977b): Effect of thymosine on brain tumor therapy. Brain Tumor Immunotherapy Conference, Durham, North Carolina.

Ono, K. and Tada, K. (1975): Metal prosthesis of the cervical vertebra. J. Neurosurg. 42: 562–566.

Onofrio, B.M. and Svien, H.J. (1976): Solitary and multiple vertebral myelomas. In Vinken, P.J. and Bruyn, G.W. (eds.): Handbook of Clinical Neurology, Vol. 20. North-Holland Publishing Co., Amsterdam, pp. 9–18.

Onuigbo, W.I.B. (1958): The spread of lung cancer to the brain. Br. J. Tub. Dis. Chest 52: 141–148.

Onuigbo, W.I.B. (1962): Lung cancer, metastases, and growing old. J. Gerontol. 17: 163–166.

Oppenheim, H. (1888): Ueber Hirnsymptome bei Carcinomatose ohne nachweisbare Veränderungen im Gehirn. Charité-Ann. (Berlin) 13: 335–344.

Order, S.E., Hellman, S., Essen, C.F. and Kligerman, M.M. (1968): Improvement in quality of survival following whole-brain irradiation for brain metastasis. Radiology 91: 149–153.

Ortega, P., Malamud, N. and Shimkin, M.B. (1951): Metastasis to the pineal body. Arch. Pathol. 52: 518–528.

Osmond, J.D., Pendergrass, H.P. and Potsaid, M.S. (1975): Accuracy of 99m Tc-diphosphonate bone scan and roentogenograms in the detection of prostate, breast and lung carcinoma metastases. Am. J. Roentgenol. Radium Ther. Nucl. Med. 125: 972–977.

Osoba, D. and Miller, J.F.A.P. (1963): Evidence for a humoral thymus factor responsible for the maturation of immunological faculty. Nature 199: 653.

Ostertag, C., Mundinger, F., McDonnell, D. and Hoefer, T. (1974): Detection of 247 midline and posterior fossa tumors by combined scintigraphic and digital gammaencephalography. J. Neurosurg. 39: 224–229.

Ottolenghi, C.E. (1969): Aspiration biopsy of the spine. J. Bone Joint Surg. 51-A: 1531–1544.

Page, R.B. and Bergland, R.M. (1977): Pituitary vasculature. In Allen, M.B., Jr. and Mahesh, V.B. (eds.): The Pituitary. A Current Review. Academic Press, New York, pp. 9–17.

Paillas, J.E. (1933): Les tumeurs cérébrales métastatiques. (Thesis) Impr. St. Lazare, Marseille.

Paillas, J.E., Constans, J.P., Roujean, J., Pellet, W. and Alliez, B. (1974a): Les tumeurs métastatiques de l'encéphale. Traitement chirurgical. Neurochirurgie (Paris) 20 [Suppl. 2]: 182–205.

Paillas, J.E., Pellet, W. and Alliez, B. (1974b): Les tumeurs métastatique de l'encéphale. Généralités. Neurochirurgie (Paris) 20 [Suppl. 2]: 7–19.

Paillas, J.E. and Pellet, W. (1975): Brain metastases. In Vinken, P.J. and Bruyn, G.W. (eds.): Handbook of Clinical Neurology, Vol. 18. North-Holland Publishing Co., Amsterdam, pp. 201–232.

Paillas, J.E., Alliez, B. and Pellet, W. (1976): Primary and secondary tumours of the spine. In Vinken, P.J. and Bruyn, G.W. (eds.): Handbook of Clinical Neurology, Vol. 20. North-Holland Publishing Co., Amsterdam, pp. 19–54.

Palma, A. (1972): Tumores metastasicos del encefalo. Neurocirugia 30: 211–218.

Paoletti, P., Walker, M.D., Butti, G. and Knerich, R. (eds.) (1979): Multidisciplinary Aspects of Brain Tumor Therapy. Elsevier/North-Holland, Amsterdam.

Papo, I. and Tritapepe, R. (1957): Considerazioni su 162 metastasi endocraniche verificate. Minerva Chir. 12: 269–274.

Parker, H.L. (1927): Involvement of central nervous system secondary to primary carcinoma of lung. Arch. Neurol. Psychiatry 17: 198–213.

Parker, J.C., Jr., McCloskey, J.J. and Jones, A.G. (1978): Prostate cancer rarely metastasizes to brain, quoted in Medical News. JAMA 239: 95.

Parsons, M. (1972): The spinal form of carcinomatous meningitis. Q.J. Med. 41: 509–519.

Patt, Y.Z., Hersh, E.M., Dicke, K., Spitzer, G. and Mavligit, G.M. (1978): Suppressor cell activity in cancer patients: A possible role for thymic hormones. Cancer Treat. Rep. 62: 1763–1768.

Pavlidis, N.A., Schultz, R.M., Chirigos, M.A. and Luetzeler, J. (1978): Effect of maleic anhydride-divinyl ether copolymers on experimental M109 metastases and macrophage tumoricidal function. Cancer Treat Rep. 62: 1817–1822.

Paxton, R. and Ambrose, J. (1974): The EMI scanner: A brief review of the first 650 patients. Br. J. Radiol. 47: 530–565.

Pazmino, N.H., Ihle, J.N., McEwen, R.N. and Goldstein, A.L. (1978): Control of differentiation of thymocyte precursors in the bone marrow by thymic hormones. Cancer Treat. Rep. 62: 1749–1755.

Pearl, R. (1929): Cancer and Tuberculosis. Am. J. Hygiene 9: 97–159.

Pearl, R., Sutton, A.C. and Howard, W.T. (1929): Experimental treatment of cancer with tuberculin. Lancet 1: 1078–1080.

Pearson, O.H. and Ray, B.S. (1959): Results of hypophysectomy in the treatment of metastatic mammary carcinoma. Cancer 12: 85–92.

Pearson, O.H. and Ray, B.S. (1960): Hypophysectomy in the treatment of metastatic mammary cancer. Am. J. Surg. 99: 544.

Pennington, D.G. and Milton, G.W. (1975): Cerebral metastasis from melanoma. Aust. N.Z.J. Surg. 45: 405–409.

Penzholz, H. (1968): Die metastatischen Erkrankungen des Zentralnervensystems bei bösartigen Tumoren. Acta Neurochir. (Wien) [Suppl. 16]: 1–205.

Perese, D.M. (1956): Brain tumors; some comments and case reports. Bull. Roswell Park Mem. Inst. 1: 91–102.

Perese, D.M. (1958): Treatment of metastatic extradural spinal cord tumors: A series of 30 cases. Cancer 11: 214–221.

Perese, D.M. (1959): Prognosis in metastatic tumors of the brain and the skull: An analysis of 16 operative and 162 autopsied cases. Cancer 12: 609–613.

Perk, K., Pearson, J.W., Torgersen, J.A. and Chirigos, M.A. (1974): An animal model for meningeal leukemia. Int. J. Cancer 13: 863–866.

Petit-Dutaillis, D., Messimy, R. and Berdet, H. (1956): Considérations sur les métastases intracranienes, d'après 107 cas histologiquement vérifiés. Rev. Neurol (Paris) 95: 89–115.

Peylan-Ramu, N., Poplack, D.G., Blei, C.L., Herdt, J.R., Vermess, M. and Di Chiro, G. (1977): Computer assisted tomography in methotrexate encephalopathy. J. Comput. Assist. Tomogr. 1: 216–221.

Peylan-Ramu, N., Poplack, D.G., Pizzo, P.A., Adornato, T. and di Chiro, G. (1978): Abnormal CT scans of the brain in asymptomatic children with acute lymphocytic leukemia after prophylactic treatment of the central nervous system with radiation and intrathecal chemotherapy. N. Engl. J. Med. 293: 815–818.

Pinsky, C.M., DeJager, R.L., Wittes, R.E., Wong, P.P., Kaufman, R.J., Mike, V., Hansen, J.A., Oettgen, H.F. and Krakoff, I.H. (1978): Corynebacterium parvum as adjuvant to combination chemotherapy in patients with advanced breast cancer: Preliminary results of a prospective randomized trial. In Terry, W.D. and Windhorst, D. (eds.): Immunotherapy of Cancer; Present Status of Trials in Man (Progress in Cancer Research and Therapy, Vol. 6). Raven Press, New York, pp. 647–654.

Pistenma, D.A., McDongall, I.R. and Kriss, J.P. (1975): Screening for bone metastases, are only scans necessary? JAMA 231: 46–50.

Pitner, S.E. and Johnson, W.W. (1973): Chronic subdural hematoma in childhood acute leukemia. Cancer 32: 185–190.

Pochedly, C. (1977a): Neurological manifestations in acute leukemia. In Pochedly, C. (ed.): Leukemia and Lymphoma in the Nervous System. C.C. Thomas, Springfield, Ill., pp. 3–40.

Pochedly, C. (1977b): How does leukemia invade the CNS? In Pochedly, C. (ed.): Leukemia and Lymphoma in the Nervous System. C.C. Thomas, Springfield, Ill., pp. 54–67.

Pochedly, C. (1977c): Pathogenesis and pathology of leukemic lesions in the CNS. In Pochedly, C. (ed.): Leukemia and Lymphoma in the Nervous System. C.C. Thomas, Springfield, Ill., pp. 68–87.

Pole, J.G. (1973): Childhood leukemia presenting in the central nervous system. Arch. Dis. Child. 48: 867–871.

Ponari, O., Cattabiani, G., Mastandrea, R. et al. (1965): Les rapports entre le système nerveux et les phénomènes de coagulation et de fibrinolyse. Revue critique et contribution personnelle. Hemostase 5: 379–387.

Pool, J.L., Ransohoff, J. and Correll, J.W. (1957): Treatment of malignant brain tumors, primary and metastatic. N.Y. State J. Med. 57: 3983–3988.

Poppen, J.L. and Hurxthal, L.M. (1934): Normal cerebrospinal fluid dynamics in spinal cord tumor suspects. JAMA 103: 391–393.

Posner, J.B. (1971): Neurological complications of systemic cancer. Med. Clin. North Am. 55: 625–646.

Posner, J.B. (1974): Diagnosis and treatment of metastases to the brain. Clin. Bull. 4: 47–57.

Posner, J.B., Howieson, J. and Cvitkovic, E. (1977): "Disappearing" spinal cord compression: Oncolytic effect of glucocorticoids (and other chemotherapeutic agents) on epidural metastases. Ann. Neurol. 2: 409–413.

Posnikoff, J. and Stratford, J. (1960): Carcinoma and metastasis to malignant glioma: Case report. Arch. Neurol. 3: 559–563.

Potter, G.D. (1970): Sclerosis of the base of the skull as a manifestation of nasopharyngeal carcinoma. Radiology 94: 35–38.

Potts, D.G. and Svare, G.T. (1964): Calcification in intracranial metastases. Am. J. Roentgenol. Radium Ther. Nucl. Med. 92: 1249–1251.

Powles, R.L., Crowther, D., Bateman, C.J.T., Beard, M.E.J., McElwain, T.J., Russell, J., Lister, T.A., Whitehouse, J.M.A., Wrigley, P.F.M., Pike M., Alexander, P. and Hamilton Fairley, G. (1973): Immunotherapy for acute myelogenous leukaemia. Br. J. Cancer 28: 365–376.

Prentice, W.B., Kieffer, S.A., Gold, L.H.A. and Bjornson, R.G.B. (1973): Myelographic characteristics of metastasis to the spinal cord and cauda equina. Am. J. Roentgenol. Radium Ther. Nucl. Med. 118: 682–689.

Price, R.A. and Johnson, W.W. (1973): The central nervous system in childhood leukemia: I. The arachnoid. Cancer 31: 520–533.

Price, R.A. and Jamieson, P.A. (1975): The central nervous system in childhood leukemia. II. Subacute leukoencephalopathy. Cancer 35: 306–318.

Price, R.A. (1979): Histopathogenesis of meningeal leukaemia and complications of therapy. In Whitehouse, J.M.A. and Kay, H.E.M. (eds.): CNS Complications of Malignant Disease. MacMillan Press, Ltd., London, pp. 3–15.

Probert, J.C., Thompson, R.W. and Bagshaw, M.A. (1974): Patterns of spread of distant metastases in head and neck cancer. Cancer 33: 127–133.

Procacci, P. and Pagni, C.A. (eds.) (1974): Recent Advances on Pain. C.C. Thomas Pub., Springfied, Ill.

Puech, P., Naudascher, J., Perrin, J. and Mallet, J. (1947): Les métastases cérébrales et médullaires dans une série de 875 tumeurs cérébro-médullaires vérifiées. Monde méd. 12: 130–132.

Purckhauer, R. (1929): Das Prostatacarcinom, seine Haufigkeit und sein Metastasen (Mit Mitteilung eines Falles von Gigantischer osteoplastische Carcinose des ganzen Skelettes bei Prostatacarcinom). Zeitschr. Krebsforsch. 28: 68–95.

Putschar, W. (1930): Pathologie und Symptomatologie der Carcinommetastasen in Zentralnervensystem. Z. Gesamte Neurol. Psychiatr. 126: 129–148.

Quinn, III, J.L., Ciric, U. and Hanser, W.N. (1965): Analysis of 96 abnormal brain scans using technetium 99m (pertechnetate form). JAMA 194: 157–160.

Raichle, M.E. (1980): Positron-emission tomography. In Weiss, L., Gilbert, H.A. and Posner, J.B. (eds.): Brain Metastasis, G.K. Hall & Co., Boston, Mass., pp. 246–253.

Rand, R.W., Dashe, A.M., Paglia, D.E., Conway, L.W. and Solomon, D.H. (1964): Stereotactic cryohypophysectomy. JAMA 189: 255–259.

Ransohoff, J. (1980): Surgical therapy of brain metastases. In Weiss, L., Gilbert, H.A. and Posner, J.B. (eds.): Brain Metastasis, G.K. Hall & Co., Boston, Mass., pp. 380–389.

Rapp, H.J. (1973): Animal models of immunotherapy of cancer. Natl. Cancer Inst. Monogr. 39: 1–2.

Raskind, R., Weiss, S.R. and Wermuth, R.E. (1969): Single metastatic brain tumors.: treatment and follow-up in 41 cases. Ann. Surg. 35: 510–515.

Raskind, R., Weiss, S.R., Manning, J.J. and Wermuth, R.E. (1971): Survival after surgical excision of single metastatic brain tumors. Am. J. Roentgenol. Radium Ther. Nucl. Med. 111: 323–328.

Rasmussen, T.B., Kernohan, J.W. and Adson, A.W. (1940): Pathologic classification, with surgical consideration, of intraspinal tumors. Ann. Surg. 111: 513–530.

Rasmussen, T.B., Harper, P.V., Yuhl, E. and Bergenstal, D.M. (1955): The destruction of the pituitary gland in metastatic carcinoma with yttrium-90 pellets. Semiannual Report to the Atomic Energy

Commission, Argonne Cancer Research Hospital, University of Chicago 3: 1–17.

Rasmussen, T. and Gulati, D.R. (1962): Cortisone in the treatment of postoperative cerebral edema. J. Neurosurg. 19: 535–544.

Rau, W. (1921): Eine vergleichende Statistik der in 5 Kriegsjahren (1914–1919) und 5 Friedensjahren (1909–1914) sezierten Fälle von Krebs und anderen malignen Tumoren am Pathologischen Institut des Stadskrankenhauses, Dresden-Friedrichstadt. Ztschr. Krebsforsch. 18: 141–170.

Ray, B.S. and Pearson, O.H. (1965): Hypophysectomy in the treatment of advanced cancer of the breast. Ann. Surg. 144: 394.

Ray, B.S. (1960): The neurosurgeon's new interest—in the pituitary. J. Neurosurg. 17: 1–21.

Ray, B.S. and Pearson, O.H. (1962): Hypophysectomy in treatment of disseminated breast cancer. Surg. Clin. North Am. 42: 419.

Ray, B.S. (1967): Hypophysectomy as palliative treatment in endocrine therapy of breast cancer. JAMA 200: 974.

Redmond, D.E., Rinderknecht, R.H. and Hudgins, P.T. (1967): The effect of total-brain irradiation on cerebrospinal fluid pressure. Radiology 89: 727–732.

Rees, J.K.H. (1979): Early experience in the use of CNS prophylactic therapy in the management of patients with acute myeloid leukaemia. In Whitehouse, J.M.A. and Kay, H.E.M. (eds.): CNS Complications of Malignant Disease. MacMillan Press, Ltd., London, pp. 97–99.

Regelson, W. (1978): Future direction of synthetic polyanions (pyran copolymer). Cancer Treat. Rep. 62: 1853–1856.

Reingold, I.M., Ottoman, R.E. and Konwaler, B.E. (1950): Bronchogenic carcinoma. A study of 60 necropsies. Am. J. Clin. Pathol. 20: 515–525.

Renoux, G., Renoux, M. and Trefouel, M.J. (1971): Immunostimulant effect of an immido-thiazole in the immunisation of mice infected with Brucella abortus. C.R. Acad. Sci. (D) 272: 349–350.

Renoux, G. and Renoux M. (1972): Levamisole inhibits and cures a solid malignant tumor and its pulmonary metastases in mice. Nature (New Biol) 240: 217–218.

Renoux, G. and Renoux M. (1973): Stimulation of anti-*Brucella* vaccination in mice by tetramisole, a phenyl-imidothiazole salt. Infect. Immun. 8: 544–548.

Renoux, G., Renoux, M., Teller, M.N., McMahon, S. and Guillaumin, J.M. (1976): Potentiation of T-cell mediated immunity by levamisole. Clin. Exp. Immunol. 25: 288–296.

Reulen, H.J., Hadjidimos, A. and Hase, U. (1973): Steroids in the treatment of brain edema. In Schürmann, K., Brock, M., Reulen, H.J. and Voth, D. (eds.): Brain Edema; Cerebello Pontine Angle Tumors (Advances in Neurosurgery, Vol. 1). Springer-Verlag, Berlin, pp. 92–105.

Reyes, V. and Horrax, G. (1950): Metastatic melanoma of the brain. Report of a case with unusually long survival period following surgical removal. Ann. Surg. 131: 237–242.

Rhodin, A.E., Larson, D.L. and Roberts, D.K. (1967): Nature of the perineural space invaded by prostatic carcinoma. Cancer 20: 1772–1779.

Rhoton, A.L., Jr., Carlsson, A.M. and Ter-Pogossian, M.M. (1964): Brain scanning with chlormerodrin Hg and chlormerodrin Hg. Arch. Neurol. 10: 369–375.

Rhoton, A.L., Jr., Eichling, J. and Ter-Pogossian, M.M. (1966): Metastatic tumors: Localization by radio-isotope scanning. Neurology (Minneap.) 16: 264–268.

Rich, A.R. and McCordock, H.A. (1933): The pathogenesis of tuberculous meningitis. Bull. Johns Hopkins Hosp. 52: 5–38.

Rich, G.J. (1930): The distribution of metastatic tumors in the cerebrum. Arch. Neurol. Psychiatry 23: 742–749.

Richards, P. and McKissock, W. (1963): Intracranial metastases. Br. Med. J. 1: 15–18.

Richmond, J.J. (1949): Cerebral tumours. J. Fac. Radiologists 1: 23–27.

Ridley, A. and Cavanagh, J.B. (1971): Lymphocytic infiltration in gliomas: Evidence of possible host resistance. Brain 94: 117–124.

Rieselbach, R.E., Morse, E.E., Rall, D.P., Frei, E., III. and Freireich, F.J. (1962): Treatment of meningeal leukemia with intrathecal aminopterin. Cancer Chemother. Rep. 16: 191–196.

Roessmann, U., Kaufman, B. and Friede, R.L. (1970): Metastatic lesions in the sella turcica and pituitary gland. Cancer 25: 478–480.

Roger, H. and Paillas, J.E. (1934): Les tumeurs cérébrales métastatiques. La Presse Med. 42: 2093–2096.

Rogers, L. (1958): Malignant tumors and the epidural spaces. Br. J. Surg. 45: 416–422.

Rogers, L. and Heard, G. (1958): Intrathecal spinal metastases (rare tumours). Br. J. Surg. 45: 317–320.

Rojas, A.F., Mickiewicz, E., Feierstein, J.N., Glait, H.M. and Olivari, A.J. (1976): Levamisole in advanced human breast cancer. Lancet 1: 211–215.

Rojas, A.F., Feierstein, J.N., Glait, H.M., Varela, O.A., Pradier, R. and Olivari, A.J. (1977): Clinical action of levamisole and effects of radiotherapy on immune response. In Chirigos, M. (ed.): Control of Neoplasia by Modulation of the Immune System (Progress in Cancer Research and Therapy, Vol. 2). Raven Press, New York, pp. 159–174.

Rokitansky, C. (1855): A manual of pathological anatomy Vol. 1., London, Sydenham, pp. 313–314.

Rose, F.C., Meikle, R. and Lord, P. (1964): Endoxan (cyclosphosphamide) in the treatment of intracerebral malignancy. J. Neurol. Neurosurg. Pychiatry 27: 470–472.

Rosemberg, J. and Passos Filho, M.C. (1970): BCG vaccination by oral technic. Critical review on vaccination studies using oral BCG in the Division of Communicable Diseases of WHO Hospital (Rio de J.)
78: 89–162. (in Portuguese)

Rosenblum, M.L., Reynolds, A.F., Jr., Smith, K.A., Rumack, B.H. and Walker, M.D. (1973): Chloroethyl-
cyclohexyl-nitrosourea in the treatment of malignant brain tumors. J. Neurosurg. 39: 306–314.

Rosenzweig, A.I. and Kendell, J.W. (1968): Diabetes insipidus as a complication of acute leukemia. Arch.
Intern. Med. 117: 397–400.

Ross, J.A.T., Leavitt, S.R., Holst, E.A. and Clemente, C.D. (1954): Neurological and electroencephalographic effects of x-irradiation of the head in monkeys. Arch. Neurol. Psychiatry 71: 238–249.

Rossio, J.L. and Goldstein, A.L. (1977): Immunotherapy of cancer with thymosine. World J. Surg. 1: 605–
616.

Roswit, B., Patno, M.E., Rapp, R., Veinbergs, A., Feder, B., Stuhlbarg, J. and Reid, C.B. (1968): The
survival of patients with inoperable lung cancer: A large-scale randomized study of radiation therapy
versus placebo. Radiology 90: 688–697.

Rottenberg, D.A., Chernik, N.L., Deck, M.D.F., Ellis, F. and Posner, J.B. (1977): Cerebral necrosis following radiotherapy of extracranial neoplasms. Ann. Neurol. 1: 339–357.

Rowan, A.J., Rudolf, N. de M. and Scott, D.F. (1974): EEG prediction of brain metastases. A controlled
study with neuropathological confirmation. J. Neurol. Neurosurg. Psychiatry 37: 888–893.

Rowinska-Zakrewsk, A.E., Lazar, P. and Burtin, P. (1970): Serum immunoglobulin levels in malignancy.
Ann. Inst. Pasteur 119: 621–625.

Roy, S., III and Johnson, W.W. (1970): Diabetes insipidus in a child with erythromyelocytic leukemia.
Am. J. Dis. Child. 119: 82–85.

Rubin, P. (1969): Extradural spinal cord compression by tumor. Part 1: Experimental production and
treatment trials. Radiology 93: 1243–1248.

Rubin, P., Mayer, E. and Poulter, C. (1969): Extradural spinal cord compression by tumor. Part II: High
daily dose experience without laminectomy. Radiology 93: 1248–1260.

Rubin, R.C., Ommaya, A.K., Bering, E. and Rall, O.P. (1965): The treatment of central nervous system
neoplasia by cerebrospinal fluid space perfusion. Proc. Am. Assoc. Cancer Res. 6: 55.

Rubin, R.C., Ommaya, A.K., Henderson, E.S., Bering, E.A. and Rall, D.P. (1966): Cerebrospinal fluid perfusion for central nervous system neoplasms. Neurology (Minneap.) 16: 680–692.

Rubinstein, L.J. (1972): Tumors of the Central Nervous System (Atlas of Tumor Pathology, 2nd Series Fasc.
6). Armed Forces Institute of Pathology, Washington, D.C.

Rupp, C. (1948): Metastatic tumors of the central nervous system: I. Intracerebral metastases as the only
evidence of dissemination of visceral cancer. Arch. Neurol. Psychiatry 59: 635–645.

Russel, J. (1876): A case of carcinomatous tumour occupying the right postero-parietal lobule of the cerebrum: Blindness from double optic neuritis. Br. Med. J. 2: 709–710.

Russell, D.S. and Cairns, H. (1934): Subdural false membrane or haematoma (pachymeningitis interna
haemorrhagica) in carcinomatosis and sarcomatosis of the dura mater. Brain 57: 32–48.

Russell, D.S. and Rubinstein, L.J. (1977): Pathology of tumours of the nervous system, 4th ed. Edward
Arnold Ltd., London.

Rustizky, J.V. (1874): Epithelialcarcinom der Dura mater mit hyaliner Degeneration. Virchow Arch. 59:
191–201.

Saenger, H. (1900): Ueber Hirnsymptome bei Carcinomatose. Neurol. Zentralbl. 19: 187–192.

Salerno, T.A., Munro, D.D. and Little, J.R. (1978): Surgical treatment of bronchogenic carcinoma with
a brain metastasis. J. Neurosurg. 48: 350–354.

Salmon, S.E. and Jones, S.E. (1974): Chemotherapy of advanced breast cancer with a combination of Adriamycin and cyclophosphamide. Proc. Am. Assoc. Cancer Res. 15: 90 (abstr.).

Sampson, D. and Lui, A. (1976): The effect of levamisole on cell-mediated immunity and suppressor cell
function. Cancer Res. 36: 952–955.

Sampson, D. (1978): Immunopotentiation and tumor inhibition with levamisole. Cancer Treat. Rep.
62: 1623–1625.

Sano, K., Sato, F., Hoshino, T. and Nagai, M. (1965): Experimental and clinical studies of radiosensitizers
in brain tumors, with special reference to BUdR-antimetabolite continuous regional infusion-
radiationtherapy (BAR therapy). Neurol. Med. Chir. (Tokyo) 7: 51–72.

Sano, K., Hoshino, T., Nagai, M., Tsuchida, T. and Sato, F. (1966): Studies on a radiosensitizer (5-bromo-2'-
deoxyuridine) in the treatment of malignant brain tumor. Neurol. Med. Chir. (Tokyo) 8: 227–231.

Sano, K., Hoshino, T. and Nagai, M. (1968): Radiosensitization of brain tumor cells with a thymidine analogue (bromouridine). J. Neurosurg. 28: 530–538.

Sano, K., Nagai, M., Arai, T. and Hoshino, T. (1971): Follow up results of BAR therapy of malignant brain
tumors. Fourth European Congress of Neurosurgery, Praha, (Abstract No. 24)

Sano, K. and Ishii, S. (eds.) (1974): Recent Progress in Neurological Surgery. Excerpta Medica, Amsterdam.

Sano, K. (ed.) (1976): Atlas of Stereoscopic Neuroradiology. University of Tokyo Press, Tokyo.

Sano, K., Manaka, S., Miyake, H., Mayanagi, Y. and Fuchinoue, T. (1979): Stationary potential of the
brain: Part II. Clinical studies. Neurol. Med. Chir. (Tokyo) 19: 655–664.

Sansone, G. (1954): Pathomorphosis of acute infantile leukemia treated with modern therapeutic agents:

meningoleukemia and Frölich's obesity. Ann. Paediat. 183: 33–41.

Saxer, Fr. (1902): Unter dem Bilde einer Meningitis verlaufende karcinomatöse Erkrankung der Gehirn-und Rückenmarkshäute. Verh. Dtsch. Pathol. Gesellsch. 5: 161–169.

Schaerer, J.P. and Whitney, R.L. (1953): Prostatic metastases simulating intracranial meningioma: A case report. J. Neurosurg. 10: 546–549.

Scholz, W. (1905): Meningitis carzinomatosa. Wien klin. Wochenschr 47: 1231–1234.

Schürmann, K., Brock, M., Reulen, H.J. and Voth, D. (eds.) (1973): Brain Edema; Cerebello Pontine Angle Tumors (Advances in Neurosurgery, Vol.1). Springer-Verlag, Berlin.

Schwab, R.B. and Weiss, S. (1935): The neurologic aspect of leukemia. Am. J. Med. Sci. 189: 766–778.

Schwarz, E. and Bertels, A. (1911): Über „Meningitis" carcinomatosa. Dtsch. Z. Nervenh. 42: 85–94.

Sciarra, D. and Sprofkin, B.E. (1953): Symptoms and signs referable to the basal ganglia in brain tumor. Arch. Neurol. Psychiatry 69: 450–461.

Scott, M. (1975): Spontaneous intracerebral hematoma caused by cerebral neoplasms: Report of eight verified cases. J. Neurosurg. 42: 338–342.

Scoville, W.B., Palmer, A.H., Samra, K. and Chong, G. (1965): The use of acrylic plastic for vertebral replacement or fixation in metastatic disease of the spine. J. Neurosurg. 27: 274–279.

Seaman, W.B., Ter-Pogossian, M.M. and Schwartz, H.G. (1954): Localization of intracranial neoplasms with radioisotopes. Radiology 62: 30–36.

Sears, E.S., Tindall, R.S.A. and Zarnow, H. (1978): Active multiple sclerosis enhanced computerized tomographic imaging of lesions and effects of corticosteroids. Arch. Neurol. 35: 426–434.

Segawa, H., Wakai, S., Asano, T. and Sano, K. (1980): Determination of regional cerebral blood flow by xenon enhanced CT. 3rd Annual Meeting of the Neuro-CT, January, Tokyo.

Selawry, O.S. and Hansen, H.H. (1973): Lung cancer. In Holland, J.F. and Frei, E. (eds.): Cancer Medicine. Lea & Febiger, Philadelphia, pp. 1473–1518.

Selawry, O.S. (1974): The role of chemotherapy in the treatment of lung cancer. Semin. Oncol. 1: 259–272.

Selker, R. (1977): Talk at Workshop on Brain Tumor Immunotherapy, North Carolina.

Sellwood, R.B. (1972): The radiological approach to metastatic cancer of the brain and spine. Br. J. Radiol. 45: 647–651.

Shantha, T.R. and Bourne, G.H. (1968): The perineurial epithelium—A new concept. In Bourne, G.H. (ed.): The Structure and Function of Nervous Tissue, Vol. 1. Academic Press, New York, pp. 380–459.

Shapiro, R. and Janzen, A.H. (1959): Osteoblastic metastases to the floor of the skull simulating meningioma en plaque. Am. J. Roentgenol. Radium Ther. Nucl. Med. 81: 964–966.

Shapiro, W.R., Young, D.F. and Mehta, B.M. (1975): Methotrexate: Distribution in cerebrospinal fluid after intravenous, ventricular and lumbar injections. New. Engl. J. Med. 293: 161–166.

Shapiro, W.R. (1980): Chemotherapy of metastatic central nervous system carcinoma. In Weiss, L., Gilbert, H.A. and Posner, J.B. (eds.): Brain Metastasis. G.K. Hall & Co., Boston, Mass., pp. 328–339.

Sharpe, W.S. and McDonald, J.R. (1942): Reaction of bone to metastasis from carcinoma of the breast and the prostate. Arch. Pathol. 33: 312–325.

Shaw, R.M., Moore, E.W., Freireich, E.J. and Thomas, L.B. (1960): Meningeal leukemia: A syndrome resulting from increased intracranial pressure in patients with acute leukemia. Neurology (Minneap.) 10: 823–833.

Shehata, W.M., Hendrickson, F.R. and Hindo, W.A. (1974): Rapid fractionation technique and retreatment of cerebral metastases by irradiation. Cancer 34: 257–261.

Shelden, W.D. (1926): Secondary tumors of the brain. JAMA 87: 650–653.

Sheline, G., Wasserman, T.H., Wara, W. and Philips, T. (1979): The role of radiosensitizers in therapy of malignant brain tumors. In Paoletti, P., Walker, M.D., Butti, G. and Knerich, R. (eds.): Multidisciplinary Aspects of Brain Tumor Therapy. Elsevier/North-Holland Biomedical Press, Amsterdam, pp. 197–218.

Shenkin, H.A., Horn, R.C. and Grant, P.C. (1945): Lesions of spinal epidural space producing cord compression. Arch. Surg. 51: 125–146.

Sherbourne, D.H., Tribe, C.R. and Varma, S. (1964): Intramedullary spinal cord metastases: A clinico-pathological report of three cases. Paraplegia 2: 100–111.

Shimizu, H., Masuzawa, H. and Sano, K. (1976): Surgical treatment for multiple metastatic brain tumors. Surgery (Tokyo) 38: 1089–1091. (in Japanese)

Shimizu, T., Kito, K., Kubota, S., Kitamura, K. and Takakura, K. (1974): Detection of tumors specific humoral antibody against brain tumors. Neurol. Surg. (Tokyo) 2: 747–756. (in Japanese with English abstract)

Shimizu, T., Kito, K., Kubota, S., Kitamura, K. and Takakura, K. (1976): The immunological diagnosis of brain tumors. Neurol. Med. Chir. (Tokyo) 16: 37–45.

Shitara, N., Kohno, T. and Takakura, K. (1976): New approach to brain tumour chemoradiotherapy with cellular synchronization by colcemid. Acta Neurochir. (Wien) 35: 123–133.

Shitara, N., Kohno, T., Nagamune, A., Takakura, K. and Sano, K. (1978): Pulse-cytophotometric studies on experimental brain tumor under the effect of chemotherapeutic agents, microwave irradiation and hyperthermia. Neurol. Med. Chir. (Tokyo) 18: 199–207.

Shuangshoti, S., Panyathanya, R. and Wichienkur, P. (1974): Intracranial metastases from unsuspected choriocarcinoma: Onset suggestive of cerebrovascular disease. Neurology (Minneap.) 24: 649–654.

Siefert, E. (1902): Ueber die multiple Karzinomatose des Zentralnervensystems. München Med. Wochenschr. 49: 826–828.

Siefert, E. (1903): Ueber die multiple Karcinomatose des Zentralnervensystems. Arch. Psychiat. Nerven Kr. 36: 720–761.

Silverberg, I.J. and Jacobs, E.M. (1971): Treatment of spinal cord compression in Hodgkin's disease. Cancer 27: 308–313.

Silverman, D. and Groff, R.A. (1957): Brain tumor depth determaination by electrographic recordings during sleep. Arch. Neurol. Psychiatry 78: 15–28.

Silverstein, A. and Doniger, D.E. (1963): Neurologic complications of myelomatosis. Arch. Neurol. 9: 534–543.

Simone, J.V., Hustu, H.O. and Aur, R.J.A. (1979): Prevention and treatment of central nervous system leukaemia in childhood. In Whitehouse, J.M.A. and Kay, H.E.M. (eds.): CNS Complications of Malignant Disease. MacMillan Press, Ltd., London, pp. 19–35.

Simionescu, M.D. (1960): Metastatic tumors of the brain. A follow-up study of 195 patients with neurosurgical considerations. J. Neurosurg. 17: 361–373.

Sinclair, V.K. and Morton, R.A. (1963): Variations in X-ray response during the division cycle of partially synchronized chinese hamster cells in culture. Nature 199: 1158–1160.

Sinclair, W. (1972): Cell cycle dependence of the lethal radiation response in mammalian cells. Current topics. Radiat. Res. 7: 264.

Siris, J.H. (1936): Concerning the immunological specificity of glioblastoma multiforme. Bull. Neurol. Inst. N.Y. 4: 597–601.

Sklansky, B., Kaplan, R.M., Reynolds, S., Rosenblum, M. and Walker, M. (1973): 4-dimethyl epipodophyllotoxin-beta d-thenylidene glucoside in the treatment of intracranial neoplasm. Proc. Am. Soc. Clin. Oncol. Cancer Chemother. Rep. 90: 57.

Smith, R. (1965): An evaluation of surgical treatment for spinal cord compression due to metastatic carcinoma. J. Neuol. Neurosurg. Psychiatry 28: 152–158.

Smith, R.B., de Kernion, J., Lincoln, B., Skinner, D.G. and Kaufman, J.J. (1978): Preliminary report of the use of levamisole in the treatment of bladder cancer. Cancer Treat. Rep. 62: 1709–1714.

Smulder, J. and Smets, W. (1960): Les métastases des carcinomes mammaires, Fréquence des métastases hypophysaires. Bull. du Cancer 47: 434–456. [cited by Hägerstrand and Schonebeck, 1969]

Sparks, F.C., Silverstein, M.J., Hunt, J.S., Haskell, C.M., Pilch, Y.H. and Morton, D.L. (1973): Complications of BCG immunotherapy in patients with cancer. N. Engl. J. Med. 289: 827–830.

Sparling, H.J., Adams, R.D. and Parker, F., Jr. (1947): Involvement of the nervous system by malignant lymphoma. Medicine 26: 285–332.

Spiers, A.S.D. (1969): Cerebral metastases from carcinoma of the lung. Med. J. Aust. 2: 178–183.

Spriggs, A.I. (1954): Malignant cells in cerebrospinal fluid. J. Clin. Pathol. 7: 122–130.

Stadelman, N.E. (1908): Zur Diagnose der Meningitis carcinomatosa. Berlin. Klin. Wochenschr. 45: 2262–2263.

Stefansson, T.A. and Rask, B.E. (1973): Acute paraplegia as the initial symptom of acute leukemia. Case report. J. Neurosurg. 39: 648–651.

Steimle, M.R., Jacquet, G. and Giqault de la Bedolliere (1970): Métastase frontale d'un épithelioma du sein ablation de la tumeur et hypophyséctomie. J. Med. Besançon. 1: 337–346.

Steimle, M.R., Jacquet, G. and Chevrier, A. (1975): Les métastases cérébrales, étude clinique et indications thérapeutiques. A propos de 37 observations. Neuro chirurgie (Paris) 21: 343–344.

Steiner, P.E., Butt, E.M. and Edmondson, H.A. (1950): Pulmonary carcinoma revealed at necropsy, with reference to increasing incidence in the Los Angeles County Hospital. J. Natl. Cancer Inst. 11: 497–510.

Stewart, C.C., Valeriote, F.A. and Perez, C.A. (1978): Preliminary observations on the effect of glucan in combination with radiation and chemotherapy in four murine tumors. Cancer Treat. Rep. 62: 1867–1872.

Støier, M. (1965): Metastatic tumors of the brain. Acta Neurol. Scand. 41: 262–278.

Stolfi, R.L. and Martin, D. (1978): Therapeutic activity of maleic anhydride-vinyl ether copolymers against spontaneous, authochthonous murine mammary tumors. Cancer Treat. Rep. 62: 1791–1796.

Störtebecker, T.P. (1954): Metastatic tumors of the brain from a neurosurgical point of view. A follow-up study of 158 cases. J. Neurosurg. 11: 84–111.

Strang, R. and Ajmone-Marsan, C. (1961): Brain metastases. Pathological-electroencephalographic study. Arch. Neurol. 4: 18–20.

Strange, L.F. (1952): Metastatic carcinoma to the leptomeninges. Trans. Am. Neurol. Assoc. 77: 181–185.

Strauss, B. and Weller, C.V. (1957): Bronchogenic carcinoma. A statistical analysis of two hundred ninety-six cases with necropsy as to relationships between cell types and age, sex and metastases. Arch. Pathol. 63: 602–611.

Suemasu, K., Watanabe, H., Kitaoka, K., Mitomi, T., Naruke, A. and Ishikawa, S. (1972): Metastasis of Cancer. Nakayama Publ. Co., Tokyo, pp. 17–19. (in Japanese)

Sullivan, R.D., Jones, R., Jr., Schnabel, T.G., Jr. and Shorey, J.M. (1953): The treatment of human cancer with intra-arterial nitrogen mustard (methyl bis (2-chloroethyl) amine hydrochloride) utilizing a simplified catheter technique. Cancer 6: 121–134.

Sullivan, R.D., Miller, E. and Sikes, M.P. (1959): Antimetabolite combination cancer chemotherapy. Effects of intraarterial methotrexate-intra muscular citrovorum factor therapy in human cancer. Cancer 12: 1248–1262.

Sullivan, R.D., Miller, E. and Duff, J.K. (1961): Effects of continuous intraarterial methotrexate with intermittent intramuscular citrovorum factor therapy in human cancer. Proc. Am. Assoc. Cancer Res. 3: 271.

Sullivan, R.D. (1962): Continuous arterial infusion cancer chemotherapy. Surg. Clin. North Am. 42: 365–388.

Symoens, J. (1974): The effects of levamisole on host defense mechanisms. Proc. of the Levamisole Meeting held at the National Cancer Institute in Bethesda, December.

Symoens, J. (1976): Levamisole, an antianergic chemotherapeutic agent: An overview. In Chirigos, M.A. (ed.): Control of Neoplasia by Modulation of the Immune System (Progress in Cancer Research and Therapy, Vol. 2). Raven Press, New York, pp. 1–24.

Symoens, J. Veys, E., Mielants, M. and Pinals, R. (1978): Adverse reactions to levamisole. Cancer Treat. Rep. 62: 1721–1730.

Taguchi, T. (1977): Mitomycin C. In Saito, T., Niitani, H. and Kanagami, H. (eds.): Chemotherapeutic Agents for Cancer. Clinic Magazine Co., Tokyo, pp. 103–111. (in Japanese)

Takakura, K., Mason, W.B. and Hollander, V.P. (1966): Studies on the pathogenesis of plasma cell tumors. I. Effect of cortisol on development of plasma cell tumors. Cancer Res. 26: 596–599.

Takakura, K. (1971): Clinical experience of application of Bleomycin to brain tumor. Bull. Bleomycin Study Group (Brain Tumor Section) 3: 237–242. (in Japanese with English abstract)

Takakura, K., Oei Kiem Sing, Sakura, M., Hasegawa, H., Ishikawa, S., Shimosato, Y., Watanabe, K., Tanaka, Y. and Yoshida, M. (1971): Metastatic brain tumors from lung adenocarcinoma demonstrating high serum LDH. Saishin Igaku (Osaka) 26: 1602–1607. (in Japanese)

Takakura, K. and Oei Kiem Sing (1972): Inhibitory role of immunologically competent cells on glioblastoma and its clinical application—in vitro studies. In Fusek, I. and Kunc, Z. (eds.): Present Limits of Neurosurgery. Avicenum, Czechoslovak Medical Press, Prague, pp. 47–51.

Takakura, K., Matsutani, M., Koyama, Y. and Oei Kiem Sing (1972): Intrathecal therapy for malignant brain tumors. Brain and Nerve (Tokyo) 24: 585–593. (in Japanese)

Takakura, K. (1974): Cellular immunity of glioma. A study with phase-contrast microcinephotography. In Sano, K. and Ishii, S. (eds.): Recent Progress in Neurological Surgery. Excerpta Medica, Amsterdam, pp. 133–138.

Takakura, K., Miki, T. and Kubo, O. (1975): Adjuvant immunotherapy for malignant brain tumors in infants and children. Child's Brain 1: 141–147.

Takakura, K. (1976): Metastatic brain tumors and metastasis of gliomata. Surgical Therapy (Osaka) 35: 57–62. (in Japanese)

Takakura, K. (1977): Immunotherapy of glioma. Cancer & Chemotherapy (Tokyo) 4: 507–513. (in Japanese with English abstract)

Takakura, K., Sano, K., Kosugi, Y. and Ikebe, J. (1979): Pain control by transcutaneous electrical nerve stimulating using irregular pulse of 1/f fluctuation. Appl. Neurophysiol. 42: 302–321.

Takeuchi, K., Atsuji, M., Ogashiwa, M. and Oda, S. (1968): Chemotherapy of brain tumors by subcutaneously inserted intracarotid continuous infusion. 11th Ann. Meeting of Japanese Chemotherapy Soc., Tokyo.

Takeuchi, K. (1971): Metastatic brain tumors. Modern Surgery 26B, Brain, Spinal Cord II. Nakayama Publ. Co., Tokyo, 117–132. (in Japanese)

Tanimura, K. (1974): Effect of OK-432 on brain tumor therapy. 12th Annual Meeting of the Japan Cancer Therapy Soc. Kyoto.

Tarnoff, J.F., Calinog, T.A. and Byla, J.G. (1976): Prolonged survival following cerebral metastasis from pulmonary cancer. J. Thorac. Cardiovasc. Surg. 72: 933–937.

Taveras, J.M. and Wood, E.H. (1976): Diagnostic Neuroradiology, 2nd ed. Williams & Wilkins Co., Baltimore. pp. 1008–1009.

Teears, R.J. and Silverman, E.M. (1975): Clinicopathologic review of 88 cases of carcinoma metastatic to the pituitary gland. Cancer 36: 216–220.

Teoh, T.B. (1957): Epidermoid carcinoma of the nasopharynx among Chinese: A study of 31 necropsies. J. Pathol. Bacteriol. 72: 451–465.

Terashima, T. and Tolmach, L.J. (1963): Variation in several responses of Hela cells to X-irradiation during the division cycle. Biophys. J. 3: 11–33.

Terashima, T. (1974): Proposals of tumor therapy based on cell cycle dependent sensitivity change. Cancer and Chemotherapy (Tokyo) 1: 533–541. (in Japanese with English abstract)

Ter-Pogossian, M., Ittner, W.B., III., Seaman, W.B. and Schwartz, H.G. (1952): A scintillation counter for the diagnosis and localization of intracranial neoplasms. Am. J. Roentgenol. Radium Ther. Nucl. Med. 67: 351–357.

Terry, W.D. and Windhorst, D. (eds.) (1978): Immunotherapy of Cancer; Present Status of Trials in Man (Progress in Cancer Research and Therapy, Vol.6) Raven Press, New York.

Thienpont, D., Vanparijis, O.F.J., Raeymaekers, A.H.M., Vandenberk, J., Demoen, P.J.A., Allewiji, F.T.N., Marsboom, R.P.H., Niemegeers, C.J.E., Schellekens, K.H.L. and Janse, P.A.J. (1966): Tetramisole (R 8299), a new, potent broad spectrum antihelminthic. Nature 209: 1084–1086.

Thomas, D.G.T., Lannigan, C.B. and Behan, P.O. (1975): Impaired cell-mediated immunity in human brain tumours. Lancet 1: 1389–1390.

Thomas, L.B., Chirigos, M.A., Humphreys, S.R. and Goldin, A. (1962): Pathology of the spread of L1210 leukemia in the central nervous system of mice and effect of treatment with Cytoxan. J. Natl. Cancer Inst. 28: 1355–1389.

Thomas, L.B., Chirigos, M.A., Humphreys, S.R. and Goldin, A. (1964): Development of meningeal leukemia (L1210) during treatment of subcutaneously inoculated mice with methotrexate. Cancer 17: 352–360.

Tinney, W.S. and Moersch, H.J. (1944): Intracranial metastasis of carcinoma of the lung. Arch. Otolaryngol. 39: 243–244.

Tokoro, Y. (1959): Meningeal diffuse metastatic carcinomatosis. In Tokoro, Y.: Brain Tumors. Igaku-Shoin Ltd., Tokyo, pp. 521–532. (in Japanese)

Tokumaru, T. and Catalano, L.W. (1975): Elevation of serum immunoglobulin M (IgM) level in patients with brain tumors. Surg. Neurol. 4: 17–21.

Tolmach, L.J., Terashima, T. and Phillips, R.A. (1965): X-ray sensitivity changes during the division cycle of HeLa cells and anomatous survival kinetics of developing microcolonies. In Anderson Tumor Institute: Cellular Radiation Biology. Williams & Wilkins Co., Baltimore, p. 376.

Tom, M.I. (1946): Metastatic tumors of brain. Canad. Med. Assoc. J. 54: 265–268.

Tomita, T., Tazima, K., Yamamoto, M. and Kikuchi, H. (1977): Surgery of metastatic brain tumors. Operation (Tokyo) 31: 469–477. (in Japanese)

Törmä, T. (1957): Malignant tumors of the spine and spinal extradural space. A study based on 250 histologically verified cases. Acta Chir. Scand. [Suppl.] 225: 1–138.

Toshima, S., Moore, G.E. and Sandberg, A.A. (1968): Ultrastructure of human melanoma in cell culture. Electron microscopic studies. Cancer 21: 202–216.

Toumey, J.W. (1943): Metastatic malignancy of the spine. J. Bone Joint Surg. 25: 292–305.

Toyokura, Y., Shiozawa, R., Mikami, R., Seki, A. and Tokoro, Y. (1957): A clinical and anatomical study on metastatic tumors of the brain. Prog. Brain Res. 2: 215–231.

Trouillas, P. and Lapras, C. (1970): Immunothérapie active des tumeurs cérébrales. A propos de 20 cas. Neuro chirurgie (Paris) 16: 143–170.

Trouilass, P. (1972): Immunologie des tumeurs cérébrales; l'antigéne carcinofoetal glial. Ann. Inst. Pasteur 122: 819–828.

Turner, O. and German, W.J. (1941): Metastases in the skull from carcinoma of the thyroid. Surgery 9: 403–414.

Upton, A.C. and Furth, J. (1954): The effects of cortisone on the development of spontaneous leukemia in mice and on its induction by irradiation. Blood 9: 686–695.

Urich, H. (1974): Neurological involvement in the lymphomas and leukemias. Proc. R. Soc. Med. 67: 979–981.

Urtasun, R.C., Band, P.R., Chapman, J.D., Wilson, A.F., Marynowski, B. and Starreveled, E. (1976a): Metronidazole as a radiosensitizer. N. Engl. J. Med. 295: 901–902.

Urtasun, R.C., Band, P.R., Chapman, J.D. and Wilson, A.F. (1976b): Radiation and high-dose metronidazole in supratentorial glioblastoma. N. Engl. J. Med. 294: 1364–1367.

Ushio, Y., Chernik, N.L., Posner, J.B. and Shapiro, W.R. (1977a): Meningeal carcinomatosis: development of an experimental model. J. Neuropathol. Exp. Neurol. 36: 228–244.

Ushio, Y., Chernik, N.L., Shapiro, W.R. and Posner, J.B. (1977b): Metastatic tumor of the brain: development of an experimental model. Ann. Neurol. 2: 20–29.

Ushio, Y., Posner, R., Kim, J.H., Shapiro, W.R. and Posner, J.B. (1977c): Treatment of experimental spinal cord compression caused by extradural neoplasms. J. Neurosurg. 47: 380–390.

Ushio, Y., Posner, R., Posner, J.B. and Shapiro, W.R. (1977d): Experimental spinal cord compression by epidural neoplasms. Neurology (Minneap.) 27: 422–429.

Ushio, Y., Posner, J.B. and Shapiro, W.R. (1977e): Chemotherapy of experimental meningeal carcinomatosis. Cancer Res. 37: 1232–1237.

Van Allen, M.W. and Rahme, E.S. (1962): Lymphosarcomatous infiltration of the cauda equina: Myelography in an unusual case. Arch. Neurol. 7: 476–481.

van Dellen, J.R. and Danziger, A. (1978): Failure of computerized tomography to differentiate between radiation necrosis and cerebral tumor. S. Afr. Med. J. 53: 171.

Van der Kogel, A.J. and Barendsen, G.W. (1974): Late effects of spinal cord irradiation with 300 kV x-rays and 15 MeV neutrons. Br. J. Radiol. 47: 393–398.

Vannucci, R.C. and Baten, M. (1974): Cerebral metastatic disease in childhood. Neurology (Minneap.) 24: 981–985.

Vaughan, H.G., Jr. and Howard, R.G. (1962): Intracranial hemorrhage due to metastatic chorionephithelioma. Neurology (Minneap.) 12: 771–777.

Venditti, J.M., Kline, I. and Goldin, A. (1964): Evaluation of antileukemic agents employing advanced leukemia L1210 in mice. Cancer Res. 24 [Suppl.]: 827–879.
Verity, G.L. (1968): Neurologic manifestations and complications of lymphoma. Radiol. Clin. North Am.
6: 97–109.
Viadana, E., Cotter, R., Pickren, J.W. and Bross, I.D.J. (1973): An autopsy study of metastatic sites of
breast cancer. Cancer Res. 33: 179–181.
Viadana, E., Bross, I.D.J. and Pickren, J.W. (1976): The metastatic spread of kidney and prostate cancers
in man. Neoplasma 23: 323–332.
Vider, M., Maruyama, Y. and Narvaez, R. (1977): Significance of the vertebral venous (Batson's) plexus in
metastatic spread in colorectal carcinoma. Cancer 40: 67–71.
Vieth, R.G. and Odom, G.L. (1965a): Intracranial metastases and their neurosurgical treatment. J. Neu-
rosurg. 23: 375–383.
Vieth, R.G. and Odom, G.L. (1965b): Extradural spinal metastases and their neurosurgical treatment. J.
Neurosurg. 23: 501–508.
Vinken, P.J. and Bruyn, G.W. (eds.) (1974): Handbook of Clinical Neurology, Vol.18. North-Holland
Publishing Co., Amsterdam.
Vinken, P.J. and Bruyn, G.W. (eds.) (1976): Handbook of Clinical Neurology, Vol.20. North-Holland
Publishing Co., Amsterdam.
Vorderwinkler, K. (1951): Zur Histogenese von Krebsmetastasen im Gehirn. Zentralbl. Neurochir. 11:
116–124.

Wagenknecht, L. (1973): Atteintes malignes du système nerveux central. Médecine et Hygiène 1080: 1837.
Wagner, J.A. (1955): Neuropathology of neoplastic metastasis to the brain. South. Med. J. 48: 302–305.
Walker, M.D. and Hurwitz, B.C. (1970): BCNU 1, 3-bis (2-chloroethyl)-1-nitrosourea; (NSC-409962) in
the treatment of malignant brain tumor—a preliminary report. Cancer Chemother. Rep. 54: 263–
271.
Walker, M.D., Alexander, E., Jr., Hunt, W.E., MacCarty, C.S., Mahaley, M.S., Mealey, J., Jr., Norrell,
H.A., Owens, G., Ransohoff, J., Wilson, C.B., Gehan, E.A. and Strike, T.A. (1978): Evaluation of
BCNU and/or radiotherapy in the treatment of anaplastic gliomas. J. Neurosurg. 49: 333–343.
Wallach, J.B. and Edberg, S. (1959): Metastases of cancer to primary intracranial tumors. Arch. Neurol.
1: 191–194.
Walter, W.G. (1936): The location of cerebral tumours by electroencephalography. Lancet 2: 305–312.
Walters, T.R., Aur, R.J.A., Hernandez, K., Vietti, T. and Pinkel, D. (1972): 6-Azauridine in combination
chemotherapy of childhood acute myelocytic leukemia. Cancer 29: 1057–1060.
Walters, T.R. (1977): Special neurological complications due to acute nonlymphocytic leukemia. In
Pochedly, C. (ed.): Leukemia and Lymphoma in the Nervous System. C.C. Thomas, Springfield,
Ill., pp. 41–53.
Walther, H.E. (1948): Krebsmetastasen. Benne Schwarbe Co., Basel.
Wanebo, H.J., Hilal, E.Y., Pinsky, C.M., Strong, E.W., Mike, V., Hirshaut, Y. and Oettgen, H.F. (1978):
Randomized trial of levamisole in patients with squamous cancer of the head and neck: A preliminary
report. Cancer Treat. Rep. 62: 1663–1669.
Wara, D.W. and Ammann, A.J. (1975): Activation of T-cell rosettes in immunodeficient patients by thy-
mosin. Ann. N.Y. Acad. Sci. 249: 308–314.
Warren, B.A., Chauvin, W.J. and Philips, J. (1977): Blood-borne tumor emboli and their adherence to vessel
walls. In Day, S.B., Myers, W.P.L., Stansly, P., Garattini, S. and Lewis, M.G. (eds.): Cancer Inva-
sion and Metastasis: Biologic Mechanisms and Therapy (Progress in Cancer Research and Therapy,
Vol. 5). Raven Press, New York, pp. 185–197.
Weibel, E.R. and Palade, G.E. (1964): New cytoplasmic components in arterial endothelia. J. Cell Biol.
23: 101–112.
Weisberg, L.A. (1979): Computerized tomography in intracranial metastases. Arch. Neurol. 36: 630–634.
Weller, C.V. (1929): The pathology of primary carcinoma of the lung. Arch. Pathol. 7: 478–519.
Westenhöffer, M. (1904): Pachymeningitis carcinomatosa haemorrhagica interna productiva mit Colicacil-
losis agonalis. Virchows Arch. 175: 364–379.
Whisnault, J.P., Siekert, R.G. and Sayer, G.P. (1956): Neurologic manifestations of the lymphomas. Med.
Clin. North Am. 40: 1151–1161.
White, W.A., Patterson, R.H., Jr. and Bergland, R.M. (1971): Role of surgery in the treatment of spinal
cord compression by metastatic neoplasm. Cancer 27: 558–561.
Whiteside, J.A., Philips, F.S., Dargeon, H.W. and Burchenal, J.H. (1958): Intrathecal amethopterin in
neurological manifestation of leukemia. Arch. Intern. Med. 101: 279–285.
Wickbom, I. (1953): Angiographic determination of tumour pathology. Acta Radiol. 40: 529–546.
Wild, W.O. and Porter, R.W. (1963): Metastatic epidural tumor of the spine. A study of 45 cases. Arch.
Surg. 87: 825–830.
Wilhyde, D.E., Jane, J.A. and Mullan, S. (1963): Spinal epidural leukemia. Am. J. Med. 34: 281–287.
Wilkins, R.H. and Wu, W.K. (1971): Spontaneous rupture of a metastatic brain tumor into the ventricular
system: Report of two cases. J. Neurosurg. 34: 412–416.

Williams, H.M., Diamond, H.D. and Craver, L.F. (1958): The pathogenesis and management of neurological complications in patients with malignant lymphomas and leukemia. Cancer 11: 76–82.

Williams, H.M., Diamond, H.D., Craver, L.F. and Parson, H. (1959): Neurological Complications of Lymphomas and Leukemias. C.C. Thomas, Springfield, Ill.

Williams, W.R. (1887): Cancer and phthisis as correlated diseases. Lancet 1: 977.

Willis, R.A. (1948): Pathology of Tumors. Butterworths, London.

Willis, R.A. (1952): The Spread of Tumours in the Human Body, 2nd ed. Butterworth & Co., Ltd., London.

Willis, R.A. (1973): The Spread of Tumours in the Human Body, 3rd ed. Butterworth & Co., Ltd., London.

Willoughby, M.L.N. (1979): Problems in management of childhood CNS leukaemia. In Whitehouse, J.M.A. and Kay, H.E.M. (eds.): CNS Complications of Malignant Disease. MacMillan Press, Ltd., London, pp. 70–79.

Wilson, C.B., Winternitz, W.W., Bertan, V. and Sizemore, G. (1966): Stereotaxic cryosurgery of the pituitary gland in carcinoma of the breast and other disorders. JAMA 198: 587–590.

Wilson, C.B., Winternitz, W.W., Rush, B.F., Walton, K.N. and Maddy, J.A. (1967): Cryohypophysectomy-indications, technic, and results. Int. Surg. 48: 28–40.

Wilson, C.B., Saglam, S., Winternitz, W.W., Norrell, H., Rush, B. and Walton, K. (1969): Indications for hypophysectomy in the management of diabetic retinopathy and endocrine-sensitive cancer. Presented at the annual AMA meeting in New York, 1969.

Wilson, C.B., Boldrey, E.B. and Enot, K.J. (1970): 1, bis (2-chloroethyl)-1-nitrosourea (NSC-409962) in the treatment of brain tumors. Cancer Chemother. Rep. 54: 273–281.

Wilson, C.B. and Fewer, D. (1971): Role of neurosurgery in the management of patients with the carcinoma of the breast. Cancer 28: 1681–1685.

Wilson, C.B. and Saglam, S. (1973): Pathophysiology of and indications for hypophysectomy. In Youmans, J.R. (ed.): Neurological Surgery, Vol. 3. W.B. Saunders Co., Philadelphia, pp. 1901–1907.

Wilson, W.L. and de la Garza, J.G. (1965): Systemic chemotherapy for CNS metastases of solid tumors. Arch. Intern. Med. 115: 710–731.

Windeyer, B. (1964): Metastases in the central nervous system. Treatment by radiotherapy and chemotherapy. Pro. R. Soc. Med. 57: 1153–1159.

Witcofski, R.L., Maynard, C.D. and Roper, T.J. (1967): A comparative analysis of the accuracy of the technetium-99m pertechnetate brain scan: follow-up of 1,000 patients. J. Nucl. Med. 8: 187–196.

Witt, J.A., Gardner, B., Gordan, G.S., Graham, W.P., III. and Thomas, A.N. (1963): Secondary hormonal therapy of disseminated breast cancer. Comparison of hypophysectomy, replacement therapy, estrogens, and androgens. Arch. Intern. Med. 11: 557–563.

Wright, R.L. (1963): Malignant tumors in the spinal extradural space: Result of surgical treatment. Ann. Surg. 157: 227–231.

Wright, P.W., Hill, L.D., Peterson, A.V., Jr., Pinkham, R., Johnson, L., Ivey, T., Bernstein, I., Bagley, C. and Anderson, R. (1978): Preliminary results of combined surgery and adjuvant Bacillus calmette-guérin plus levamisole treatment of resectable lung cancer. Cancer Treat. Rep. 62: 1671–1675.

Wolfson, S.A., Reznick, S. and Gunther, L. (1941): Early diagnosis of malignant metastases to the spine. A clinical syndrome. JAMA 116: 1044–1048.

Wooley, G.W. and Peters, B.A. (1953): Prolongation of life in high-leukemia AKR mice by cortisone. Proc. Soc. Exp. Biol. Med. 82: 286–287.

Wood, S., Jr., Holyoke, E.D. and Yardley, J.H. (1961): Mechanisms of metastasis production by blood-borne cancer cells. Can. Cancer Conference 4: 167–223.

Wu, W.Q. and Hiszczynskyj, R. (1977): Metastasis of carcinoma of cervix uteri to convexity meningioma. Surg. Neurol. 8: 327–329.

Youmans, J.R. (ed.) (1973): Neurological Surgery. W.B. Saunders, Philadelphia.

Young, D.F., Pasner, J.B., Chu, F. and Nisce, L. (1974): Rapid-course radiation therapy of cerebral metastases: Results and complications. Cancer 34: 1069–1076.

Young, H.F. (1976): Inhibition of cell-mediated immunity in patients with brain tumors. Surg. Neurol. 5: 19.

Young, H., Kaplan, A. and Regelson, W. (1977): Immunotherapy with autologous white cell infusions ("lymphocytes") in the treatment of recurrent glioblastoma multiforme. Workshop on Brain Tumor Immunotherapy, North Carolina.

Zachrisson, L. (1963): Angiography of cerebral metastases. Acta Radiol. [Diagn.] (Stockh.) 1: 521–527.

Zbar, B., Bernstein, I., Tanaka, T. and Rapp, H.J. (1970): Tumor immunity produced by the intradermal inoculation of living tumor cells and living mycobacterium bovis (strain BCG). Science 170: 1217–1218.

Zbar, B. and Tanaka, T. (1971): Immunotherapy of cancer: Regression of tumours after intralesional injection of living mycobacterium bovis. Science 172: 271–273.

Zelen, M. (1973): Keynote address on biostatistics and data retrieval. Cancer Chemother. Rep. 4: 31–42.

Zervas, N.T. (1969): Stereotaxic radiofrequency surgery of the normal and the abnormal pituitary gland. N. Engl. J. Med. 280: 429–437.

Zimmerman, H.M. (1971): Malignant lymphomas. In Minckler, J. (ed.): Pathology of the Nervous System, Vol. 2. McGraw-Hill, New York, pp. 2165–2178.

Zimmerman, H.M. (1974): Malignant lymphomas of the nervous system. Brain and Nerve (Tokyo) 26: 1153–1170.

Zimmerman, H.M. (1975): Malignant lymphomas of the nervous system. Acta Neuropathol. (Berl.) [Suppl. 6]: 69–74.

Zucker, D.K., Katz, R., Koto, A. and Horoupian, D.S. (1978): Sarcomas metastatic to the brain: Case report of a metastatic fibrosarcoma, and review of literature. Surg. Neurol. 9: 177–180.

INDEX